THE HEALTH DETECTIVE'S
456
MOST POWERFUL
Healing Secrets

NAN KATHRYN FUCHS, PH.D.
Editor in Chief, *Women's Health Letter*

**Basic
Health**
PUBLICATIONS, INC.

The information contained in this book is based upon the research and personal and professional experiences of the author. It is not intended as a substitute for consulting with your physician or other healthcare provider. Any attempt to diagnose and treat an illness should be done under the direction of a healthcare professional.

The publisher does not advocate the use of any particular healthcare protocol but believes the information in this book should be available to the public. The publisher and author are not responsible for any adverse effects or consequences resulting from the use of the suggestions, preparations, or procedures discussed in this book. Should the reader have any questions concerning the appropriateness of any procedures or preparation mentioned, the author and the publisher strongly suggest consulting a professional healthcare advisor.

Basic Health Publications, Inc.
www.basichealthpub.com

Library of Congress Cataloging-in-Publication Data

Fuchs, Nan Kathryn.
    The health detective's 456 most powerful healing secrets / Nan Kathryn Fuchs.
    p. cm.
    Includes bibliographical references and index.
    ISBN: 978-1-59120-187-8 (Pbk.)
    ISBN: 978-1-68162-810-3 (Hardcover)

1. Medicine, Popular. 2. Self-care, Health. 3. Naturopathy. I. Title.

    RC81.F83   2006
    615.5'38—dc22

                                                    2006004349

Typesetting/Book design: Gary A. Rosenberg
Cover design: Mike Stromberg

Contents

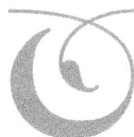

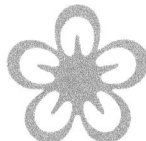

PART 9

New Breakthroughs to Prevent and Fight Cancer

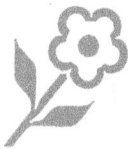

Introduction

When I was a child I drove my parents crazy, asking "why?" about everything. I know. Many children do this. But I took questioning to an extreme. No matter what they replied, I remember feeling another question bubbling up inside me that just wouldn't go away. "But why is that?" I would ask in response to their original answer. I never grew out of this.

My curiosity turned into an asset when I became a nutritionist more than twenty-five years ago. While some of my colleagues trusted the information they heard or read from supplement companies and other vested interest groups, I questioned everything. This led me to read scientific studies. When there were few studies on certain therapies, I sought out doctors with keen observational skills and asked them about the newer therapies they were using in their treatments. I wanted to know what these doctors were finding in their clinics. When I became a nutritional consultant, I called my practice "The Nutrition Detective" because it echoed my questioning style.

My first book, published in 1985, reflected this approach to women's health. It, too, was called *The Nutrition Detective.* The same month it came out, a study on premenstrual syndrome, for which I was the primary author, was published in the *Journal of Applied Nutrition.* This study found some nutritional solutions for both the physical and emotional symptoms of PMS that have become familiar to many doctors of integrative medicine.

It was no accident that I authored a scientific study and a popular book on nutrition at the same time. My interest has always been to combine science with digging around for more information. Whether in my books, my research, or my nutritional counseling practice, I have always looked for clues that lead to the underlying causes for women's health problems.

Now I've expanded my focus to include a person's lifestyle (exercise, stress reduction, etc.), as well as their use of pharmaceutical drugs and traditional diagnostic tools. I've become the Health Detective to the many thousands of women who read *Women's Health Letter,* my monthly national newsletter. This expansion has given me a wider view of the health problems that face all of us as we grow older. It has also helped me look at both sides of an issue.

There's a tug-of-war going on and your health is at risk. Business interests are pulling on one end, and science is tugging at the other. I'd be amazed if you're not confused and frustrated. To tell you the truth, I've found that most doctors are as well. It takes time to sift through current information and separate the hype from the real deal. Who has the time to read through technical scientific studies? Who calls up researchers and doctors to better understand the validity of their conclusions? Well, I do. In fact, this is precisely what I've been doing for the past twenty-five years as a nutritionist and health writer.

During this time, I discovered that there are good scientific studies that draw sound conclusions about drugs or nutrients. And then there are poorly designed studies that are meaningless if you read them carefully. These studies are often designed to help sell a drug or a supplement. But the science behind them is so faulty that the study is meaningless except as a sales tool.

If only you had the time and the expertise to separate the wheat from the chaff, you'd know that there are truly miraculous substances and diagnostic tools out there that could help improve your health dramatically. I've uncovered a number of these health secrets over nearly a dozen years of writing for *Women's Health Letter.* And I decided to put the most relevant ones I've come across in one place to make it easy for you to use. You may have heard of a few of them already. But I'll guarantee there are many you've never heard of.

Did you know that a common garden herb can often stop the hot flashes that accompany menopause? You may not need to take hormones at all if this is your primary menopausal complaint.

Are you aware that an overlooked mineral deficiency could be responsible for both an underactive thyroid and breast cancer? Not only is there a way to test for this deficiency, it isn't expensive and you don't need a doctor's prescription to get it.

What can you do when you can't get a yearly flu shot or it doesn't work? I found a supplement that has kept my patients and me free from colds, flu, bronchitis, and pneumonia for the past four years.

I could go on and on. But instead of listing more of the health secrets I found, put aside your confusion and let go of your frustrations. Turn to the Table of Contents and pick a chapter or two to read that could improve your health for the rest of your life. Or read the book straight through. It doesn't really matter. This book is here to help you live life as healthily as you can.

How to Find
the Information You Want

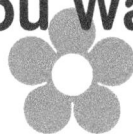

Congratulations on deciding to read my latest book. *The Health Detective's 456 Most Powerful Healing Secrets* has been written specifically to help people like you find the answers to their most pressing health questions.

Here are three suggestions to help you get the greatest value from this book.

First, for information on a specific topic or question, start with the Table of Contents. This should help you locate the *general topic* you're looking for. To look up a specific word or phrase, please turn to the index, where you'll find an alphabetical listing of hundreds of items.

Next, once you've found the information you're seeking, you'll want to know where can you purchase the product or service that is best for your needs. That's where our unique Resource Guide comes in. On pages 383–400, you'll find a complete listing, by chapter, of all the products and services recommended in these pages.

Finally, for the latest up-to-date health information, please go to my website, www.womenshealthletter.com. There you can sign up to receive my free Health Alerts, learn about subscribing to my one-of-a-kind health newsletter, and research hundreds of health topics, and much, much more.

I know that finding the answers you seek is the first step in having the kind of health (and life) you want. I've dedicated my life to helping people like you learn about their best solutions.

Nan Kathryn Fuchs, Ph.D.
Editor in Chief, *Women's Health Letter*

PART 1

FIGHT DISEASE and REVERSE CHRONIC ILLNESSES

There are more therapies and diagnostic tools available today to keep you healthy than ever before. Some are so powerful that they can reverse or reduce the severity of chronic illnesses.

Still, you'll hear about most of them here for the first time. Why is that? Quite simply, many of them are secrets that even your doctor doesn't know about. There are studies to back up their effectiveness, but not as many as those funded by pharmaceutical companies and big suppliers of diagnostic tools.

Whoever shouts the loudest gets heard. Giant corporations shout loudly with their advertising dollars. That's why you've heard about their products. But you've also heard about their drugs that were recalled because government agencies gave them the go-ahead too quickly—after people died or became sicker.

Well, over the past twenty-five years, I've discovered a number of natural therapies that are both safer and more effective than their drug counterparts. In this section, I'd like to share with you some of the most powerful health secrets I've ever found to fight chronic illnesses.

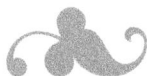

CHAPTER 1

This Hidden Deficiency Could Be Causing Your Health Problems

Thyroid problems are among the most prevalent underdiagnosed and mistreated types of chronic illness. That's because they're so hard to test. I first looked at a potential solution for low thyroid back in 2001. Since then, I've found a link between breast cancer and a common mineral that's found in seaweed.

That's not all. It could be that this mineral is the first non-plant adaptogen—a substance that helps to regulate many body functions including the thyroid. This means it can work for people with an underactive or overactive thyroid. If you read all of the secrets surrounding this particular nutrient, I think you'll see why I call it the best-kept health secret of all.

SECRET #1 Your thyroid could be low even when your tests are normal.

You may have been told that your thyroid tests are normal. Yet, if you are frequently cold and constipated and have brittle hair and unexplained fatigue, your thyroid gland may not be functioning optimally.

The problem with thyroid blood tests is that they are notoriously poor indicators of thyroid function. At a meeting I attended recently, dozens of doctors who use integrative medicine were asked how many of them used thyroid tests to determine whether or not their patients had an underactive thyroid.

Not one of them did!

Instead, they performed a thorough examination and asked detailed questions of their patients about thyroid-related symptoms. Then they treated their thyroid based on their findings. Their patients' symptoms improved.

You may not be aware of this, but hypothyroidism is an epidemic. One in ten women in this country have been diagnosed with thyroid problems. Some endocrinologists believe that as many as one in four women have either an underactive or overactive thyroid.

7

Why is this? A simple reason may be because our thyroid glands are twice as large as those in men, creating a greater need for iodine—a mineral essential to thyroid function. When we're under stress, our thyroid glands become even larger and more active. This further increases our need for even more iodine.

After investigating this subject and reading a number of studies, I've come to the conclusion that today's thyroid epidemic seems to be caused to a great extent by a decline in dietary iodine. In 1940, the typical American diet contained 500–800 micrograms a day of iodine. By 1995, that daily intake had dropped down to 135 mcg. Thyroid problems can also be caused by exposure to substances that interfere with iodine levels, as well as to an increased exposure to harmful radio-active iodine.

Why are our diets lower in iodine than ever before? In the 1960s, we got more iodine from the bread we ate. Iodine-containing dough conditioners added 150 mcg of iodine to each slice! But over the past twenty years, food processors have substituted this conditioner with bromine, a substance that opposes iodine and actually contributes to goiters. So instead of getting a little iodine in every slice of bread you eat, you're now getting a little bromine. The problem is that bromine lowers your iodine levels even further.

What about just using iodized salt to increase your iodine intake? Simply put, it won't work. Iodine was originally added to salt to prevent goiters. Iodized table salt contains 74 mcg of iodine for every gram of salt. Sea salt, soy sauce, and Bragg's liquid amino acids are all salty condiments that contain no iodine. To get sufficient iodine you'd need to eat 168 grams of salt every day! A healthy Western diet contains less than 0.500 *milligrams* (mg) a day—including whatever is naturally found in our foods. You can't safely eat enough iodized salt to reverse an iodine deficiency.

Substances That Interfere with Iodine

If you don't get enough iodine in your diet, it allows other substances that interfere with thyroid function and the central nervous system to wreak havoc. These include chlorine, fluoride, and bromide. Their ability to cause problems depends on how much iodide (a form of iodine) your body contains. Sufficient iodine and iodide compete with bromide. This means that bromide can't be utilized in the thyroid. Iodide also reduces the toxicity of fluoride.

Water that contains chlorine, fluoride, or bromine interferes with iodine molecules and causes your body to excrete the iodine it needs so much. It doesn't matter if you drink this water or bathe in it. And there's no way to escape at least some of these chemicals. Chlorine is present in most city water supplies. Unless you de-chlorinate your water, you are being exposed to thyroid-lowering gases whenever you bathe, shower, or have a drink of water.

Fortunately there are products available that can quickly and easily remove chlorine in your shower. I even discovered one that removes chlorine from your bathtub. See the Resources section at the end of this book for more information.

If you have a hot tub, you probably use chlorine or bromine as a disinfectant. Both can lower your iodine levels. Bromine is also found in some pesticides—another reason to eat organic food whenever possible.

Aspirin, blood-thinner medications, and steroids all increase iodine excretion and can result in iodine deficiency thyroid problems. If you're taking any of these medications, ask your doctor to check your thyroid function.

SECRET #2   Not all forms of iodine are safe.

Getting enough iodine in your diet is vital to preventing many health problems. But you have to make sure you're getting the right type of iodine. There are two forms of iodine: iodine 127 (safe, natural dietary iodine) and iodine 131 (a harmful, radioactive byproduct of nuclear energy). Your body absorbs and retains any kind of iodine to which it is exposed. Most of it is deposited in your thyroid gland or breast tissues. These are the two places that use the highest amounts of iodine.

If you're already deficient in iodine, your body will absorb more radioactive iodine 131. But if you have enough dietary iodine, you won't absorb as much of the radioactive kind. The good iodine blocks the harmful type (just as it does bromide, fluoride, and chlorine).

If you think you haven't been exposed to radioactive iodine, you're wrong. All of us have. Radioactive material has been released into the air from nuclear testing and nuclear power plants since 1945. The ordinary day-to-day operations of these nuclear plants put harmful radioactive iodine into our atmosphere. Since you can't avoid it, you need to block its absorption. This exposure to iodine 131 is very possibly the origin of many thyroid disorders we're seeing today.

SECRET #3   Seaweed improves low thyroid function.

The good news is, there's an easy way to get dietary iodine and fight off all these dangerous substances. Seaweed provides a safe form of dietary iodine for better thyroid function and healthier breast tissues. It also protects you from the harmful effects of radioactive iodine. The regular consumption of seaweed could even restore your thyroid function.

I first heard about using seaweed for an underactive thyroid several years ago at a health conference. The speaker, Ryan Drum, Ph.D., was talking about the probable causes, and possible cures, for low thyroid function. Dr. Drum is a former university professor and researcher in cell biology and chemistry. He teaches herbology in workshops and at John Bastyr University, a naturopathic college near Seattle, Washington. He is also a practicing medical herbalist. Dr. Drum is an expert on seaweed's role in thyroid function. His talk on seaweed and the thyroid captured my attention.

Boost Your Iodine Level with Seaweed

You may not realize seaweed is an excellent food, especially if you don't live near the ocean. But seaweed is a delicious and very healthy food.

You can eat as much of it as your body wants. There are red and brown seaweeds (although they don't all look either red or brown). Brown seaweeds are highest in iodine. They include all forms of kelp. *Fucus*, also known as Bladder-wrack, is considered to be the best for underactive thyroids because it contains the most iodine. Hijiki and *Sargassum* are two other forms of brown seaweeds. Red seaweeds include dulse, nori, Irish moss, and *Gracilaria*.

Since toasting doesn't affect seaweed's iodine content, you can eat it dried or dried and toasted. Toast some in the oven or in a dry frying pan to see if you prefer that taste. You can also add powdered seaweed to your food or add larger pieces of seaweed to soups, grains, or vegetables. Seaweed should be an enjoyable addition to your diet, not an unpleasant experience. If you simply don't like its taste, you can get it powdered, in capsules.

Dr. Drum uses 5–10 grams of mixed brown and red seaweeds daily for people with thyroid problems. This translates to about one and one half teaspoons a day. Each variety of seaweed contains different amounts of iodine. Nori, a type of kelp, is a popular form of seaweed that's used to make sushi. It's available in all Oriental markets and many health-food stores. Nori is delicious, but it's not particularly high in iodine. Most forms of kelp have 500–1,500 ppm (parts per million) of iodine; nori has only 15 ppm!

Not all seaweeds are safe to eat. Some come from polluted waters. I buy mine from reliable sources—directly from people who harvest them from the cleanest available waters. Check the Resources section at the end of this book for a list of companies that carefully harvest and dry various types of seaweed.

If you've been told that your thyroid is borderline-low, eating seaweed makes sense. But remember, if you're iodine-deficient, you need to eat seaweed every day or take iodine in a different form.

If you're taking thyroid medication and want to try seaweed, you may want to call Dr. Drum first for a consultation. The protocol for taking seaweed while on thyroid hormone replacement is different from the one I've described.

Instead of using seaweed to boost your iodine levels, you might consider using an iodine supplement. Some contain iodine alone, while others have both iodine and iodide.

SECRET #4 An iodine supplement should also contain iodide.

The form of iodine you take determines where it will go and which parts of your body it can help. While both thyroid and breast tissues need iodine, your thyroid gland prefers it in a form called iodide. Iodide is a reduced form of an iodine compound containing potassium. Textbooks on endocrinology say that iodine by itself is sufficient since it is converted into iodide in the intestines. But a study using both iodine and iodide indicates our thyroid gland functions better when iodide is included. Research endocrinologist, Guy E. Abraham, M.D., developed both a test to determine iodine sufficiency and an iodine product designed to reverse this deficiency.

His supplement is a high-potency iodine/potassium iodide tablet containing 5 mg of iodine and 7.5 mg of potassium iodide. Doctors will recognize this as a tablet form of an iodine solution called Lugol's solution, a well-absorbed form of iodine that has been used for 180 years. The tablet is called Iodoral, and it's available through several sources to anyone who has been found by their doctors or by Dr. Abraham's test to be iodine-deficient.

Studies show that women who weigh about 110 pounds need at least 5 mg of iodine a day for normal breast function. If you're heavier, you may need more. To get a better idea of how much iodine is best for you, you'll want to first take advantage of Dr. Abraham's iodine-loading test.

SECRET #5 Your iodine level can now be measured accurately.

At one time, people would paint a circle of tincture of iodine on their inner arm to see whether or not they were iodine-deficient. The thought was that if you were not deficient in iodine, this iodine patch would disappear in from twenty minutes to two hours. But if it was visible for more than four hours, your iodine level was just low. It's not a particularly accurate way to measure your iodine level. But until recently, it was all that was available.

Now there's a simple twenty-four-hour urine test developed by Dr. Abraham that measures the amount of iodide in your urine using an ion-selective electrode (ISE) following an oral intake of iodine/iodide. The ISE method to measure urinary iodide has been tested effectively on more than 4,000 Japanese men and women by Japanese researchers.

Of all the people in the world, the Japanese, whose diets are high in iodine, have some of the lowest incidence of iodine-deficiency diseases like goiter, hypothyroidism, and cancers of the reproductive system (breast, ovaries, and uterus). The Japanese eat a lot of seaweed and are very interested in its effects on health.

Without getting into the scientific details of Dr. Abraham's test, let me just say that it's a fast, inexpensive, and accurate way of evaluating how much or how little iodine a person has in their urine. The percent of an oral dose excreted in your urine over twenty-four hours helps determine the iodine sufficiency in your tissues. I spoke with a number of doctors who were using this iodine test in their practice. Almost all of them found that the majority of patients they tested were low in iodine.

Why then do most doctors say we're getting enough—or too much—iodine?

It's what they're taught.

Doctors learn about iodine from reading such textbooks as *The Thyroid* edited by Baverman and Utiger (Lippincott, 2000). These books say that excessive iodine is any amount greater than 500 mcg (.5 mg). But this amount is 100 times less iodine than healthy Japanese get. While the recommended dietary allowance (RDA) for iodine is 150 mcg a day, the average consumption of iodine from seaweed by the mainland Japanese is nearly 14 mg. As our intake of iodine has declined, breast cancer has increased. Coincidence? I don't think so.

SECRET #6 A deficiency of iodine can increase your risk for breast cancer.

I first wrote about seaweed in my newsletter the *Women's Health Letter*. Shortly after I wrote the article, I received a call from Dr. Abraham. "Your article was very good," he said, "but there's more to the subject of iodine than its role in thyroid function. There's strong evidence that women who are deficient in iodine are more prone to breast cancer!"

This is because iodine is highly concentrated in breast tissues. When radioactive iodine breaks down in your breasts, it can contribute to breast cancer. And, if you remember, dietary iodine blocks the absorption of this harmful iodine.

Low iodine can increase the production of estrogens, and your lifetime exposure to estrogens increases your risk for breast cancer. Iodine normalizes the effect of estrogens on breast tissues.

Remember what I said earlier about the time when our bread contained traces of iodine? Our risk for breast cancer was then one in twenty. Now that bromine is being used instead of iodine, our risk for breast cancer has jumped to one in eight.

In a study on iodine in the thyroid and breast tissues of rats, Dr. B. Eskin, who has been researching this subject for more than thirty years, found that when rats became deficient in iodine they became hypothyroid. Then, when they were given thyroid hormones—the usual treatment for hypothyroidism—an excessive number of cells grew in their breast tissues.

It's important that you follow this next concept carefully.

When estrogen was given to these rats, these breast cells became pre-cancerous. But when iodine was given to the rats, this abnormal cell growth stopped. You see, iodine turns down or turns off estrogen receptors in the breast. So with an iodine deficiency, the breast tissues respond abnormally to estrogen. This can lead to pre-cancer and then to cancer.

While thyroid experts and most endocrinologists keep telling us that we need only 150 mcg of iodine a day, Dr. Abraham believes we need 100 times that amount! He has found evidence from the Japanese diet and health to back up his claim. Getting 150 mcg of iodine a day may be enough to prevent you from having a goiter, which is a sign of frank iodine deficiency. But you could need as much iodine as the Japanese get in order to support your thyroid gland and protect you from breast cancer.

Thyroid imbalances and breast cancer are not the only health consequences of an iodine-deficient diet. Evidence is mounting to suggest that iodine affects a number of important body functions.

SECRET #7 Iodine is more than a mineral. It is an adaptogen.

Adaptogens are substances that help normalize various bodily functions. Usually, adaptogens are herbs like *Rhodiola rosea* or *Cordyceps* mushrooms. Now we're seeing that iodine, so crucial to good health, may in fact be the ultimate adaptogen. Studies show that if you take enough iodine—100 to 400 times the RDA—it helps regulate other body functions as well.

You Heard It Here First

I was the first person to write about Dr. Abraham's test for iodine insufficiency several years ago, before it was even available to the public. And I've been talking about iodine ever since. It's the most exciting nutritional breakthrough I've discovered in the past decade!

Dr. Abraham found that more than 90 percent of us are low in iodine. He's not alone in this finding. Drs. Jorge Flechas and David Brownstein, who have tested for iodine and used iodine/iodide supplementation for years, are convinced that whole-body iodine insufficiency is contributing to numerous health problems from hypothyroidism to breast cancer and fibromyalgia.

The RDA for iodine is 0.15 mg (150 mcg), but Dr. Abraham found that when we take 50 mg of iodine/iodide a day, it acts as an adaptogen, regulating various body functions. Here are some ways iodine affects your health.

- *Iodine normalizes hormone receptors:* Hormones have "parking spaces" called receptors that are reserved for them. These receptors need to have iodine attached to them for optimal function. Without enough iodine, your hormones won't work at their best. If you're taking any hormones at all and they're not working as well as you and your doctor think they should, the reason could be iodine insufficiency.

• *Iodine regulates the thyroid:* Your thyroid gland needs iodine whether it's working normally, is underactive (hypothyroidism), overactive (hyperthyroidism), or enlarged (goiter). Enough iodine normalizes all these conditions.

• *Iodine reduces fibromyalgia in patients with low thyroid function:* Dr. Jorge Flechas observed some improvement in his fibromyalgia patients who were taking iodine supplementation. One reason for this could be because excess bromide often displaces iodine. Fibromyalgia patients often have high levels of bromide. Dr. Abraham has reported that iodine removes bromide from the body, improving fibromyalgia.

• *Iodine protects your breasts:* When bromide gets into breast tissues, it displaces iodine. Some women with fibrocystic breast disease find their cysts and tenderness disappear after iodine supplementation.

• *Iodine supports your adrenal glands and helps reduce stress:* Your adrenal glands need sufficient iodine to function properly and respond to life's many stresses.

• *Iodine helps your digestion:* Your stomach makes HCl (hydrochloric acid) to help you digest protein. HCl is an acid that also helps you break down and use calcium, magnesium, and iron. Low HCl production can be caused by iodine insufficiency. Our bodies need iodine to pump chloride into our stomach cells in order to help make hydrochloric acid.

• *Iodine improves immunity:* Iodine protects us from two toxic elements, fluoride and bromide, by competing with them for their place in our tissues. These toxins are in our water, hot tubs, non-organic foods, and some soft drinks. Bromide is even used in some asthma drugs. If you don't have enough iodine, chances are you have too much fluoride and bromide. Sufficient iodine pulls these toxins out of your body.

SECRET #8 You may need iodine even if you're healthy.

If you suffer from any chronic illness, including cancer, you need to have Dr. Abraham's twenty-four-hour urine test performed to measure your iodine levels. I even suggest this test for healthy individuals, as it may help prevent disease from occurring.

I took this test several years ago and discovered I was low in iodine—and I'm very healthy. After taking his iodine supplement, Iodoral, for several months I noticed more mental clarity, increased energy, and a better complexion. These positive effects disappeared when I stopped taking it.

Needless to say, I'm back on Iodoral. I was tested five times in one year to see the correlation between different doses of Iodoral and my symptoms, and can feel the difference. I'm more energetic, sharper, and look younger when I take enough of it. But everyone is different. You may find other benefits.

The implications for getting sufficient iodine are vast. Forward-thinking doctors are seeing that iodine may hold the key to their patients' health problems. Until you have been tested, and have achieved iodine sufficiency, you won't know how vital iodine is to your own health. What are you waiting for?

Health care professionals can contact Dr. Abraham for a free PowerPoint presentation on iodine and this iodine-loading test. You can contact Dr. Flechas for the 24-hour urine kit and find out if you, too, are low in iodine. You will find their contact information in the Resources section.

CHAPTER 2

How the Right Bacteria Can Protect Your Health

Our intestines are filled with bacteria. Some are beneficial to our health, while others cause disease. Helpful bacteria fight everything from undigested pieces of food and staph infections to the bacteria that causes food poisoning *(E. coli)*.

You may have heard of acidophilus, and possibly even bifidus. They're friendly bacteria that help keep bad (pathogenic) bacteria in check. As you may already know, your populations of friendly bacteria, called "probiotics," become depleted after a bout of diarrhea or a course of antibiotics. This is when you're more vulnerable to bacterial infections and have a lower immunity. It's no secret that taking probiotic supplements can reverse this deficiency. What you may not know is that not all probiotics are equally effective or even safe. Some could put your health at greater risk.

There are hundreds of species of bacteria. Within each species are many different strains. Some of them are naturally found in our bodies while others are not. Just how important are probiotics?

SECRET #9 The right probiotics can save your life.

I had heard miraculous stories attributed to probiotics, but none were more impressive than the one my friend's mother experienced. An extremely strong formula of herbs and friendly bacteria literally brought her back from death.

The doctor told my friend Joan that her ninety-five-year-old mother, Bernice, was unlikely to survive the night. The massive doses of antibiotics she had been given for her severe bacterial infection were not working. Joan wanted to give her mother some probiotics I had supplied her with, but Bernice's doctor advised against them. Why? Because he didn't know what they were. "She has a bacterial infection, so I don't want her to take any bacteria," he said.

But Joan felt there was nothing to lose. She knew that probiotics were beneficial bacteria that fight harmful ones, so she gave her mother two of these strong probiotic perles. The next morning, her mother was sitting up in bed and eating breakfast!

"I saw a tunnel," she told Joan. "At the end of it was a white light and lots and lots of white clouds." She had also seen her parents and long-dead husband. Bernice had been very close to death. Now she was back for a while, thanks to a probiotic product so strong it's been shown in university-based studies to kill antibiotic-resistant superbugs.

Don't expect results like this from just any probiotic. Many actually have very little activity. They may help your digestion or reduce an overgrowth of *Candida albicans* (a yeast infection), but they won't turn your health around like the best formulas can. And other formulas may not be safe at all. Before I tell you about some excellent products, I'd like you to know about the limitations of the probiotics that are being marketed as soil-based organisms.

SECRET #10 Some probiotics could be harmful to your health.

If you already have immune problems, be careful about taking any probiotics that come from the soil. Some claim to be superior to more commonly known organisms. But not only is their superiority unproven . . . they could possibly contribute to major health problems!

The most widely used soil-based organisms used in probiotic formulas are several species of *Bacillus*. The people who make and sell these formulas tout their virtues and list dozens of testimonials. But Dr. Hamilton-Miller, a medical microbiologist at a major London medical school, is worried. *Bacillus* is not considered to be part of the normal flora in the intestines of people or animals, and some species are known to cause serious health problems. Anthrax, for instance, is a species of *Bacillus*.

SECRET #11 There are more than 100 *Bacillus* species and they are notoriously difficult to identify.

Because some species of *Bacillus* can be harmful, you need to know exactly which ones are in any formula you intend to take. Unfortunately, this isn't always possible because the various species are so hard to identify.

You should also know whether there have been long-term, double-blinded, randomized studies on the safety and effectiveness of each species, published in peer-reviewed medical journals, before taking any product that contains them.

I read more than fifty studies, papers, and textbooks, and spoke with experts in the field of probiotics to research this subject. I couldn't find sound studies on people to back up the claims for soil-based bacteria for human health anywhere!

I know that my stand on soil-based bacteria is likely to make me very unpopular with anyone who has read articles or ads about them. Especially since some well-known doctors have endorsed them and many people feel better after taking them. But I can't help it. If there isn't good science behind a product, I need to tell you. Then, when the science exists, I'll help you understand what it means. When I can, I'll change my opinion and give that product the green light. Unfortunately, I can't do this yet with soil-based bacteria. They may be safe for you to take, or they may not be.

Safety First

The Food and Agriculture Organization of the United Nations and the World Health Organization asks that all probiotic producers prove that any particular species they use in their products is safe. To my knowledge, this has not been done with soil-based bacteria. Often, the specific strain within the species is not identified.

I spoke with Ted Sellers, the vice president of Life Science Products, Inc., a multilevel marketing company that sells a probiotic formula including soil-based organisms. He's convinced they're safe. Ted is passionate about *Bacillus* based solely on its anecdotal use. His comfort level comes from his product's history and its reported long-term safety over twenty years. And there's no doubt in my mind that soil-based probiotics do help some people.

Ted understands that some people would feel more comfortable with double-blinded studies, but is concerned that this might put probiotics under the scrutiny of the Food and Drug Administration (FDA), complicating matters for some companies. At the same time, it would identify each species and strain and assure its safety. Personally, I vote for more information on safety.

Some Problems with *Bacillus*

It's very possible that the people who need probiotics the most should avoid those containing soil-based bacteria. Probiotics are particularly valuable for people who have serious immune problems. I explained the potential problem of using soil-based products for people with immune problems to one doctor. He looked at me with concern. "That's all of my patients!" he said. "I'd rather not take a chance with people who are already sick."

One nutrition expert I spoke with originally embraced the concept and philosophy of these organisms until receiving dozens of calls from people who complained that they became severely sick after using them. This person no longer recommends them.

Each expert I interviewed had had a similar change of mind. They are concerned about the lack of quality control, lack of identification of the species and their strain on a product's label, and lack of studies on the safety and effectiveness of these particular strains of bacteria.

Two of the most commonly used soil-based organisms found in probiotic formulas are *Bacillus subtilis* and *Bacillus licheniformis*. A paper from the Graduate School of Biomedical Sciences at the University of Texas Medical Branch states that both "are periodically associated with bacteremia/septicemia, endocarditis, meningitis, and infections or wounds, (in) the ears, eyes, respiratory tract, urinary tract, and gastrointestinal tract." Let's take a closer look at these two bacteria.

Bacillus subtilis: If you ever need to take an antibiotic, you may not want to take *B. subtilis* with it. It could cancel out any benefits from the drug. Some strains of *B. subtilis* are resistant to many antibiotics and can even cause an infection in the blood (septicemia) in people with a suppressed immune system. In one case, it contributed to a patient's death.

A man in his seventies with leukemia had been taking an Italian formula of soil-based bacteria until he was admitted to the hospital with a high fever from a bacterial infection. His condition deteriorated, and he was given a number of antibiotics. The antibiotics didn't work. His blood tests showed high levels of *B. subtilis*, and further lab tests found it was resistant to every antibiotic he had been given. Unfortunately, he died.

> Some *Bacillus* "may be problematic and should be accepted only for clearly defined strains, which have been tested negative for toxicity and pathogenicity in vitro and in vivo."
>
> —EUROPEAN COMMISSION HEALTH & CONSUMER PROTECTION DIRECTORATE-GENERAL, UPDATED OCTOBER 17, 2002

A group of London researchers attempted to evaluate the effectiveness of a group of soil-based organisms. They were dismayed to find that only one out of five products were correctly labeled. In most cases, the bacterium labeled *B. subtilis* was not that species at all. All were resistant to antibiotics including penicillin and ampicillin. Most microbial laboratories throw out *B. subtilis* or report it as a contaminant.

Bacillus licheniformis: Food poisoning, antibiotic resistance, and infections have all been associated with this species of *Bacillus*. A group of mice with low immunity were given thirteen different strains of *B. licheniformis*. Every single one of these strains caused infections in their brains and lungs.

That's not all. A committee on animal nutrition found that one strain of *B. licheniformis* was unsafe in animal feed because it caused antibiotic resistance. A Finnish research team found that other strains caused food poisoning and infections. These scientists question the safety of *B. licheniformis* in general. A third study conducted at the University of Maryland Cancer Center on *Bacillus* infections in cancer patients concluded that these *Bacillus* species are "now being recognized as a bacterial pathogen for compromised hosts."

The Right Strain

Most companies list the species of probiotics used in their formulas, but not the strain. Saying that a product contains *Lactobacillus acidophilus* is not enough. The strain appears after the type of probiotic (*Lactobacillus*) and species (*acidophilus*), like *L. acidophilus* (R0052) or *L. acidophilus* (NAS).

You need to be a good detective to separate the safe from the questionable probiotics. There are more than 400 species of protective and harmful bacteria in your digestive tract and hundreds of strains within each species. Some strains are harmful and some are ineffective. Others may be safe with little activity, or both safe and potent. There's no way to know unless the strains are identified. Every strain of probiotics you take should be listed and tested for safety and effectiveness. Testimonials alone just won't do for me. If the label doesn't list the strain, ask the manufacturer.

Clearly, we need more studies to show which species, and strains of a species, are both safe and effective in humans. This is especially important for anyone who is sick or has low immunity. I'd like to see a number of double-blinded tests over a longer period of time with each species and strain of bacteria clearly identified.

The FDA agrees. It issued a warning letter to one company that sells soil-based bacteria. The company advertised that its products have "been shown to drastically reduce populations of yeast, parasites, and bad bacteria in the intestines." The FDA said, prove it.

Which Probiotics Should You Take?

Some companies, in an attempt to be upfront about the limitations of soil-based bacteria for severely immune-compromised people, have a warning printed on the label of their products for them. I commend them for doing this. But not everyone reads the small print on bottles. If you have any reservations about using soil-based bacteria to enhance your health, understand that you have other options.

Many probiotic formulas contain species and strains that have been found safe and effective in hundreds of good double-blind tests published in peer-reviewed medical journals. Each species is clearly marked on its label or in its literature so you can find the studies on that particular species. And the particular strain of the species is also identified and proven to be safe. Unfortunately, you can't judge probiotics by the company that sells them. Some good supplement companies sell friendly bacteria that don't do much. Let me explain how to identify the best.

SECRET #12 Good digestion could destroy your probiotics.

In order to be effective, friendly bacteria need to stay alive after passing through your stomach. But live bacteria often don't survive the trip to your intestines because stomach acid (HCl) kills both good and bad bugs. If you have good digestion, you probably have enough HCl to destroy the probiotics you're taking.

To help them survive better, take probiotics after meals when your stomach contains less acid. Or you take them on an empty stomach the first thing in the morning and before going to bed at night. But there's an even better, simpler way. Only take probiotics that have been coated to survive stomach acids. Use powders, liquids, or capsules only if they have been shown to get past acids.

Don't be fooled by potency claims. Probiotics don't necessarily contain the amount of bacteria listed on their labels. They may have when they were manufactured, but many may have died off in the bottle. Look for a guarantee of potency *after* the bottle has been opened. Here are some of the best probiotic formulas available.

SECRET #13 This little-known probiotic formula can kill superbugs.

The strongest, most effective probiotic product I've ever found is Dr. Ohhira's 12-Plus Probiotic Formula. This formula is made in Japan and distributed in the United States by Essential Formulas. It's an enteric-coated product that contains twelve strains of lactic acid bacteria as well as micronutrient byproducts such as vitamins, minerals, amino acids, FOS (probiotic food), and bacteriocins (nature's own antibiotic).

The manufacturer ferments ninety-two plant products together for five years to produce this formula. It also contains organic acids that perform an important function. They help the probiotics stick to the intestinal walls and colonize. No other company I know of has done research on the adhesion ability of its particular formula like Dr. Ohhira, a Japanese researcher.

He also developed a special strain of bacteria, *Enterococcus faecalis* TH10, from a fermented soy food (tempeh). This strain is more than six times stronger than any other naturally occurring lactic acid bacteria. This is the formula I gave Joan for her mother. I also used it with patients whose intestinal problems did not respond to other probiotics. In every case it worked, and it worked quickly.

Studies show Dr. Ohhira's formula is effective against *H. pylori* (a source of ulcers and migraines), *E. coli* (food poisoning), and even the superbug that causes staph infections (methicillin-resistant *Staphylococcus aureus*). It helps regulate the bowels like no other formula I've heard of. And an added bonus is its ability to help increase bone density in women over forty.

Dr. Ohhira's formula does not need to be refrigerated and has a three-year shelf life. If you have a serious problem, or a condition that isn't responding to other probiotics, try it for at least one or two months. When your condition is under control, as evaluated by your doctor, you can either take a maintenance dose of one capsule a day or switch to a good, less-potent, and less-expensive formula.

SECRET #14 This probiotic trio can't be destroyed by stomach acid.

Natren is a company that has always produced excellent probiotic products backed with sound scientific research. I've used their products for nearly twenty years. Healthy Trinity is my favorite. It's Natren's strongest formula and contains three well-studied super strains, *Lactobacillus acidophilus*, *Lactobacillus bulgaricus*, and *Bifidobacterium bifidum*. Not only does it contain strong strains of probiotics, but stomach acid won't break them down.

One of the super strains, *Lactobacillus acidophilus* NAS, sticks well to the intestinal lining. But what I like best about Healthy Trinity is how it's designed to keep the friendly bacteria alive until they get into your intestines. A special oil matrix separates each of the three probiotics in this formula. This oil matrix has two functions. It keeps the three strains of bacteria from competing with one another. And your stomach acid can't break down the oil and destroy the bacteria after its gelatin capsule dissolves in your stomach. This means that the friendly bacteria in this formula can easily pass through your stomach untouched until they get to your intestines.

Healthy Trinity is particularly helpful for people with acid reflux (heartburn), *H. pylori*, chronic candida, and diarrhea caused by *Clostridium difficile* (from taking antibiotics). If you have any persistent diarrhea, or if you've had diarrhea for a week or more, talk with your doctor. Then, consider taking Healthy Trinity for two weeks to a month to replenish your depleted stores of friendly bacteria.

Natren guarantees the potency of Healthy Trinity through the expiration date on its label. It needs to be refrigerated, so look for it in the refrigerated section in your health-food store.

SECRET #15 This inexpensive probiotic works well and needs no refrigeration.

Dr. Ohhira's 12-Plus Probiotic Formula and Healthy Trinity are two potent probiotic formulas with good, sound science behind them. The biggest problem with them is that they're rather expensive. Let me say here that they're well worth the price if you have severe digestive or immune problems. But not everyone does.

Many of us are looking for a good probiotic formula to take once a year to repopulate our intestines. Or a good friendly bacteria formula to take after food poisoning or the flu. For everyday use, consider using a less-expensive probiotic formula. Just make sure that it contains effective, well-studied strains of friendly bacteria that are enteric-coated and are guaranteed to be strong. Unfortunately, few fall into this category.

The formula I like in this category is Women's Preferred Advanced Probiotic Formula. It contains six strains of friendly bacteria normally found throughout the intestines. Each strain works alone and with the others to stick well to the intestines. These strains have been shown to fight infections like food poisoning or candida, help regulate bowel movements, and support the immune system. If you have a serious or long-standing problem, you may want a stronger formula. Otherwise, this one should work well at less than half the price of the first two.

In the Advanced Probiotic Formula, 100 percent of the coated bacteria survives a full hour's exposure to stomach acid. That's impressive! Capsules that are not coated have only a 5-percent survival rate. Since you don't have to refrigerate this product like most others, pack a bottle in your suitcase when you travel and keep some in your purse. (For order information on these three probiotic formulas, see the Resource section.)

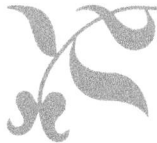

CHAPTER 3

Boost Your Immunity with an Ancient Oriental Secret

If you suffer from annual bouts of bronchitis, pneumonia, severe colds and flu, or just have a severely weakened immune system, there's an ancient secret from the Orient that will boost your immune system and fight off all types of infection.

Ever since I was a child exposed daily to secondhand smoke, I was prone to frequent colds and flu. They never remained simple head colds. They would settle in my lungs and turn into bronchitis. As an adult, they often became full-blown pneumonia. I couldn't remember the last time I had a simple head cold with a runny nose.

In spite of being healthy most of the rest of the time, I had to be extra careful during fall and winter months to avoid getting sick. Seasonal weather changes were typically when I (and thousands of other people) were most vulnerable to viruses. Through the years, I tried many dietary plans and supplements to enhance my immune system, but none really worked consistently.

Until a few years ago, that is! During a serious bout of pneumonia, I realized that I had to solve the problem of my lifelong lung weakness. If I didn't, it could eventually cost me my life. Respiratory illness is one of the leading causes of death in seniors, especially those with congestive heart failure. I didn't want this to be my future. I was determined to find an answer—and I did! But it wasn't anything I thought it would be.

The solution to my lung problems was given to me at a health convention, of all places. Coughing away with an unexpected spring cold, I spied an old friend, Janet Zand. Janet is an experienced acupuncturist and herbalist with an encyclopedic mind filled with herbal information. At one time, she founded a large herbal company. I asked Janet what she'd suggest and without hesitation she replied, "*Cordyceps* and shiitake mushrooms. They stimulate the immune system and strengthen the lungs."

Not only did the mushrooms work at that time, they have continued to work ever since. Mushrooms are particularly valuable because they boost immunity and many of them also give specific support to the lungs.

Janet Zand's advice started me on a search for more information on medicinal mushrooms. What a surprise it was to find that the oldest grower of medicinal mushrooms for the supplement industry had a plant in my little hometown. In fact, I could walk to it! David Law, president of Gourmet Mushrooms, introduced me to the fascinating world of medicinal mushrooms, a realm based on thousands of years of usage and a number of sound scientific studies.

Today, medicinal mushrooms are one of the best-kept health secrets I've ever discovered. In my opinion, they support the immune system better than any herb or herbal formula. The Chinese know this. They've used mushrooms as medicines for centuries.

Out of more than 100,000 species of fungi, over a dozen varieties have been used in China for more than 3,000 years to increase immunity, strengthen the lungs and other organs, and as part of cancer therapy. They are included in traditional Chinese medicine and used extensively by acupuncturists under their Latin names.

Lately, medicinal mushroom sales have been . . . well . . . mushrooming. I've been shouting their praises loudly since 2000, and they've become one of the main supplements I both take and recommend.

SECRET #16 These "sponges" can either help you detoxify or make you sicker.

Medicinal mushrooms are one of nature's best detoxifiers. They act like sponges, absorbing and removing toxins like chemotherapy agents, pharmaceutical drugs, and heavy metals. In fact, their role in removing heavy metals like mercury is one of their greatest benefits.

But this blessing can also be a curse. You see, some mushrooms that are grown in China contain high amounts of heavy metals. This contamination comes from the water used in their growing process. Mushrooms containing heavy metals or other contaminants could cause more harm than good. Be sure that any medicinal mushrooms you buy are grown organically with water tested for heavy metals. Many of those grown in this country meet these specifications.

But detoxification is just one way medicinal mushrooms work to keep you healthy. They also have a profound effect on the immune system.

SECRET #17 Mushrooms work by reminding your immune system to fight.

When I first learned how medicinal mushrooms acted on the immune system, I was astonished. The more I learn about them, the more it seems like they were designed specifically to help us stay healthy. Perhaps the most significant key to staying healthy is having a strong immune system. Mushrooms are a great help. Here's how they work.

Mushrooms are made up from various-sized molecules. The smaller molecules contain nutrients, while the larger ones are used by the immune system to make antigens. Antigens, in turn, produce antibodies to fight disease-producing substances. The large mushroom molecules have a unique shape that your immune system somehow remembers. When you are exposed to bacteria or viruses that have similar shaped molecules, your body remembers that mushrooms can produce the antibodies you need to fight these harmful invaders. This is amazing to me.

You see, as long as you have mushroom molecules circulating in your body, your immune system is on alert, ready to take action at a moment's notice. This is why so many healthcare practitioners now believe it is best to take medicinal mushrooms more than once a day—so those molecules are always present in your blood.

The part of your immune system that remembers the size and shape of these large mushroom molecules are your T cells, a group of cells living in the thymus gland. Your thymus gland protects you against harmful bacteria, viruses, and parasites, but it shrinks as we age, reducing our army of T cells. This is why it's so important to boost your immune system as you get older, especially before changing winter weather increases our susceptibility to cold and flu viruses. I decided to take a mushroom formula every morning and evening. They've kept me healthy for years.

There are a number of mushroom formulas available in health-food stores and through the mail. Here are a few of the most helpful mushrooms you'll find in them.

Shiitake (*Lentinus edodes*)

If you've ever cooked with dried Chinese mushrooms, you've eaten shiitake mushrooms. Fresh shiitake are becoming more common in some grocery stores and health-food stores. They have a rich earthy flavor that I find more satisfying than the common button mushrooms. Their medicinal use goes back to the Ming Dynasty in China where they were used for lung problems and to increase stamina.

Shiitake are now being used as part of a nutritional program for people with cancer. They contain a chemical called lentinan that has been shown to reduce tumors. Currently, lentinan is under investigation as a potential cancer-fighting drug. Early studies are indicating, however, that there are other substances in shiitakes besides lentinan that fight cancer. For this reason, it may be best to use the whole mushroom.

When you use a powder or extract made from whole mushrooms, you're taking a food that supports your health. When you use a product made from one ingredient in the mushroom, it's more like taking an over-the-counter drug. If pharmaceutical companies find benefits from lentinan, or any other single nutrient in a mushroom, the result is likely to be an expensive prescription drug. It makes sense to me to use the whole product.

Let food become your medicine, as Hippocrates suggested centuries ago, by adding shiitake mushrooms to your diet. You can buy a pound of dried shiitake mushrooms at an Oriental market and soak a handful of them in warm water until they're soft. Add slices of them to a stir-fried dish or soup. Don't throw away the water they soaked in since it contains important immune-stimulating substances. If you like, you can freeze this mushroom-water in ice cube trays and add some to soups and sauces. If you can find fresh shiitake, use them as well.

In addition to improving stamina and possibly fighting cancer, shiitake mushrooms help the body make interferon. Interferon is a powerful antiviral substance that's been used in the treatment of hepatitis C. Shiitake mushrooms have been used for an overgrowth of *Candida albicans*, and for bronchial inflammation including asthma, environmental allergies, and frequent colds and flu.

Reishi (*Ganoderma lucidum*)

Reishi mushrooms strengthen the immune system by increasing white blood cells and cells that fight tumors. Some studies indicate that they specifically help the lungs by regenerating lung tissue. Reishi also appear to prevent bronchitis, strengthen the adrenal glands (the glands that handle all types of stress), and have antiviral effects through their production of interferon. In his practice, Christopher Hobbs, an herbalist who specializes in medicinal mushrooms, has found reishi mushrooms to be particularly effective for nervous or anxious people suffering from adrenal exhaustion. He often prefers to use them instead of relaxing herbs like valerian root or scullcap.

Reishi are becoming more widely used in cancer treatment. In fact, the Japanese government has formally listed reishi as a supplement to be used specifically for people with cancer. They have conducted studies that show reishi protects against radiation. If you have had radiation treatments, or if you should decide to have them in the future, you may want to consider taking a supplement that includes reishi. I would also recommend this mushroom as part of any cancer protection plan.

Maitake (*Grifola frondosa*)

Maitakes were used in ancient China for respiratory problems, poor circulation, liver support, weakness, exhaustion, and to strengthen the life force (*chi*). But that's not all. We're finding that maitakes have even more applications than the Chinese identified. One Japanese study using rats showed that powdered maitake lowered cholesterol and increased the excretion of bile, a substance we need to digest fats. This means that maitakes could help with fat digestion.

Now maitakes are becoming popular for one isolated substance they contain called D-fraction. D-fraction is a powerful substance. It has been shown to have antitumor activity and also supports the immune system in general. But so does the complete mushroom. One study found that maitakes blocked the growth of tumors in 86 percent of mice. People and mice are different, of course. But the history of medicinal mushrooms indicates that once again, the whole mushroom may contain cofactors that either enhance the absorption of D-fraction or add to its usefulness as an immune supporter.

It appears that using D-fraction may be more like using an over-the-counter medication, while taking the complete mushroom is more like eating a food that enhances immunity and helps the body function more effectively. Each has its place.

SECRET #18 Nature's most unusual mushroom turns back the aging clock.

Cordyceps (Cordyceps sinensis)

This mushroom grows high in the mountains of Tibet and China and has been prized for centuries for its amazing, energizing, and restorative properties. So many of the conditions it supports are associated with aging that it's recognized as a potent antiaging nutrient.

At one time, only emperors and the very wealthiest people in Asia could afford it. Even now, it's the highest priced of all Chinese herbs.

What is it?

Without a doubt, it's the most unusual supplement you've ever heard of. *Cordyceps* is a rare, finger-shaped, capless mushroom. But this is not just another medicinal mushroom. It is a fungus known as the caterpillar mushroom that actually grows out of a caterpillar.

All mushrooms and fungi are nature's recyclers. They absorb nutrients and toxins from the debris and plants around them. *Cordyceps* is a special type of fungus that grows on insect larvae and caterpillar cocoons. It absorbs proteins and other nutrients from its host. The result is a fungus with amazing qualities.

How *Cordyceps* Grows

The life cycle of *Cordyceps* is a fascinating story of chance meetings and interdependence. A small Asian caterpillar, foraging for food, either brushes up against some *Cordyceps* spores or eats them accidentally. When the weather gets colder, the caterpillar burrows underground and wraps itself in a silken cocoon. The mushroom spores germinate while the caterpillar sleeps. When the caterpillar dies, the mushroom spores grow, taking their nourishment from the caterpillar. In spring, the mushroom grows above ground and out of the caterpillar's head, releasing some of its spores for other caterpillars to find. And the cycle continues.

Today, *Cordyceps* is grown on brown rice under strict conditions where tissues from an original caterpillar and particularly potent mushroom are duplicated. The result is a safe product with the same properties as wild *Cordyceps*.

Of all the mushrooms I've ever used and researched, *Cordyceps* is the most remarkable for anyone over the age of forty. It truly is an antiaging mushroom.

What Does Antiaging Really Mean?

To me, antiaging means staying healthy and vigorous with an absence or minimum of disease and discomfort. A strong immune system helps us stay healthy.

Our immune systems weaken over time, and *Cordyceps* regulates immunity. We become more easily fatigued as we get older. *Cordyceps* not only increases energy, it helps you recover more quickly after exercising. High cholesterol, high triglycerides, frequent colds and bronchitis, irregular heartbeat, and kidney failure are all signs of aging. We know from more than 1,000 years of use and numerous studies that *Cordyceps* helps all of these conditions.

How can any one substance do so much? It's because *Cordyceps* is an adaptogen. An adaptogen helps regulate—not stimulate—your body's functions. Here are just a few of the areas where *Cordyceps* excels in turning back the aging clock:

Immunity: Your immune system is your doorway to health. *Cordyceps* can either activate a sluggish immune system or calm it down when it's overstimulated. This means that it has the ability to improve both immune and autoimmune disorders including diabetes, lupus, and cancer.

Lungs: Cordyceps helps relax smooth muscles. This may be why ancient Chinese texts found it to be especially effective for respiratory problems like chronic bronchitis, asthma, and pulmonary and congestive heart diseases. I have never felt so old as when I had bronchitis and was coughing day and night for weeks without relief. I haven't had one serious cold, much less bronchitis or pneumonia, since I began taking a mushroom formula high in *Cordyceps*.

As we grow older, we become more at risk for complications from the flu. Pneumonia and bronchitis are the real dangers, not just the flu. Now is the time to strengthen your lungs and regain your health and youthfulness. Don't wait until flu season approaches.

Heart Health: Heart disease is the number one killer of postmenopausal women. Anything that improves symptoms or prevents disease turns back our aging clocks.

The Chinese use *Cordyceps* for difficult cases of high cholesterol when other treatments don't work. Several studies show it reduces the oxidation of fats. It's oxidized cholesterol (fats), not cholesterol itself, that's the real health hazard. Oxidation promotes free radicals—and free radicals contribute to aging and disease.

Cordyceps improved the quality of life and health in a number of studies of seriously ill patients with chronic heart failure and pulmonary heart disease. It showed remarkable results in resolving or reducing arrhythmias (heart palpitations) in just two weeks in more than 80 percent of patients. *Cordyceps* is a valuable nutrient whether you have heart disease or want to prevent it.

In the past, some wild Chinese *Cordyceps* imported from China contained lead or were contaminated with harmful bacteria. Always buy medicinal mushrooms grown under strict conditions from reputable companies.

SECRET #19 This mushroom improves athletic performance and recovery from exercising.

Cordyceps has been used in Asia for hundreds of years to restore vitality in older people. The energy you get from it comes from its ability to enhance adrenaline without causing anxiety. But this capless mushroom also improves athletic performances. In fact, a group of Chinese athletes broke five world records at an international competition after taking *Cordyceps* during their training. But it not only works for high-performance athletes, it works for ordinary people who exercise, as well.

Let me give you an example from my own experience. One day I over-exercised (I was kayaking for an hour against the wind and had no choice but to continue). My muscles were exhausted when I finished and I could hardly drive home. I immediately took a double dose of medicinal mushrooms containing high amounts of *Cordyceps*. The next morning my arms were still very fatigued and I didn't know when they would feel strong and rested. But that afternoon, barely twenty-four hours later, I was ready to go paddling again. My muscles had recovered much more quickly than they had before when I was many years younger.

Where to Find *Cordyceps*

You can buy *Cordyceps* alone or in combination with other medicinal mushrooms in most health-food stores. Plain *Cordyceps* is more expensive than a combination product because the fungus is so tiny and difficult to grow. I take a variety of medicinal mushroom products depending on the results I want. For maintenance, I suggest taking one capsule of mushrooms that includes *Cordyceps* twice a day. If you have problems you want to correct, you can take as many as four to six capsules twice a day for at least a few months.

SECRET #20 Mushrooms can be enhanced for even greater effectiveness.

Just as mushrooms can absorb toxic heavy metals from the soil or water in which they grow, they also absorb beneficial nutrients. That's what David Law, president of Gourmet Mushrooms, realized. He was growing medicinal mushrooms for a well-respected physician and acupuncturist, Dr. Isaac Eliaz. The two men began talking about the possibility of growing mushrooms with enhanced properties by growing them on herbs and organic rice, rather than on rice alone. But Dr. Eliaz didn't choose just any herbs. He selected a variety of herbs that have been found to regulate immunity. The theory worked and a super nutrient was born.

The two men discovered that the mushrooms did, indeed, take on some of the properties of the herbs on which they were grown. The result was an enhanced mushroom formula unlike any other. This product is now being used successfully as an important part of treatment programs for cancer and other immune problems. In the future, Dr. Eliaz plans to design additional mushroom/herb combinations to target other specific health problems. For now, I use it as part of my daily supplement program.

Growing mushrooms on medicinal Chinese herbs is a blending of ancient wisdom and current scientific information. It's a new technique that creates a whole food with specific enhanced medicinal qualities. It makes sense biochemically and energetically since the body can't heal itself without both the proper nutrients and the energy to support and detoxify. This supplement does both. Part of the reason for its success is that it uses the whole mushrooms.

The Whole Is Greater Than the Sum of Its Parts

Often, a whole-food supplement out-performs one that emphasizes a single ingredient because it contains cofactors and "minor" nutrients that increase its effectiveness. These cofactors often haven't been studied or understood. Any of them could be responsible for the supplement's safety and effectiveness.

Whenever a single nutrient is emphasized, the natural balance is destroyed. The result is often a "natural" supplement that acts like a drug. It may work, but it can more easily upset your body's natural balance and lead to side effects. Mushrooms grown on herbs provide two types of whole foods that combine into one enhanced whole-food product.

SECRET #21 Taxol comes from a fungus, not from Yew trees.

Taxol is a potent—and expensive—anticancer drug found on the bark of the Pacific yew tree that unnecessarily threatens the extinction of these trees due to overharvesting. You see, Taxol doesn't come from the yew tree itself. Andrea and Don Stirele, along with Gary Strobel, of Montana State University, made a startling discovery. They found that Taxol is actually manufactured by a fungus that grows on yew trees!

The yew tree provides nutrients needed by this fungus, but it is the fungus that contains the active anticancer ingredients. In exchange for its food, the fungus produces a substance like a fungicide or insecticide that protects the tree from infectious diseases. The yew tree provides mushrooms with raw materials, and the fungi are the factories that process these raw materials into another product.

This is true for other medicinal mushrooms. Mushrooms grow on, and eat, dead tissues. In nature, they grow in soil rich in decomposed leaves and other materials. Cultivated medicinal mushrooms need nourishment, also. The quality of their food determines their beneficial qualities.

Like the fungus on yew trees, mushrooms can increase the potency of other compounds and create new ones. The rate at which mushrooms grow, the amount of heat they generate, and the quantity of food they eat, all factor into their beneficial qualities. Many medicinal mushrooms are grown on simple carbohydrates like brown rice. These carbohydrates help make immune-enhancing compounds. But when you feed the mushrooms on a base of brown rice and medicinal herbs, their growth increases by 30 percent!

A supplement made from mushrooms grown on herbs is more potent, and less expensive, than if the mushrooms and herbs were taken separately.

Combining Mushrooms with Chinese Herbs

Dr. Eliaz is a creative-thinking, science-based medical doctor well versed in Chinese herbs. He designed a proprietary blend of Chinese herbs that have the ability to increase the immune system, reduce cancer, detoxify, and act as adaptogens (nutrients that help restore the body's natural balance). Each medicinal mushroom is grown separately on a base of these Chinese herbs, then harvested, dried, and blended into the final formula. This formula, MycoPhyto Complex, is currently being studied at Amitabha Medical Clinic & Healing Center, Dr. Eliaz's clinic, in Sebastopol, California.

MycoPhyto Complex has been found to work well with many cancer patients. Dr. Eliaz, along with a number of other doctors and acupuncturists, is evaluating the formula for a widening number of conditions including chronic fatigue, hepatitis and other viral infections, and congestive heart failure. I expect to hear of more applications for this new and unusual process in the future.

Medicinal mushrooms, like shiitake and *Coriolus versicolor*, enhance the effectiveness of chemotherapy and radiation while removing the toxic debris left in their aftermath. They also strengthen the immune system and act as antitumor agents while destroying small tumors, often preventing them from growing into dangerous cancers. At the same time, they increase resistance to stress, enhancing overall health. One early observation found that cancer patients on chemotherapy were dramatically less fatigued after using this formula. When they stopped taking it, their fatigue returned.

In my opinion, anyone who uses pharmaceuticals of any kind should take a strong formula of detoxifying herbs and mushrooms to avoid future problems caused by any remaining impurities. Mushrooms help you detoxify, but this detoxification process doesn't have to make you tired if you are being strengthened at the same time. Many of the herbs in this formula are also tonifying.

SECRET #22 This combination of a lichen and a fungus works miracles on lung problems.

All mushrooms are fungi, but not all fungi are mushrooms. In my search for an answer to my many years of chronic bronchitis and pneumonia, I stumbled across a lichen called *Usnea barbata*. Lichens are a combination of an algae (a one-celled plant) and a fungus that live off one another so closely that they look and act like a single plant. Usnea grows on many oak trees throughout the country and looks like a short version of Spanish moss. Native American Indians, who called it "the lungs of the Earth," knew it was a very valuable plant. It was effective against pneumococcus, *Mycobacterium tuberculosis*, and other gram-positive bacteria that cause lung problems. Usnea also has antiviral activity, which makes it particularly useful if you don't know whether or not you have a bacterial infection or a virus. Hippocrates suggested Usnea for uterine problems many centuries ago, and the Chinese have included it in their repertoire of herbs as well.

The active ingredients in Usnea are usnic and barbatic acids, two acids that are soluble in alcohol, but not in water. The dried herb has considerably less activity. This is why you'll find more Usnea tinctures than teas or capsules.

Some Usnea tinctures are stronger than others because of the way they're made. Some are prepared using a hot alcohol extraction, while others use a cold alcohol-extraction method. Obviously, the easiest and cheapest method is cold extraction. But I spoke with several herbalists and discovered that the hot extraction method is superior. The finished product contains more usnic and barbatic acids. The result is a tincture with a higher antibiotic and antiviral activity. A cold extraction method will give fewer of these beneficial acids and more polysaccharides.

Now, there's something to be said for polysaccharides. They do support the immune system. However, you can get polysaccharides from any fresh or dried mushroom. Or you can make your own simple extraction. Buy some dried marshmallow root from a health-food store. Put the marshmallow root in a jar and add room temperature water to cover and let it stand for a day or two. Then, for the best of both worlds, remove enough of the water from the jar to put in your Usnea.

I haven't found any products that keep me healthy and stave off colds and flu as well as various forms of fungi. Just last year a medical-doctor friend of mine called to ask me, "What do you know that's as good as Usnea? It works so well for my patients!" At the time, I didn't have anything new to offer. But this year I'm going to tell her, "A mushroom combination like MycoPhyto Complex *and* Usnea!"

HAVE CANDIDA OR SEVERE ALLERGIES TO YEAST AND MOLDS? READ THIS . . .

I've been asked whether or not people with a *Candida albicans* yeast overgrowth can take medicinal mushrooms. After speaking with doctors and herbalists, I discovered that it's safe. If you have a severe allergy to yeasts and molds, talk with an acupuncturist or doctor of integrative medicine before using medicinal mushrooms. They may be fine, but this is one time when it's smart to ask someone who knows your condition.

CHAPTER 4

Battle Infections
with Herbal Antibiotics

Antibiotics are saving lives and costing thousands of people their health at the same time. This is truly a double-edged sword. If only doctors had originally dispensed them judiciously for conditions they could affect, perhaps we wouldn't be where we are today: in need of an antibiotic that works.

In case you hadn't noticed, antibiotics are not as effective as they once were. When you understand a little more about bacteria you may marvel, as I do, that any of them still work at all! I constantly see patients with chronic bacterial infections and suppressed immune systems from overusing, or misusing, antibiotics. Unless we can find an alternative to conventional antibiotics—one that won't result in antibiotic resistance—our health will be in even more jeopardy.

SECRET #23 Your antibiotic could kill you if you take it with certain foods or drugs.

You may think that the worst problem associated with taking antibiotics is that they kill off friendly bacteria in the intestines. Wrong! Although overusing antibiotics can lead to problems such as lowered immunity, digestive complaints, and yeast overgrowth, there are much more serious consequences.

In fact, taking one of the most popular antibiotics being used today could be fatal!

If you're taking the specific drugs I'll list for you, don't ever combine them with erythromycin. And pass along this information to everyone you know who is taking medications. It could save their life.

Erythromycin has been used for the past fifty years and has always been considered to be safe. But Wayne A. Ray, professor of preventive medicine at Vanderbilt University School of Medicine in Nashville, Tennessee, found that when you combine this antibiotic with certain drugs or foods the antibiotic stays in your body longer. The result is a five times greater risk for cardiac death.

Here's what's happening in your body: Erythromycin should stay in your bloodstream for a fixed period of time and then break down. That's why you take it several times a day. But certain drugs slow down this breakdown making the antibiotic much stronger.

What happens next is the potential killer. High amounts of erythromycin cause salt to be trapped in resting heart-muscle cells. This lengthens the time until the next heartbeat. Sometimes it actually triggers a deadly abnormal rhythm, and that's that.

If you're not taking medications, erythromycin has a very low risk of causing sudden death. But if you're taking any of the following drugs, ask your doctor for a different antibiotic, such as amoxicillin, which was found to be safe when taken with the medications that were studied.

Avoid erythromycin if you're taking any of the following:

- AIDS drugs that are protease inhibitors

- Antibiotic: clarithromycin (Biaxin)

- Antifungals: ketoconazole (Nizoral) and itraconazole (Sporanox)

- Blood pressure meds: verapamil (Verelan, Isoptin) or diltiazem (Cardizem, Tiazac)

- Grapefruit juice (it also raises blood levels of the antibiotic)

If you're taking any medications, check with your pharmacist before adding any new prescription. The safest medication when taken alone could be harmful when taken with others.

SECRET #24 Antibiotics won't help your colds or flu.

Antibiotics work by interrupting bacterial growth. They are only effective against bacteria, not viruses. Don't ask your doctor to give you a prescription for an antibiotic when you have a cold or the flu. They're both viruses. Don't take an antibiotic unless your doctor has done a culture to determine that you have a bacterial infection. According to researchers at the Center for Disease Control and Prevention, about one-third of the 150 million prescriptions written annually for antibiotics are unnecessary. The problem is that repeated exposure to antibiotics results in even more resistance.

SECRET #25 Antibiotic resistance is caused by gossiping bacteria.

Not very long ago, the FDA announced that feeding antibiotics to chickens and turkeys was causing antibiotic resistance in humans. Then the FDA turned around and recommended approval for still another antibiotic, linezolid (Zyvox). Zyvox, they said, is more effective against staph infections than our most potent antibiotics. But how long will it take before we become resistant to Zyvox? Not long at all, I predict.

Each year 100,000 people die from drug-resistant bacteria because their antibiotics didn't work. To find out why, I spoke with Stephen Harrod Buhner, an herbalist and the author of *Herbal Antibiotics*. He told me that one reason is that bacteria are actually ganging up on us.

Buhner calls bacteria the biggest gossips on earth. This is because they communicate silently from one organism to another. When bacteria are exposed to antibiotics, they create solutions that are antagonistic to them. In fact, they secrete chemicals called pheromones that attract other bacteria and help them communicate with one another. What do they "talk" about? How to stay alive by resisting antibiotics.

Spreading the Word

Resistance to bacteria spreads quickly through a species and even crosses species' boundaries from animals to humans. Buhner tells a chilling story about chickens fed small amounts of antibiotics in their feed. One to one and a half days afterwards, their feces contained bacteria resistant to *E. coli*. Three days later, chickens in adjacent cages were resistant to *E. coli* as well as other antibiotics that they had not even been exposed to. Three months later, chickens never fed antibiotics that lived outside the barn containing the antibiotic-fed chickens became resistant. And six months later, people living in a nearby house who had no contact with these chickens whatsoever became resistant to multiple antibiotics.

SECRET #26 Herbal antibiotics don't cause antibiotic resistance.

We can't escape bacteria or some resistance to them. They live in us and on all living things. Right now, about one to two pounds of your weight come from bacteria. Some are good guys (like *L. acidophilus* and *B. bifidus*), some are pathogenic (disease-causing). If colonies of pathogenic bacteria are not kept in check by beneficial bacteria, you may need to take some kind of antibiotic. The question is, can we find an antibiotic that doesn't cause antibiotic resistance? And the answer is, "Yes"!

Pharmaceutical antibiotics are usually made from one chemical that fights bacteria while herbs contain hundreds of compounds. It's easier to develop a resistance to one chemical than to many. This is why I prefer herbal antibiotics whenever possible. It's just about impossible to develop resistance to a plant-based antibiotic consisting of so many different compounds. Doctors may prescribe broad-based antibiotics, but there's nothing as broad-based as an herb with antibiotic properties. And there are times when herbs may be a safer answer that works just as well as a drug—or even better.

SECRET #27 There are six common herbs with antibiotic properties.

Grapefruit seed extract (GSE)—GSE is an extract made from the seeds of ordinary grapefruit. It contains a powerful broad-spectrum antibiotic that is used throughout the world. GSE fights bacteria, yeasts, and fungi when it's used in very small doses. It can be used internally and externally to kill off intestinal or skin bacteria. But be careful. If you take too much of it, you could kill off some good bacteria as well. Buhner suggests taking three to fifteen drops of GSE in citrus juice two to three times a day, but I find that one or two drops twice daily is often enough.

Garlic (Allium sativum)—Garlic has been studied more than any other herb, and is second in usefulness to GSE as an herbal antibiotic. It is antimicrobial and fights a wide number of conditions including pathogenic bacteria, fungi, viruses, and protozoa. It also can be used on skin infections including athlete's foot. Garlic is effective against both gram-positive and gram-negative bacteria, as well as most major infectious bacteria. It can be used in food or taken in capsule form. If you're already taking any blood thinner, don't use more than one clove of garlic a day. Garlic is a powerful anticoagulant, and high amounts could thin your blood too much. Other than this, garlic is very safe.

Aloe vera juice—Use the juice or gel externally as an antibacterial, antimicrobial, or antiviral. It is effective against staph infections as well as burns.

Goldenseal (Hydrastis canadensis)—The active ingredient in goldenseal root that has antibiotic properties is berberine. This is why some products are labeled "high in berberine." Goldenseal has been used for tuberculosis, *H. pylori*, and diarrhea resulting from *E. coli*. It can also be used if you have skin, vaginal, or eye infections. Goldenseal can be found in tinctures, capsules, salves, or tablets. All work well. Many people use it at the first sign of a cold or infection and take it for a week or two. Avoid using it every day. There are not enough long-term studies on its safety and effectiveness when it is used constantly. Goldenseal relaxes smooth muscles, so don't use it if you're pregnant.

Lemon balm (Melissa officinalis)—This is an excellent antiviral and antibacterial that is now being used in some over-the-counter ointments to treat cold sores (herpes simplex virus). I have found it works beautifully. Use it at the first tingling sign that a cold sore may be starting. You can often prevent a sore from occurring by using it immediately. Ointments for cold sores can be found in health-food stores and pharmacies. If your "cold sore" is actually a little bacterial infection, it will work for that, also.

Ginger (Zingiber officinale)—Ginger root has both antibacterial and antiviral properties. It is effective against foodborne illnesses caused by bacteria of *Shigella*, *E. coli*, and *salmonella*. It also acts as an expectorant and antihistamine, and works well for upper respiratory infections. You can use it as a tea, in capsules, or in food in any amounts due to its low toxicity. Ginger is also a blood thinner, but to a lesser degree than garlic.

What to Use When

Use all antibiotics appropriately. Pharmaceutical antibiotics don't work for viruses, so make sure your doctor has identified a bacterial overgrowth and that any prescribed antibiotic is both necessary and appropriate against that particular bacterium.

Take friendly bacteria (probiotics) like *L. acidophilus* and *B. bifidus* for several weeks after using any kind of antibiotic. Probiotics fight pathogenic bacteria and keep them under control.

Use antibacterial soaps and cleaners appropriately—not all the time. They kill good bacteria as well as pathogens. Keep your kitchen and bathroom low in bacteria by keeping them clean, but don't scrub your hands with antibacterial soap throughout the day—just when you've been exposed to something nasty.

If your infection is not serious, try using herbs with antibiotic properties, or ask your doctor if you can try this natural approach for a few days to see if herbal antibiotics are effective. With a little trial and error you'll find which herbs work best for you. And by having them on hand, you can begin treating yourself at the first sign of discomfort—when it's easiest to control. Always see your doctor if symptoms progress or don't improve within a few days.

A Word of Caution

Ingredients in plants have the potential to interact adversely with medications. Always check with your doctor or pharmacist before using any herbs if you are also taking prescription or over-the-counter medications. This includes hormones. Herbal antibiotics may be appropriate for uncomfortable, non-life-threatening conditions like bladder, skin, or sinus infections. They can be useful at the first sign of a cold, since bacterial infections may be present with viruses. Be smart. Always get a medical diagnosis before you treat your condition. If you have a fungal infection, use an antifungal. If you have a bacterial infection, use antibiotic herbs. If it's a virus, choose a plant with antiviral properties.

CHAPTER 5

Improve Circulation and Reduce Plaque with This Herbal Formula

I'd like to tell you about an herbal formula that's no secret to the many doctors throughout Europe who have been using it successfully for thirty years, or to their patients who no longer suffer from leg pain or heart disease. But it's still a secret to mainstream doctors in this country. They continue to give their patients pharmaceutical drugs like statins, shown to have serious side effects, rather than trust the experience of European doctors and use a natural product. This is a secret you just must know about.

SECRET #28 This Tibetan herbal formula dramatically increases circulation.

I'm talking about an ancient Tibetan formula called Padma Basic, or Padma. It's a combination of nineteen herbs that can be extremely helpful for anyone with circulatory problems. I first heard about Padma several years ago when I was asked to write a small book about it. What I discovered changed the way I work with patients.

Padma is just one of a number of classical herbal formulas that originated in Tibet. It was hand-carried through Mongolia to Siberia by followers of Tibetan Buddhism and Tibetan medicine during the Communist invasion. The fascinating story of how it was discovered by a Tibetan doctor and brought to Russia, along with more detailed information on its many other valuable uses, can be found in my book *Padma: An Ancient Tibetan Herbal Formula*.

More than fifty well-designed scientific studies show it's both safe and effective. In fact, Padma is the most well-known and widely researched of all Tibetan herbal formulas in the world. Originally made high in the Himalaya Mountains, it is now manufactured under strict quality-controlled conditions in Switzerland by Padma, Inc. The current Padma Basic formula has been carefully evaluated and found to be accurate by the Tibetan doctor who founded Tibet's premier medical school and was also the personal physician of the Dalai Lama.

What's in It

Padma consists of nineteen different plants along with camphor and calcium sulfate. These ingredients are rich in antioxidants, containing plant compounds including polyphenols such as bioflavonoids and tannins, as well as other plant chemicals. The antioxidants (chemicals that protect cells from damage caused by oxidation) promote good circulation and a healthy heart, while the combination of ingredients reduces inflammation and supports the immune system. In this chapter, I'll talk about Padma's usefulness in increasing circulation and dissolving plaque. Later in Chapter 38, I'll talk about its applications in reducing inflammation—the initial cause of many chronic illnesses.

Each of the ingredients in Padma has at least one of the following actions:

1. Causes the main effect, such as increasing circulation or reducing inflammation;

2. Supports the primary effect;

3. Counteracts any negative side effects from any other ingredients.

One problem with Western medicines is that they often have side effects. To counteract these side effects, patients are given other medications. These new medications may have side effects, also. And on and on it goes. But traditional Tibetan formulas are different. They contain within them the properties needed to balance any side effects. The result is formulas that rarely have any side effects.

Asian herbal formulas are categorized by their properties. Some create heat while others, like Padma, are cooling. All types of inflammation, and circulatory disorders like peripheral artery disease, arteriosclerosis, and intermittent claudication, are considered to be "hot diseases" and can benefit from Padma's cooling effects.

But poor circulation not only contributes to diseases, it accelerates aging as well.

SECRET #29 These herbs can slow down aging.

Do you feel rundown for no apparent reason? The reason may be poor circulation. Your circulatory system carries blood throughout your body, through your veins and arteries, nourishing your tissues with oxygen and nutrients. But poor circulation reduces the ability of these nutrients and of oxygen to reach your cells.

You probably know that a healthy diet and regular exercise can help support good circulation. And that smoking, a poor diet, and inactivity can lead to a buildup of plaque that results in blockages in your veins and arteries. What you may not realize is that this buildup of plaque can contribute to circulatory problems that affect your legs and heart. You want to prevent these blockages to stay healthy, and to look and feel young for as long as you can.

Blockages cause arteries to become narrow and stiff, thus, reducing circulation.

When less oxygen and nutrients are supplied to waiting cells, the result is that you feel tired and rundown. Often, feeling blah is the first subtle sign that you may be heading toward heart disease. If this feeling persists, see your doctor for a thorough evaluation.

Supporting good circulation is vital in both slowing down your aging process and increasing longevity. This is why many doctors of integrative medicine are now using Padma in their antiaging nutritional programs.

SECRET #30 You can prevent and reverse atherosclerosis and blockages with these herbs.

The idea is to prevent a buildup of plaque in your arteries. Studies show that Padma is particularly effective in keeping veins and arteries free from plaque. While surgery and chelation therapy are two modern methods of reversing atherosclerotic plaque, Padma has been found to be effective both in helping to prevent and treat this buildup at a fraction of the cost and without side effects. Oral chelation therapy is not nearly as effective as intravenous chelation. If you want to use an oral therapy to reduce plaque, Padma may be much more effective than the many advertised chelation pills.

When atherosclerotic plaque builds up in the legs, it is called peripheral artery disease or peripheral vascular disease (PVD). Sometimes, leg pain develops intermittently from this buildup of plaque. This condition is called intermittent claudication. Intermittent claudication is a huge problem. It affects 12 percent of all adults over the age of fifty. This leg pain from intermittent claudication usually changes people's lives, and their health, forever. It limits their ability to get the exercise they need for a healthy heart, for muscle strength, and for weight control. Both peripheral artery disease and intermittent claudication are complications of atherosclerosis.

When you're sitting down, your blood vessels carry two cups of blood a minute to your legs. But when you're exercising, your body's need for oxygen increases. In fact, the quantity of blood that's needed to meet these needs jumps to three or four quarts of blood every minute. When your arteries have become obstructed with plaque, they just can't carry enough blood or oxygen to your legs. The result is muscle pain that begins after even mild exercise—like walking one or two blocks—and disappears with complete rest. The good news is that current studies show Padma to be well suited to both peripheral artery disease and intermittent claudication.

In fact, it was a particularly difficult case of intermittent claudication that brought Padma to the attention of doctors throughout Europe in the mid-1900s. Dr. Charles, a Swiss medical doctor, had a high-profile patient who suffered from intense leg pain. His patient, the municipal president of a neighboring town, was in such pain from advanced obstructions in the arteries of his legs that he was barely able to walk.

Dr. Charles had tried every medication he could think of for his patient, but nothing helped. Then he remembered being given a Tibetan herbal formula by a pharmaceutical representative. The representative had told the doctor that this formula was effective in relieving leg pain. With no other options available for him to try, Dr. Charles gave his patient the herbal formula. To his surprise and delight, it worked beautifully. After taking Padma for a number of weeks, his patient was able to walk a considerable distance without any pain.

Dr. Charles was delighted to find an answer for his patient. But could this success be duplicated? Anxious to know, he tried the formula on several of his patients with atherosclerosis. Their conditions improved, as well. Word spread about Dr. Charles' successes, and more and more doctors began to experiment with Padma. Eventually, it was used in double-blind placebo-controlled studies at the Zurich University Clinic and then throughout the world.

Currently, there are more studies showing the effectiveness of Padma for peripheral artery disease and intermittent claudication than for reducing a buildup of plaque in the arteries of the heart. This is because it's quicker and easier to test the arteries in the legs. But it's important for you to know that the principle is the same. If Padma can reduce the buildup of plaque in arteries in your legs, it stands to reason that it also can remove a buildup of plaque from other arteries in your body, including coronary and cerebral arteries. Clinical trials have already demonstrated this to be so.

SECRET #31 You could reduce your leg pain in just one month.

It's already been done. A German study published in 1985, gave patients with intermittent leg pain Padma for only one month. They had a 100 percent increase in the distance that they could walk without pain. Clearly, this is an herbal formula that not only works well, but also has the ability to work quickly.

A randomized, double-blind study published in the medical journal *Angiology* in 1993 took a bit longer. But it still had excellent results. Three dozen patients in their sixties who suffered from intermittent leg pain for five years either took a placebo or two tablets of the Padma formula twice a day for four months. At the end of the study, the patients who took Padma were able to walk twice as far as before without leg pain, while those who took the placebo had no improvement. Whether it takes one month or four months, this herbal formula can outperform many drugs.

How Padma Works

Just how does Padma prevent this buildup of plaque? A Polish study found it increases the helpful cholesterol (HDL) and reduces the harmful cholesterol

(LDL). HDL, or high-density lipoprotein, is the slick form of cholesterol, while LDL, or low-density lipoprotein, is sticky. When you have enough HDL, it keeps the sticky fats from adhering to the arterial walls. If, on the other hand, you have too much LDL, these fats can cause a buildup of plaque that often leads to poor circulation and leg pain. Here's what the study found.

Fifty patients with arteriosclerosis and intermittent claudication were given Padma or a placebo for four months. At the end of this study, the patients taking the herbal formula were able to walk further without pain than those who took the placebo, just as in previous studies. But this study went beyond pain measurement. It examined lipid levels in all of the participants as well. It discovered that Padma reduced cholesterol and triglyceride levels. It also lowered LDL cholesterol, reducing the stickiness that can lead to more plaque buildup. Once again, the placebo group had no change in their pain or in lipid levels.

SECRET #32 You could reduce your angina pain in just two weeks.

That's what most of the fifty participants in a research study found. In this study, all of them were given a placebo for two weeks. Then all of them took Padma for another two weeks. The researchers compared the severity and frequency of their angina attacks, their response to therapy, their ability to exercise without any pain, the ability of their blood to clot, and their levels of cholesterol and triglycerides. Eighty percent of the participants had either a good or excellent response to Padma. Afterwards, they could work harder and longer before feeling any pain. And there was a significant decrease in their cholesterol, triglycerides, and clotting time. I like this study because it was so thorough and compared placebos to Padma in each person.

What causes angina? When you understand its origin, you'll be able to better understand better why you may want to try Padma to reduce heart pain. When atherosclerotic plaque builds up in the coronary arteries it is called atherosclerosis or arteriosclerosis—hardening of the arteries. The arteries, which originally were flexible, become stiff and hard. Blockages caused by plaque leave less room for blood to travel through them. This slows down your circulation. When your circulation is reduced, less oxygen can be pumped through the blood and into your tissues. Padma decreases the plaque that gums up arteries.

Both exercise and eating heavy meals can cause your heart to pump faster than usual. At these times, your blocked arteries can't carry enough oxygen to your heart. The result is pain, and the condition is known as angina pectoris. Angina pain is not an indication of a heart attack as some people think. But it is a signal of insufficient oxygen. If you ignore it, angina often can eventually lead to heart attacks.

SECRET #33 This formula may prevent and stop the progression of Alzheimer's disease.

I don't know anyone over the age of sixty who isn't at all concerned about getting Alzheimer's disease. It's a fear that often lurks in the recesses of our mind. Alzheimer's disease is the most common form of senile dementia. It affects 10 percent of people over age sixty-five and nearly half of the population over the age of eighty-five. What you may not realize is that many times Alzheimer's disease is characterized by a buildup of plaque on nerve endings. This buildup causes the nerves connecting segments of the brain to die. A lack of blood supply to the brain, often caused by constricted arteries, appears to be a vascular form of Alzheimer's disease that may be closely associated with coronary artery disease. Padma could be ideal for preventing and stopping the progression of this type of Alzheimer's disease.

I discovered the association between plaque, Padma, and Alzheimer's disease when I was researching for my book on Padma. The connection had never been publicly made before. Quite by accident, I came across an article in a medical journal that talked about Alzheimer's disease and a buildup of plaque in veins and arteries. I quickly put the doctor who is organizing studies on Padma in contact with the authors of this article to see if there could be a connection. They all felt there was a good possibility that Padma could benefit people with memory loss who had this plaque buildup.

Here's something I found to be extraordinary. More than 85 percent of people with coronary artery disease have plaque in their brain tissues that looks just like the plaque found in people with Alzheimer's disease. Remarkably, when these people have coronary artery surgery, the plaque in their brain tissue often clears up. As we've seen in the studies on peripheral artery disease, Padma reduces arterial and vascular plaque. This appears to be the same mechanism responsible for the improvement in people with a vascular form of Alzheimer's disease.

In a small observational study on older adults with Alzheimer's disease conducted in the mid-1980s, thirty-four people were given 1 gram of Padma a day in divided doses for six months (equivalent to 1 tablet, three times a day). At the end of the study, the majority of them had significant improvements in memory, mental alertness, energy, attitude, and general well-being. Of course, we need double-blind studies to further determine Padma's effectiveness. But is there any need to wait before you try this safe herbal formula? All I can say is, I'm not waiting.

I'd like to leave you with a final note on Padma and Alzheimer's disease. Cell damage caused by oxidation also contributes to this progressive illness. Padma is filled with antioxidants. They provide a second line of defense in preventing and slowing down the progression of Alzheimer's disease.

CHAPTER 6

Save and Restore Your Memory with These Two Powerful Nutrients

Alzheimer's disease aside, the sad truth is that as we age we forget things more. Little things like where we left our keys. Or what we ate for lunch yesterday. Unfortunately, these changes in memory tend to affect most of us to varying degrees.

My memory has never been perfect, so after menopause when I thought I was forgetting more than usual, I began taking a memory formula containing a number of nutrients that support brain function. I also took one of the safest hormones that has been linked to memory. Both helped, but eventually they were not enough.

One day, I realized that my short-term memory had suddenly dropped dramatically. Names, events, and "to do" lists were hard to remember. I could see an image in my mind but couldn't find the word to match this image no matter how hard I tried.

I was so upset that I focused my full attention on this problem and looked for its cause. If I could find out why my memory had suddenly declined, I could find a solution. After all, I am the Health Detective! My determination paid off. Within two weeks I had found two supplements essential for good brain function. They were both included in my memory formula, but I discovered that my body needed more of one of them. This nutrient quickly returned my lost memory to me. Now, while people around me complain about their memory, mine appears to be better than ever.

Don't think that everyone will get results this quickly. I was already doing a lot of other things to support my memory. But when I added this missing link the results were almost immediate. We are not alike in our needs for memory-boosting nutrients. Some formulas and particular nutrients will work well for you while others won't. Ginkgo biloba, an herb that increases circulation and is known for its effect on memory, is sufficient for many people. It wasn't enough for me, and many of my patients find they need to do more than take gingko. I suggest you do what I did: begin at the beginning. First, look at whether or not your forgetfulness is a sign of hormone deficiencies.

If you're peri- or post-menopausal, your declining memory may simply be due to lowering levels of hormones that begin to decline some time after menopause. At one time, it was thought that low estrogen was the culprit. Doctors gave women estrogen to help their memory. Now there are studies—and women who used estrogen—that say it doesn't work. More and more women are looking for solutions that don't include estrogen. I found one that helps the brain and is quite safe.

SECRET #34 This safe hormone, made by your adrenal glands, can improve your memory.

Pregnenolone is a safe hormone that usually helps memory. It's produced by the adrenal glands, small glands that handle all our stress. That is, the adrenal glands make pregnenolone if they're not too exhausted. So many women have adrenal exhaustion that it's no wonder they have low pregnenolone by the time they reach menopause!

I began my investigation into improved memory function by getting my pregnenolone level checked with a blood test. Indeed, it was low. Pregnenolone drops dramatically after we reach fifty, so I wasn't particularly surprised. My memory improved after I began taking a low dose of this hormone (25 mg). It was not my final solution, but it certainly helped. Dr. Uzzi Reiss, author of *Natural Hormone Balance for Women,* suggests that women take 50–100 mg of pregnenolone in the morning. He's my doctor and a good friend whose information I have always been able to trust. Why didn't I take more pregnenolone? Because Dr. Reiss found that my blood test indicated I didn't need more than 25 mg.

Pregnenolone can be found in health-food stores, through compounding pharmacies, and from a number of good supplement companies. Please check with your doctor first to see if you need it. It's best to be monitored when taking any hormones at all, even the safe ones. You can find more specific information on natural hormones including estrogens and pregnenolone in Part 6.

Thyroid hormone production also declines with age, and hypothyroidism can contribute to memory loss. Ask your doctor to thoroughly check your thyroid, or take your temperature under your armpit before you get out of bed in the morning. This at-home test is known as the Broda Barnes' Basal Body Temperature Test. Shake down the thermometer the night before. Next morning place the thermometer in your armpit and keep it there for a full ten minutes. If your temperature is lower than 97.8 every day for a week, chances are that your thyroid is low. If so, your memory loss may be due, at least in part, to hypothyroidism (see Chapter 1). But the connection between hormones and memory is not limited to the thyroid.

Your brain needs more than hormones to function properly through the years. It needs antioxidants like coenzyme Q_{10}, vitamin C, vitamin E, and zinc. You can get many of these in a good quality multivitamin/mineral combination. Or take an antioxidant formula designed to boost memory. Many of them include ginkgo biloba, as well. I was already taking all of these.

The nutrients that can turn your memory around are phosphatidyl serine (PS) and acetyl-l-carnitine (ALC). One of them was my solution.

SECRET #35 PS, this secret really works to restore memory.

Phosphatidyl serine is a naturally occurring fat that is found in cell membranes. It's one of the most plentiful fats in your brain tissue, and is a key building block in helping your cells communicate with one another. It also stimulates the production of brain chemicals like serotonin and dopamine.

PS is found in food such as organ meats and fish. There's some in whole grains and white beans, as well, but not enough to improve your memory.

THIAMINE AND YOUR BRAIN

Thiamine (vitamin B1) is one of the B vitamins with antioxidant properties. It's found in whole grains, brewer's yeast, molasses, and meats. While blood tests may not show a thiamine deficiency, a study with 120 women college students indicates a deficiency may not even be necessary for thiamine supplementation to be beneficial.

The women in this study, who were around twenty years of age, were given either 50 mg of thiamine a day for two months or a placebo. The women who took thiamine noticed significant improvements in their mood, as well as in their mental acuity. Multivitamins contain from 5 to 100 mg of thiamine. If you're taking a low-potency vitamin, you may want to boost your thiamine and see if your memory improves.

Taking the right supplements isn't the complete solution to a fading memory. Don't forget daily exercise. It's good for your brain! An eight-year study conducted with 6,000 women over sixty-five who walked regularly and moderately had the least amount of cognitive decline and memory loss. And while many of these brain-boosting nutrients are expensive, walking won't cost you a dime.

Your body can make PS if it has enough folic acid, vitamin B_{12}, and essential fats. But as we age, we get less of these nutrients in our diets and our absorption is often poorer. In these cases, supplemental PS made from soy lecithin may be helpful.

More than 65 human studies on PS and brain function showed it stimulates the memory in people with age-related memory loss. At the same time, it relieves age-related depression. When a group of people took 300 mg of PS a day for three months, they reported an improvement in mental clarity and the ability to remember names, faces, and telephone numbers. Some studies called the results "astounding."

How much PS should you take? Some doctors recommend beginning with 300 mg until you notice improved clarity and recall. Then taper down to 100 mg a day for maintenance. Dr. Reiss recommends 100 mg with breakfast and 200 mg with dinner.

SECRET #36 This nutrient improves memory by transporting fuel to your brain.

Acetyl-l-carnitine (ALC) is a derivative of carnitine, a vitamin-like compound that carries slow-burning, long-chain fats into your cells. Chemically, ALC is a combination of acetic acid and carnitine bound together in a single molecule. This combination seems to be more effective than carnitine alone for good brain function, since ALC crosses the blood-brain barrier more easily than carnitine. The whole idea is to get nutrients into your brain. If they can't get past the blood-brain barrier, they're useless.

Your brain needs energy in order to function, and ALC is like a train that carries fuel to your brain cells so they can work better. ALC improves communication among neurons in the brain and is also an antioxidant that protects your brain from aging. It removes toxic byproducts formed during brain metabolism, acting as a "brain detoxifier." Studies have shown that ALC improves energy production in brain cells and delays the progression of Alzheimer's disease. In animal studies, it even prevented animals from developing Parkinson's disease. This is a very powerful brain nutrient.

Your brain makes ALC, but once again, it's often not enough as you age. The recommended dose for ALC is between 500 and 1,500 mg a day in divided doses. This doesn't mean you need as much as 500 mg, but you may. Neurologist David Perlmutter, M.D., uses a formula with 400 mg of ALC, while many brain formulas that are effective use less of this expensive nutrient.

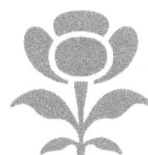

CHAPTER 7

This Antioxidant in Spinach and Beef Can Prevent Cataracts

Cataracts are not an inevitable result of aging. A number of antioxidants may keep them from forming. Yet out of all the antioxidants, one found in spinach and beef could be the most beneficial.

But don't think you can get enough of this super antioxidant from your food. You can't. Your eyes need too much of it.

This particular antioxidant is found not only in some common foods, but it's also manufactured inside your body. The problem is that when you're young, your body makes enough to meet your needs. As you get older, your body makes less while your need for it increases.

All antioxidants are considered to be antiaging nutrients because they neutralize harmful free radicals that lead to a number of degenerative diseases. But some antioxidants are more protective for the eyes than others.

SECRET #37 This antioxidant protects your eyes inside and outside.

Most antioxidants are either soluble in water or in oil. They fight harmful free radicals on the surface of cells. This particular antioxidant is different. It is both oil-soluble and water-soluble. This means it can protect the cells in your eyes from both the inside and outside. It can get into the watery tissues of your eyes and destroy the free radicals that contribute to cataracts.

Preliminary research suggests that it also binds to metals in the eye. These metals could be an additional factor in the formation of cataracts, especially in diabetics.

The antioxidant I'm talking about that appears to be a key nutrient in protecting us from cataracts is alpha-lipoic acid (ALA). You may have heard that ALA is useful in treating diabetes, cancer, and heart disease. It's also been used to repair liver damage. Now we have studies showing that ALA can save your sight. It's an important preventive for all types of cataracts: those from aging, from exposure to chemicals, and from the progression of diabetes.

SECRET #38 ALA protects you from cataracts by keeping antioxidants in your eyes longer.

ALA finds and destroys free radicals: A defective antioxidant defense system inside the lens of the eye often leads to cataracts. ALA is a powerful antioxidant that hunts down free radicals in the eye and destroys them. It also increases the presence of the following key antioxidants:

• *ALA regenerates antioxidants:* After an antioxidant neutralizes a free radical, that antioxidant becomes oxidized and stops working. ALA turns it back into an active antioxidant that can continue to fight free radicals. ALA is particularly effective in regenerating some key antioxidants that protect your eyes from forming cataracts. These include vitamins C and E. The longer these anti-cataract antioxidants remain in the lens of your eye, the more protective they are. You don't necessarily need more antioxidants. You need the antioxidants you're taking to remain in your eyes longer.

• *ALA increases glutathione:* Cataracts form when there's not enough glutathione in the eyes. If you aren't familiar with glutathione, it's a powerful immune booster and detoxifier. Like ALA, it's able to get into the cells of the eye, not just remain on their surface. ALA increases glutathione levels and helps it work better. This is particularly important since oral glutathione needs cofactors, such as N-acetyl-cysteine, to work best. When ALA was given to laboratory animals, it not only increased the quantity of glutathione in their lenses, but it also decreased the amount of chemicals that help form cataracts.

• *It binds to heavy metals:* We're beginning to see a connection between diabetic cataracts and the presence of heavy metals. Since heavy metals cause oxidation, I think we're going to find that they play an important role in forming all types of cataracts. ALA attaches itself to heavy metals and pulls them out of the body.

Antioxidants Fight Cataracts

I think ALA is a particularly valuable and overlooked nutrient that can protect your eyes. I say this because of its own antioxidant properties, as well as its ability to recycle and promote the production of other anticataract antioxidants.

A number of researchers share my opinion and see the value in boosting antioxidant levels to prevent cataracts even without conclusive evidence. Nearly fifty women, aged fifty-three to seventy-three, were followed over thirteen years and had their vitamin consumption carefully monitored. The women who took vitamin C supplements over the longest period of time had the least number of cataracts. Since ALA extends the life of vitamins C and E in tissues, anything that helps keep these antioxidants in your eyes longer seems to help prevent cataracts.

If vitamin C can prevent cataracts, just think of the added protection you'll get by adding ALA.

If you want to include ALA in your supplement program to protect your eyes, I'd suggest you take a minimum of 25–50 mg per day. How much is in your food? Not enough to flood your eyes with helpful nutrients. It's highest in organ meats, and three ounces of beef liver has just 14 mg of ALA. A cup of raw spinach contains 5 mg. And a large egg yolk has only 0.3 mg of ALA. Don't depend on your diet for adequate amounts. The formula I take, Women's Preferred Advanced Vision Formula, has 25 mg of ALA in a daily dose.

But you could need more. Before ALA can function as an antioxidant, you may need 50–400 mg per day (600 mg has been shown to be very safe). One study found that 600 mg a day for four months significantly reduced oxidative stress in healthy people. You can find ALA supplements in most health-food stores, or check the Resources section at the end of this book for products I've found to be of good quality. Be sure to include a multivitamin high in other antioxidants as well.

ARE YOU OVER FIFTY WITH BLUE EYES?

If so, you're more prone to retinal disease than brown-eyed people. This is because your retinas contain half as much lutein, one of the hundreds of carotenoids found in vitamin A. Beta-carotene, essential for good eye health, needs lutein before it can be absorbed. If you take extra beta-carotene without extra lutein, you may be at more risk for eye problems as you age. Most vitamin pills have plenty of beta-carotene and no lutein. To get the amount of lutein it takes to use the beta-carotene in your vitamins, you would need three to five servings of spinach or kale a week. This may be easy in the summer when spinach salads taste good, but difficult other times of the year.

CHAPTER 8

Which Supplements Work— And Which Don't

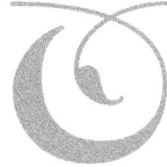

There are so many secrets surrounding the subject of nutritional supplements that even doctors of integrative medicine and knowledgeable nutritionists are often confused. If a supplement contains a proprietary formula, there's no way you can know exactly what's in it. When you don't know the difference between several forms of a nutrient, you can't know whether or not one will be better absorbed than another. Some of the studies quoted to sell products are good studies, while others prove nothing. This is one confusing mess for the consumer! Doctors who read my newsletter constantly approach me and say, "I didn't know that! Your information is going to change the way I practice medicine."

The quality and appropriateness of a supplement determines whether or not it can help you get and stay well. Nutritional supplements have become big business and not all companies that distribute them are ethical. Some will say just about anything to make a sale. Others are more concerned with the ability of their products to help people. How in the world can you hope to separate the good ones from those you'd rather leave alone? Let me help you understand some of the problems—and solutions—that can lead you to buy those supplements that work and avoid those that don't. This investigation begins by first looking at why they're called supplements.

I've always maintained that supplements are just that: *supplements* to a good diet. There's a reason they're called supplements, not *instead-ofs*. A good, healthy diet is the essential foundation for good health. Diets rich in fresh produce are high in fiber, antioxidants, and immune-building nutrients. They are your first line of defense against serious illnesses. It's unfair to expect supplements alone to keep you healthy. This is especially true in today's world.

SECRET #39 A healthy diet may have been enough in the past to stay healthy. Now it's not.

Many people believe that a healthy diet provides all the nutrients they need. If only

53

that was true! At one time it may have been the case. Now, environmental toxins from smog and polluted water, foods containing residues of antibiotics, pesticides and herbicides, and the additional stresses that come from living in the twenty-first century, all impact our nutritional needs. A diet that once was enough is now sadly deficient.

Few people today are consistently eating a healthy diet. They're too busy to prepare and eat three balanced meals a day. Some get their energy boosts from caffeine, alcohol, or sugar, all of which deplete the body of one or more nutrients. To digest sugar, for example, you need to eat and digest more B vitamins than you can get in a typical diet. Whenever you eat foods high in sugar, you need extra B vitamins.

If you think you can take supplements and still eat a lot of fast foods or highly processed foods—filled with fats, animal protein, and sugar, and low in fresh produce, whole grains, and beans—you're fooling yourself. If you think that eating a lot of sugar is just a minor dietary discretion with no lasting consequences—you're wrong. Stop playing Russian roulette with your health. It's just not going to give you the results you want. Begin by cleaning up your diet. Then begin building a foundation of nutritional supplements. Just don't expect them to be complete.

SECRET #40 Not all important nutrients can be put into supplements.

The idea is to take supplements that are as complete as possible. Sometimes, however, you can't. Take beta-carotene, for instance. It's just one of around 600 fat-soluble carotenoids that are part of the vitamin A family. Some supplements contain mixed carotenoids, but they don't include all of them. That's because you can't put all of the nutrients in a food into pills. This is why you need to eat a diet with plenty of fruits and vegetables that contain the whole vitamin A family.

After hearing so much about the benefits of the complete carotenoids, I spoke with the president of a large, natural supplement company and asked her when she would be coming out with a complete carotenoid product. "Never," she told me. "Some of them are very unstable. And there are too many of them. If we came out with a product that contained a dozen or so carotenoids, we might well be missing just the ones that make a difference in someone's health. It just won't happen." You can't fool Mother Nature, and you can't duplicate her, either.

In our culture we think that more is better. This isn't true when it comes to some nutrients. In fact, taking too much of one of the most popular categories of supplements can actually hurt you. Not very many people know about this. It is a secret that supplement companies don't want you to know.

SECRET #41 Too many antioxidants can be harmful.

The fats you eat oxidize (spoil) and form dangerous free radicals. This is a good reason to keep your dietary fats low. The more oxidants there are in your diet, the more antioxidants you need in your diet and supplements to fight these free radicals. So this means that the more antioxidants you take, the healthier you'll be, right?

Wrong!

Very high levels of antioxidants can actually cause a harmful *pro-oxidant* effect and suppress your immune system. In fact, the antioxidant function in healthy people has been shown to decrease when their antioxidant intake is too high.

This is why I'm so disturbed about an antioxidant test that one multilevel marketing company is using to help them sell more supplements.

This test is misleading. There are dozens of important antioxidants including vitamin C and its bioflavonoids, vitamin A and its carotenoids, vitamin E, vitamin D, coenzyme Q_{10}, resveratrol, superoxide dismutase (SOD), selenium, alpha-lipoic acid, and such amino acids as cysteine, glutathione, methionine, and taurine.

Nu Skin is a company that uses a biophotonic scanner to determine a person's level of a single group of antioxidants—carotenoids—by shining a very low-power laser on the skin. The company says, "The scanner can help consumers determine whether they are consuming adequate amounts of antioxidant-containing nutrients. . . ."

No, the scanner doesn't measure antioxidants, plural, as the literature says. It measures one type only. Different antioxidants have different chemical structures, and their effects on your health vary, as well. Measuring one group of antioxidants does not let you know the balance of antioxidants in your body. It also doesn't tell you whether or not these antioxidants are functioning. Remember that large, long-term randomized trial that concluded that taking beta-carotene supplements raised the risk of lung cancer in smokers? More is not always better.

In my opinion, it's irresponsible to suggest that taking high levels of a single group of antioxidants is an indication of good health. So why is this test being used? In Nu Skin's *2002 Annual Report*, they said: "The ability to measure carotenoid antioxidant levels provides our distributors a tremendous competitive advantage—demonstrable proof of the ability of LifePak [a line of supplements from Nu Skin] to improve overall health by increasing antioxidant levels. . . . As customers track their skin carotenoid content, we believe they will be motivated to consistently consume LifePak for longer periods of time."

This test is a marketing tool, plain and simple. And it's not giving you the information you need. It doesn't tell you whether the antioxidants in your body are protecting you or not. That depends on how they function.

SECRET #42 You may have high antioxidant levels and low antioxidant function.

Antioxidants are valuable only if they help protect you. Just ask anyone at Spectra-Cell Laboratory, a company that measures how antioxidants and other nutrients function—not just how much are present in your blood or tissues. These folks know that if you have a high amount of an antioxidant, but your cells can't use it to defend themselves, the amount you have is meaningless. What matters is how your cells function. And the people at SpectraCell also know that some people may have high antioxidant levels, but poor antioxidant function. This may be one reason why taking beta-carotene increased lung cancer in smokers.

You may have enough of a nutrient in your body, but if it's not activated, or if it doesn't have enough cofactors, it may not function normally. Zinc is one example of an important cofactor that's often too low to allow your immune system to respond. Antioxidants support your immune system by fighting free radicals, but without sufficient zinc, some antioxidants can't respond. Zinc is often low as we age because of reduced intake and absorption.

Then there's the matter of genetics and biochemical individuality. Each of us is unique in our genetic makeup and in how we utilize various nutrients. So the amount you need may be different from what works for someone else.

Developing an Accurate Test

Dr. William Shive wanted to identify a person's limiting nutritional and biochemical factors, so he developed SpectraCell's test at the University of Texas. This test, the Functional Intracellular Analysis (FIA), evaluates how well an antioxidant or its cofactor functions within lymphocytes. Lymphocytes are protective immune-system cells. Dr. Shive decided to test nutrients within these cells since lymphocytes carry your genetic identity and have the same metabolic pathways as most of your other cells. This means that what works with lymphocytes is likely to work with other cells in your body.

One advantage of using lymphocytes is that they represent our nutritional status over a period of three to twelve months. They don't only indicate nutritional levels over the past several weeks.

The SpectraCell test has been developed and refined over the past eighteen years. Here's how it works. You have your blood drawn at your doctor's office or at a laboratory and the blood is sent overnight to SpectraCell in a special collection kit. There they isolate your white blood cells and grow them in a patented media in culture plates. They're first grown in one culture that acts as a control media, containing optimal amounts of various micronutrients. Then each micronutrient is removed one at a time and the cells are stimulated to grow in the culture. If the lymphocytes don't grow well, you're deficient in that micronutrient. If they do, you have enough of that micronutrient to help your immune system function well.

Oxidative Stress and Disease

Oxidative stress caused by an overabundance of free radicals contributes to heart disease, stroke, aging, reduced cognitive abilities associated with aging, cancer, complications from diabetes, and low immunity. You may feel relieved after getting a more limited test, or falsely assume that since you're taking vitamins that you're protected. However, this may not be true. Taking high quantities of antioxidants, or emphasizing (or testing) one of them, may not be protecting you.

There are a number of functional tests offered by SpectraCell. One measures antioxidants alone, while the others add a variety of nutrients such as B vitamins and minerals as well as glucose/insulin metabolism and fructose sensitivity. The SpectraCell FIA test is the only test that measures the function of antioxidants and other nutrients—and it's function that counts.

The beauty of a test like this one is that you can discover whether or not you're taking enough or too many antioxidants. Some blood tests will give more information on the need for other nutrients. The better you know your body's specific needs, the healthier you can be and the more money you can save.

SECRET #43 **You're healthier when you know as much about your body as you do about your car.**

Your car came with an owner's manual. Your body didn't. And yet, an owner's manual is precisely what we all need, especially since everyone's body is a little different. It's important to learn which nutrients you need to replenish depleted stores of vitamins and minerals and how you can meet your body's individual needs. Unfortunately, you know what kind of gas your car needs better than you know which nutrients you need to feel better.

Vitamins and minerals feed all the cells in your body. Without them, your cells would starve and you would die. When you have too few of one or more nutrients, you run the risk of not feeling completely well and energetic. Eventually, you could get a nutrient-deficiency disease. Many nutrient-deficient diseases, such as scurvy from a lack of vitamin C, are no longer a health problem in developed countries. Others, like anemia, which can be caused by either iron or B_{12} deficiencies, may cause extreme fatigue. Sometimes, nutrient deficiencies lead to PMS (often caused by a lack of sufficient B_6 or magnesium), restless leg syndrome, unexplained fatigue, or skin problems and never lead to serious illness.

SECRET #44 Professional help can save you money.

Learn as much about your body's nutritional needs as possible. It will cost you far less to meet once or twice with a healthcare practitioner who uses nutrition in his or her practice than to try to figure this out on your own. Whether a medical doctor, acupuncturist, naturopath, or nutritionist . . . find someone who can help determine just which vitamins, minerals, and herbs are best suited for you at this time. Look for someone who doesn't sell supplements, or who gives you options to buy them on your own with a little direction.

Many patients come to me with a huge box filled with nutritional products. They don't need half of them! They're just listening to every advertisement on the radio and television, to the salesperson at their health-food store, and to each friend who discovered a miracle product.

A good health practitioner will look at your family's health history and look at yours. They will ask what you've done to yourself over the years that may have caused a nutritional imbalance, like drinking a lot of alcohol or caffeine, or eating a lot of fried foods or sugar. They will examine your health and ask about any uncomfortable symptoms. And they will recommend changes in your lifestyle as well as suggestions for appropriate supplementation. A list of organizations that can help you find a qualified practitioner are in the Resources section at the end of this book.

Whether you work with someone or on your own, find a diet that's the most healthful one for you. A high complex-carbohydrate diet may be better for you than one high in protein. Or vice versa. You may do well eating more raw foods, or have better digestion when the meals you eat are cooked. Next, add the supplements you and your health practitioner believe would boost your nutrient levels to the needed amounts. Use the best-quality, natural (not synthetic) supplements you can find. Take nutrients with any needed cofactors (like lutein with beta-carotene or vitamin C with bioflavonoids). Take a little less rather than a little more. Err on the side of caution. Be careful. Be well. Be happy.

Take enough vitamins and minerals for a reserve your body can tap into when they're needed. You need extra amounts of nutrients when you're under stress, exercising, fighting off a cold or flu, smoking, exposed to environmental pollutants, or taking medications. Can you get enough of the vitamins and minerals you need from your diet? And when you take vitamin or mineral supplements, how do you know they are getting into your cells and doing their job?

All vitamins are not created equal. Some are higher potency than others, some have better ratios of particular nutrients, and some are better absorbed. You usually get what you pay for, so the least expensive supplements are often not the best.

First, they tend to be lower in potency. Frequently, their formulas are based on older studies and are not the balance that current scientific research suggests your body needs. Most important, they are not particularly well absorbed.

Look for a complete multivitamin/mineral formula that will fit your needs rather than buying bottle after bottle of individual nutrients and making your own mixture. Some formulas are put together in such a way that they break down and are absorbed without competing with one another. Others are so low in potency that they have little benefit.

SECRET #45 Your multi may be too low in nutrients to work.

If you're taking one of the many "one-a-day" formulas, you may not be getting much bang for your buck. That's because they're so low in potency. Most fall into the "less well absorbed" category. I'm qualifying this statement because the form of nutrient used is not even listed in numerous popular one-a-day supplements like Theragram M, Geritol, and Centrum. One-a-day formulas frequently contain synthetic colorings, waxes, and other ingredients that bind the tablet together. You could be sensitive to these ingredients. And they certainly don't add to your health.

The biggest problem with one-a-day formulas is that they can't give you high potencies of nutrients. There just isn't room to put a lot of nutrients into a single tablet or capsule. Supplements with therapeutic amounts need to be taken in larger quantities—from four to six tablets or capsules daily.

This may seem like a lot, but it's not. These therapeutic formulas usually contain plenty of vitamin C, so you don't need to take any extra. They also have 200 to 400 international units (IU) of vitamin E. All of the antioxidants they contain are in higher amounts, so you don't need an extra formula to protect your eyes or heart—unless you specifically want a little more lutein, coenzyme Q_{10}, or other nutrient.

Good quality vitamins and minerals can be found in health-food stores and through many healthcare practitioners. Some offer a 100 percent money-back guarantee. If you can't find formulas with this guarantee in your local store, check the Resources section at the end of this book for several companies that will refund your money if don't like their supplements or don't benefit from them. Frankly, you're wasting your money if the supplements you take are too low in potency, poorly absorbed, contaminated, mislabeled, or not appropriate for your condition. Let me explain why.

SECRET #46 You are not what you eat.

I've been saying for more than twenty years, "You are not what you eat. You are what you eat, digest, and absorb." This applies to supplements as well as to foods. Supplements are worthwhile only when the nutrients they contain get into your cells. It doesn't matter what the label says if the particles in a supplement are too large to get into your bloodstream and cells. Or if they can't dissolve quickly enough. Well-absorbed nutrients often cost more to be manufactured than cheaper supplements.

ConsumerLab.com's *Guide to Buying Vitamins and Supplements* is a book you can use as a guideline for highly absorbable and safe forms and amounts of nutritional supplements. Or you can take the information from companies that make high-quality supplements to your local health-food store to compare the form and composition of each nutrient and formula. Here are a few valuable tips to get you started.

Calcium, magnesium, and many other minerals are best absorbed when they are bound to an acidic carrier such as citrate, aspartate, picolinate, or amino acid chelate. Minerals need an acidic base to break down and get used. If your stomach does not produce enough stomach acid (hydrochloric acid) to help break down these nutrients into particles that are small enough to be absorbed, they won't get into your cells. Calcium carbonate and magnesium oxide are the poorest absorbed forms of those two minerals. You'll find them in a lot of supplements because they're inexpensive.

Scientific studies show that natural vitamin E is much better absorbed than the synthetic form. How can you tell the difference? Simple. Your vitamin supplement will either say d-alpha tocopherol or dl-alpha tocopherol. You can remember which is natural and which is synthetic by thinking, the extra "l" is for limited absorption. Dl-alpha forms of vitamin E are synthetic. Look for a vitamin E with mixed tocopherols to get a broader form of this nutrient.

Vitamin B_6 is called pyridoxine. It is metabolized through the liver. Pyridoxal-5'-phosphate, or P5P, is a coenzyme form of vitamin B_6. That is, it turns into B_6 in your body, and does so without going through your liver. So it's easy to absorb and is well tolerated. Coenzyme B vitamins are best absorbed. If you think you want coenzyme Bs, look for pyridoxal-5'-phosphate on the label as an indicator of the form of the B vitamins it contains.

Are Capsules or Tablets Best?

It depends on the quality of the supplement. Cheaper tablets may not disintegrate properly, while good quality ones do. Because some nutrients are best utilized in the stomach and some in the small intestines, the better brands are formulated so that the ones that need to be released first, in the stomach, are. Nutrients in capsules are released in the stomach.

It may surprise you to learn that no supplements are absorbed 100 percent. The cheaper ones tend to be much less absorbable than those that are more expensive. For instance, calcium citrate is 45 percent absorbed, while calcium carbonate is only 4 percent absorbed! If you don't buy supplements that break down and get used by your body, you're wasting your money and fooling yourself about how much you body is actually getting. The form of vitamin or mineral you take is even more important than how much you take. The higher the quality, the more it is likely to get absorbed.

Poor-quality products are not limited to poorly absorbed nutrients. The supplements you take could actually contain contaminants.

SECRET #47 Some of your supplements may be contaminated.

High-quality supplements are not contaminated. This may sound obvious, but it's not necessarily anything you'd think about. Calcium from dolomite often contains lead—although, of course, it doesn't say so on the label. Lead toxicity can affect brain function and lead to depression, loss of memory, and senility.

Fish oils may contain pesticide residue and mercury. After all, the oils come from fish that swim in polluted waters. And pesticides get trapped in the fat cells of fish as well as in ours. It costs more to remove these contaminants and test each batch of fish oils. Still, I'm pleased to say that there are more supplement companies today that are spending the extra money to provide a better-quality product. Only buy fish oils guaranteed to be free of contaminants.

Herbs can be contaminated, as well. Some herbal formulas from China were contaminated with pharmaceutical drugs. Some medicinal mushrooms from China contained high amounts of lead. Heavy metals have been found in some green teas. For this reason, I recommend buying organic products whenever possible.

It's possible to find supplements that are guaranteed to be pure. Always choose them over similar products that come with no guarantees. Make sure that the supplements you take are worthwhile, not worthless.

SECRET #48 Some advertising claims are more fiction than fact.

Perhaps the biggest piece of misinformation about supplements was telling women who are tired to take more iron. The manufacturer of a synthetic vitamin product bombarded the airwaves and print ads claiming that tired women had "iron poor blood." How unfortunate. Iron oxidizes. If you take too much iron, it can lead to cancer. This is why there are few multivitamin/mineral formulas for postmenopausal women that contain iron.

If you have had cancer, or if there is a high incidence of cancer in your family, you may want to take a formula without added iron unless a blood test determines that you are iron deficient.

Unfortunately, there are still a lot of claims for supplements based on wishful thinking and strong marketing. Look for well-conducted studies to support the claims made for any supplement you're taking. Sometimes the claims seem to be made out of air, not from any substantial data. Coral calcium is one example that comes to mind.

In my opinion, and one that's shared by many of my colleagues, coral calcium from Okinawa was a huge scam. Promoters claimed that more than 200 diseases can be cured with coral calcium, yet when I researched my book *User's Guide to Calcium and Magnesium*, I found that more illnesses are caused by a need for magnesium than for calcium.

Coral calcium cures arthritis and joint pains? False. Both are caused by excessive calcium and insufficient magnesium. Coral calcium is touted as being well absorbed? False. Takuo Fujita, M.D., founder of the Calcium Research Institute and author of hundreds of scientific papers on calcium says, "The hardest calcium compound for the human body to break down and absorb is calcium carbonate— the very form in coral calcium."

Why were so many people claiming health benefits from coral calcium? It's simple. Coral calcium was big business. It contains trace minerals along with its poorly absorbed calcium, so if you're low in any trace mineral, you'll feel better by getting even a little more of it. Most people who felt better after taking this product were likely to be mineral deficient. There are no human studies to support the claims that were being made. And the FDA and FTC (Federal Trade Commission) knew this.

Sometimes there are studies to back up advertising claims. But they're not always good studies.

SECRET #49 And some studies are flawed and worthless.

I've heard in the past about studies that showed smokers with lung cancer got worse or developed coronary heart disease when they took a lot of beta-carotene, a carotenoid found in vitamin A. I've also seen studies that show that beta-carotene levels are low in many people who have lung cancer. So what's going on? Who should we believe? Do we take extra beta-carotene or shun it? Is this a case of antioxidant function versus quantity, or is something missing from the studies?

I read a meta-analysis on vitamin E saying that taking too much of it could kill you, but the conclusion was inconclusive because it was based on studies that used only one form of vitamin E and participants who were already sick.

The problem with many studies is that they tend to be limited. They often leave out more information than they contain. What about people who took the entire spectrum of carotenoids or vitamin E through a diet high in fresh fruits and vegetables, rather than taking just one or a few of them in a pill? Does an imbalance of nutrients contribute to health problems? Probably the greatest mistake we're making about taking vitamins and minerals is that we're treating them like drugs.

A letter in the British medical journal, the *Lancet,* talks about early studies done by two research scientists, Pauling and Robinson (yes, that's Linus Pauling, winner of two Nobel prizes). Apparently, these two scientists had major feuds, so some of their studies were never published—including animal studies that showed that a normal diet with high doses of vitamin C promoted cancer in mice exposed to carcinogens. But mice whose diet consisted of large amounts of raw fruits and vegetables—with the same amount of vitamin C and the same exposure to carcinogens—had much fewer cancers. In one case, vitamin C promoted cancer; in another, it inhibited it. Diet, not supplementation, made the difference. (Since then, many good scientific studies on humans have found that vitamin C supplementation is beneficial, not harmful.)

Before you believe the latest headlines either for or against a supplement, find out whether or not the study was a sound one. Frequently, follow-up articles on the Internet will give you this information.

What You Can Do

Choose supplements from companies with a good reputation. Do some price-comparison shopping. The least expensive product you find may or may not be as good in quality as the most expensive, but you can usually find one in the mid- to upper-range that is well absorbed and high enough in potency to give you the results you're looking for.

If a company is making claims about an exciting new formula that no one else has, their clams might be true. Some business people, however, are selling formulas whether or not they work. When possible, get input from your healthcare provider or pharmacist who may have experience with patients using various brands, and know which ones have a consistent pattern of working. If you're in doubt and have no one to ask, buy the best-quality supplement you can afford and try it for three to four months. If it works but cost is a significant issue, try one that's less expensive. Continue with the less expensive brand as long as it works for you.

Remember that there's a thirty-day placebo effect. This means that anything, even a sugar pill, could appear to work for you as long as one month. If a supplement appears to work for more than a month, it probably is working for you. Finally, if you're confused, you're in good company. I am at times, too, and need to investigate further.

All new products are not scams or high-priced versions of other formulas that work just as well. For example, I heard about a product that was said to be protective against breast cancer—calcium D-glucarate. It sounded too good to be true. I pursued the information and found that a reputable medical doctor at a cancer center in Denver had discovered this nutrient and patented it, and was selling it through Wieder Nutrition and Schiff supplement companies. Then I spoke with a medical doctor associated with Wieder, who I have known for decades by reputation as being a good scientist knowledgeable in nutrition. After a lengthy conversation, I was convinced of the science behind this product. You can now find calcium D-glucarate in health-food stores either alone or in combination with other nutrients. (I'll tell you more about this valuable nutrient in later chapters.)

Women tend to live longer than men, so our money—and our health—has to last longer. Since money isn't stretching as far as it used to, I thought this would be a good time for you to reevaluate your supplements. Don't just stop taking them or reach for the least expensive ones you can find. Vitamins, minerals, and other nutrients are either a wise investment or a waste of money.

Don't buy from MLMs (multilevel marketing companies) even if your best friend or a family member is selling them. They use a marketing approach that "eliminates" the middleman and sells their products through word-of-mouth. MLMs allow people to set up their own company and work from home while promoting the products they sell. While the overhead is low, the cost of these supplements is always higher than normal because many levels of participants are being paid from the sale of a single item. MLM supplements are always more expensive than other similar formulas, and not always the best quality.

Bottom-line

- Don't stop taking supplements, they're part of your health insurance.
- Take the supplements you need as long as you need them.
- Consolidate separate nutrients into a multivitamin/mineral formula.
- Buy high-quality supplements for best absorption and results.
- Look for sales or buy in large quantities to cut costs.

PART 2

END STOMACH PAIN, HEARTBURN, and INDIGESTION

You can't be healthy if you have digestive problems. Nutrients from your food and supplements simply have to get into your cells before they can do any good. At the same time, you can't continue eating a particular food if it causes your stomach to hurt no matter how beneficial it may be. Heartburn, gas, constipation, and diarrhea all limit your food choices.

A better solution would be to eliminate these uncomfortable symptoms. There are plenty of drugs designed to do just this. The problem with them is twofold: They only treat the symptom, not its cause, and many of them have side effects. There are better solutions. Some are extremely well-kept secrets, like taking acid instead of antacids to get rid of your heartburn. I'm serious. This is a new therapy backed by sound scientific studies. It's not just a wild theory. Some very talented medical doctors of integrative medicine are now using it.

Are your food choices limited to foods that cause you the least amount of discomfort? If so, I've got good news for you. You may be able to reduce or eliminate your digestive problems without resorting to drugs or a severely limited diet.

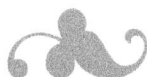

CHAPTER 9

Take Acid—Not Antacids—
To End Your Heartburn

If you're taking antacids or acid blockers for your heartburn, you're not solving your problem. You're only treating its symptoms. What's more, you may be giving your body the exact opposite treatment it needs to heal.

SECRET #50 If you have heartburn you probably need more acid, not less.

Are you surprised? I was astonished at first to discover that heartburn and gastroesophageal reflux disease are often caused by *too little acid,* not too much! I know this sounds crazy, but it's not. Bear with me while I explain it to you.

Heartburn affects 25 million people every day, and the medications they're taking are making pharmaceutical companies rich to the tune of $7 billion a year. Instead of treating the source of the problem, doctors are treating its symptoms by prescribing antacids and acid blockers. These drugs will not make you better and they could contribute to serious diseases.

Whether you're taking Tums, Maalox, Rolaids, or a prescription drug like Prilosec or Tagamet, taking them over a long period of time contributes to rheumatoid arthritis, gastrointestinal disorders, asthma, allergies, depression, and osteoporosis.

Let me begin by telling you why too much stomach acid can't possibly cause heartburn. It's simple. As we age, our stomachs produce less and less acid. This is often why we get bloating and indigestion. Foods we used to eat don't "agree" with us because we're not digesting them completely.

SECRET #51 Your heartburn is being caused by a valve that isn't working properly.

What's going on is not excessive acid. It's the malfunctioning of a valve between the esophagus and stomach called the lower esophageal sphincter, or LES. This is what causes your heartburn. When the LES is working properly, it opens up to allow food and liquids into your stomach and then it closes.

With acid indigestion, the LES opens briefly and allows a little acid to back up. If this happens frequently enough, the acid can irritate your esophageal lining. This can lead to an inflammatory condition called reflux esophagitis. Eventually, it can cause gastroesophageal reflux disease, otherwise known as GERD, and even ulcers.

It doesn't matter how much acid you have in your stomach as long as it stays where it belongs. All you're doing when you take an acid neutralizer or acid blocker is reducing the amount of leaking stomach acid. You're not repairing the LES. And you need acid not only to help digest proteins and some very important minerals, but to kill bad bacteria as well.

SECRET #52 You can't be healthy if you keep taking antacids.

Chances are that if you live on acid suppressors or neutralizers, you'll end up with some kind of intestinal problem like diarrhea or constipation. But there are additional consequences. Some vitamins (B_{12}), minerals (including calcium, magnesium, and iron), and proteins need stomach acid for good digestion and absorption. If you can't digest your foods, you can't get all of the nutrients they contain. Insufficient calcium and magnesium leads to osteoporosis. Not enough vitamin B_{12} can contribute to anemia. In addition to selective malnutrition, you may not feel satisfied after eating. This can contribute to overeating and weight gain.

You need to have sufficient stomach acid before you can digest protein. When hydrochloric acid (HCl) is released in your stomach, it signals your body to make pepsin, an enzyme needed to digest various amino acids (parts of proteins). Some of the amino acids that are dependent on pepsin—and HCl—do even more than help you digest proteins. They help prevent depression, anxiety, and insomnia as well. So your mood can be directly related to insufficient stomach acid, and antacids just add to this problem!

But there's still more.

Bacteria live and colonize in the mouth, esophagus, and intestines. They can't, however, survive in a healthy stomach. The bacteria that cause food poisoning, like *E. coli* and *salmonella*, can't live in an acid environment. We produce less HCl and become more susceptible to food poisoning as we age.

As stomach acid declines, all kinds of low acid-related disorders increase. These run the gamut from dermatitis to ulcerative colitis, gallstones, lupus, rosacea, stomach cancer, and all of the conditions mentioned earlier. Insufficient stomach acid is a huge problem. Too much stomach acid isn't.

ACID NEUTRALIZERS

Acids and alkalis cancel out one another. When you combine alkaline dairy products with an acid neutralizer (like Maalox or Rolaids), or if you take a calcium-based acid neutralizer like Tums, you can end up with milk-alkali syndrome. This condition is caused by too much alkali and not enough acid, and can lead to kidney failure and malignant tumors.

Check It Out First

The more I investigated this subject, the more I concluded that we need hydrochloric acid, not antacids. That said, I don't recommend that you stop taking your heartburn medication and begin taking HCl without first checking with a doctor—one experienced in treating heartburn with natural substances. HCl supplementation rarely causes problems, but anti-inflammatory drugs like steroids, aspirin, ibuprofen, or other NSAIDS may not interact safely with it. Talk with a doctor who can evaluate your gastric acid secretion and supervise your supplemental HCl regime. At the very least, talk to your pharmacist about any possible negative interactions with any medications you're taking.

In the meanwhile, there is something you can safely do to reduce your heartburn. Stop eating any foods that can weaken your LES. These foods include: chocolate, coffee, any variety of mint, alcohol, refined sugar, and onions. A diet high in any kinds of fats can also weaken your LES. Hydrochloric acid may be an integral part of your healing program, but it's not the entire solution.

SECRET #53 You need more than HCl to stop heartburn.

To restore balance to your intestinal tract, strengthen your LES, and provide a healthy environment for good digestive function, you need to include particular nutrients into your program. They begin with HCl, but they don't end there.

HCl with pepsin: Stomach acid triggers the production of an enzyme called pepsin. Make sure any HCl supplement you consider taking contains this enzyme. TwinLab sells HCl with pepsin through health-food stores. Talk with your doctor about the amount to take. When it's not possible to take HCl, you can try an approach used by Dr. Jonathan Wright, a doctor of integrative medicine who knows this subject well. In fact, he wrote a book on the subject. He suggests taking a gradually increased amount of either vinegar or lemon juice. While this form of acid won't work as well as HCl, it should help.

SECRET #54 When you should never take HCl.

If you have an ulcer, or a pre-ulcerous condition, you shouldn't take anything that stimulates stomach acid secretion. Nor should you take digestive enzymes or hydrochloric acid. But licorice root may be just your solution. Studies show it is very useful in treating peptic ulcers. Don't overdo licorice, either in an herbal tea or in licorice candy, since too much can cause headaches, water retention, loss of potassium, and high blood pressure. The German *Commission E Monographs* (an authoritative therapeutic guide to herbal medicine) suggest that licorice be used for ulcer treatment for no more than four to six weeks. If you have heart disease, liver or kidney problems, or a potassium deficiency, do not use this herb unless you are under the care of a physician.

DGL: Deglycyrrhizinated licorice (DGL) is a substance found in natural food stores that comes from licorice root (the herb, not the candy). It repairs the stomach and intestinal linings. In addition, it often works as well as antacids and acid-blockers for many people with heartburn. Chew two DGL tablets in between meals from three to four times a day. If HCl with pepsin causes pain in your stomach, taking DGL for a few months could help repair your stomach lining to the point where you can tolerate the acid you need.

Pancreatic enzymes: Stomach acid activates pancreatic enzymes. If you have low stomach acid, your enzyme production is most likely low. You can find digestive enzymes at health-food stores. The best time to take enzymes is after a meal, no matter what the bottle says. Papain, made from papayas, is rarely strong enough. I prefer either pancreatic enzymes or a strong vegetarian formula.

Turmeric: This herb is used extensively in Asia for a number of digestive-related complaints. One of its actions is to stimulate digestive juices that protect against irritation from acid. Take two tablets (250 milligrams each) after meals and before bedtime for symptoms of indigestion and heartburn.

Probiotics: Since stomach acid kills off bad bacteria; low stomach acid means you probably have more bad bacteria and fewer beneficial ones. Take a good quality probiotic with several strains of friendly bacteria (lactobacilli and bifidobacteria).

Heartburn is not the only uncomfortable digestive problem that causes people to reach for an antacid or other medication. Bloating, accompanied by intestinal gas, is a common and embarrassing complaint. Once again, there are safe and effective alternatives to pharmaceuticals.

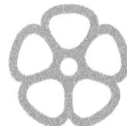

CHAPTER 10

Better Than Tums—
Herbs to End Your
Gas and Bloating

Enzymes, hydrochloric acid (HCl), and probiotics can help your body function better, but that doesn't mean that everything's working optimally. If you suffer from gas and bloating, don't despair. Herbs can once again come to your rescue. Since they affect various stages of digestion, choose the ones that best match your symptoms.

SECRET #55 These common herbs can help keep gas from building up.

You may have noticed that many Indian restaurants have a little dish of *fennel seeds* by the cash register. This is because fennel helps eliminate gas. When you eat these seeds, they can prevent bloating after eating a rich meal. Herbs that have this property are called carminatives.

Carminatives have several properties. They help you belch up trapped air; they increase the secretion of stomach acids that help digestion; and they relax your intestines, allowing gas to be passed. Some carminatives act as cholagogues, promoting the flow of bile from the gallbladder. They promote fat digestion and absorption.

Peppermint oil is the most well known and widely used of all carminatives. Most of its activity comes from the menthol it contains. Scientific studies, including the German *Commission E Monographs*, have found peppermint oil effective in reducing upper intestinal spasms, in stimulating bile flow, and in promoting stomach secretions. I have used enteric-coated peppermint oil capsules that don't open until they get into the lower intestines to treat irritable bowel disease for more than a dozen years. To help your digestion, drink a cup of peppermint tea half an hour before your meal and repeat this three or four times a day.

German chamomile flowers, the species commonly sold in this country, contain an oil that reduces inflammation and spasms. Chamomile is different from peppermint. It has anti-inflammatory properties. Many people drink a tea combining both peppermint and chamomile for their digestion. To make chamomile tea, steep the chamomile flowers for fifteen minutes and drink between meals the same as peppermint. Since chamomile flowers contain the active oil, whenever possible buy small amounts of chamomile flowers in your health-food store, rather than powdered chamomile. All varieties of chamomile are members of a plant family that include asters and ragweed. Rarely, someone allergic to ragweed cannot tolerate chamomile.

Ginger root is both a carminative and antispasmodic. It is well known in India and other countries for its digestive properties. You can use fresh ginger root in cooking, drink ginger tea (found in health-food stores and some supermarkets), or eat an occasional piece of candied ginger. All can help improve your digestion.

Other carminatives include spearmint, anise, caraway, and coriander. Their activity is weaker than peppermint or chamomile, but if you are sensitive to either of the first two, these plants offer a safe substitution. Take a teaspoon of spearmint leaves or any of these seeds, crush them, and steep in a cup of boiling water for fifteen minutes.

SECRET #56 Poor fat digestion? These herbs can solve the cause of your gas.

If you have pain in the upper part of your stomach that gets worse after you eat fatty foods, you may not produce enough bile to digest fats. If this is the case, you can either take a digestive enzyme after eating or turn to an herb known as a cholagogue. A cholagogue either helps empty your gallbladder of bile or helps your liver produce more of it. Cholagogues help correct the cause of your gas rather than alleviate its symptoms.

Turmeric root, an ingredient in curry powder, contains a volatile oil along with a substance called curcumin. Curcumin acts specifically on bile and also has significant anti-inflammatory properties. Recent studies indicate it may also protect the liver and guard against cancer, but it's too early to say for certain. The authoritative German *Commission E Monographs* say that turmeric is a safe and effective digestive aid. The active ingredients in turmeric are not water soluble, so buy this herb in an alcohol tincture from your local health-food store and take it according to directions.

Milk thistle seed increases the secretion of bile from the liver and gallbladder. It also detoxifies the liver and is used to reverse liver damage from exposure to toxic chemicals. To make milk thistle tea, steep 1 teaspoon of ground seeds in a cup of boiling water.

Dandelion root is often used to promote bile flow, and is a diuretic high in potassium. Since it's used to counteract liver and gallbladder congestion, your parents or grandparents may have used tender young dandelion leaves (either fresh or steamed) as a spring tonic. You can drink dandelion root tea or eat fresh dandelion leaves.

CHAPTER 11

Two Important Steps
to Improve Your Digestion

There are two steps you need to take to improve your digestion. Either one by itself is not enough. First, look at how you eat. Second, look at what you eat. Your lifestyle habits, as well as the foods you choose, determine whether or not you'll have good or poor digestion. Let's begin with the most frequently overlooked factor of all and take Step #1: Look at how you eat.

SECRET #57 **Cut your digestive problems in half with this one lifestyle change.**

I can't overemphasize the importance of this simple step. The first and most critical stage of digestion starts in your mouth. So you'll never have good digestion if you don't chew your food well. Ideally, we should all eat slowly and chew each bite till it is liquid before swallowing and taking the next. You may not do this, but the better you chew, the easier it is for your body to digest—and use—your food. In my nutrition counseling practice, I've found that simply chewing your food well can eliminate over 50 percent of digestive complaints. Sometimes, good old-fashioned common sense is a miracle worker!

Here's why chewing well is so important.

The first stage of digestion for carbohydrates (starches and sugars) begins in your mouth. Saliva contains an enzyme called amylase that breaks carbohydrates down into smaller, digestible sugars. If you're eating quickly, chances are you're not chewing your food well. This sets the stage for painful and embarrassing gas. Larger particles of undigested food make their way to your intestines and begin to ferment. Also, if you're not properly chewing, you could be low in important nutrients—even if the foods you're eating are healthy!

Protein digestion, on the other hand, begins in your stomach. This could give a false impression that you don't have to chew your chicken or tofu well. Nothing could be further from the truth. Chewing breaks everything into smaller particles. Since all food stays in your stomach until it's partially liquefied, the better you chew proteins, the easier they are to digest.

When you chew, your taste buds send a signal to the stomach and pancreas to produce other digestive juices, like HCl, pancreatic enzymes, and bile. Bile is a substance that helps break down fats. So all foods are broken down into more usable particles when you chew your food thoroughly.

We know that different foods contain different amounts of various vitamins, minerals, fatty acids, and other nutrients. Somehow we think that because we eat foods that contain these nutrients, they automatically get into our body and provide us with nourishment. Unfortunately, this is not the case. Unless foods are well digested, some of their nutrients will not be freed from fibers and other material and these nutrients can't be used.

SECRET #58 You could be diluting your digestive juices too much.

It's probably fine to sip a glass of water or another beverage with your meal. But if you drink glass after glass of anything, you could be diluting the HCl you need to digest proteins. This is especially true if you're over fifty. As we age, we naturally produce less HCl.

Reduce the liquids you drink at meals to one glass. This isn't difficult if you chew your food well. The exception is red wine. It actually helps stimulate the production of HCl. This is not a suggestion to drink too much wine. All you need is one glass.

Some people drink large quantities of liquids with their meals because they're thirsty. This is because they don't drink enough throughout the day. By the time they sit down to a meal they realize they're thirsty. If this sounds like you, make a concerted effort to drink more water throughout the day.

Do you drink a lot with meals because your food is dry and hard to swallow? Then chew your food better and eat moist foods like soup or salads along with a sandwich or entrée.

SECRET #59 Eat light at night.

High-fat snack foods such as nuts, cheese, ice cream, and chips are hard to digest. They're not a good choice for a late night snack. It's difficult to get a good night's sleep when you lie down with a stomach full of partially digested food. If you're not ready to give up these foods at night, at least reduce their fat content, limit your portions, and chew them well!

For a few weeks, switch to non-fat yogurt with applesauce, a piece of fruit, a few whole grain crackers, or fat-free corn chips. Temporarily avoid nuts after dinner. See if this makes a difference in your sleep patterns or in your digestion.

Instead of eating foods high in fats, make a small amount of low-fat or air-popped popcorn. Be sure to chew it well. Fresh fruit, carrots, or slices of jicama (a sweet, crunchy root vegetable that's eaten raw) make good evening snacks.

Make a pot of herb tea—something with relaxing herbs like chamomile, passionflower, or skullcap—and sip a cup or two of tea instead of eating. These herbs will relax you and give you something to do with your mouth at the same time.

Now you're ready for Step #2: Look at what you eat. Some of this is obvious. Some, less so. Perhaps you've been eating more dairy products than usual. Or maybe over time your body's ability to digest milk sugars changed. If so, your gas and stomach pain may be caused by lactose intolerance.

SECRET #60 Dairy could be causing problems now even if it never bothered you in the past.

Lactase is an enzyme that helps you digest lactose, a sugar found naturally in milk and other dairy products. Your body needs to make lactase before lactose can be digested. But if you're over the age of five, your body may be making very little lactase. Seventy-five percent of the world's population stops producing lactase after they're weaned. That's almost everyone! This is nature's way of telling us we don't need to drink milk to be healthy.

If you can't digest lactose, you're considered to be lactose intolerant. This condition can be extremely painful. It can cause a lot of intestinal gas and pain. Some ethnic groups like Asians, African Americans, and Jews have a high predominance of lactose intolerance. But just about anyone from any nationality can suffer from it. Lactose intolerance is actually an enzyme deficiency. It's not an allergy. It increases with age as our enzyme production decreases.

Basics of Lactose Intolerance

If you don't have enough lactase, lactose can't be digested well enough to get into your bloodstream. Instead, it remains in your intestines. The lactose in your intestines attracts water, which leads to bloating. When lactose makes its way into your large intestines (colon), intestinal bacteria eat this undigested sugar creating gas and acid. The gas and acid produce cramps, more gas, and, frequently, diarrhea.

SECRET #61 You don't have to guess whether or not you are lactose intolerant. You can know.

You may be lactose intolerant if you get any unpleasant symptoms either immediately or for up to twelve hours after eating dairy. There are tests that can confirm or rule out a lactose-digesting problem. One you can do on your own. The others require the help of a savvy doctor.

Lactose challenge test: The simplest way to test for lactose intolerance is to stop eating any dairy except for butter for two weeks. Read the labels of all foods carefully. If any foods contain milk solids or are creamy, they may contain dairy. Some creamed soups available in health-food stores contain no dairy. Otherwise, most creamed foods in supermarkets do.

At the end of these two weeks, drink a little milk or eat some ice cream. Wait up to half a day and see what happens. If you have no digestive problems, try eating more dairy the following day. Still feel fine? Chances are you don't have a problem with lactose. Feel more bloated or have diarrhea? Dairy is likely the culprit.

Lactose tolerance test: Your doctor needs to administer this test. First, you fast overnight and in the morning before being tested. Your doctor will take a blood sample and then give you a drink with 50 grams of lactose (milk contains about 12 grams a glass). Two hours after you drink the lactose-laced beverage, your doctor will take another blood sample. If you are not lactose intolerant, your blood-sugar level will rise because your body is able to break down the sugar. If you are lactose intolerant, your blood sugar either won't rise or will not rise completely. If you have a lactose problem, you're also likely to have bloating, cramps, and diarrhea.

Hydrogen breath test: This is another test your doctor can perform. You simply breathe into a bag to collect a sample of the gasses in your breath. Then you drink a solution containing a little lactose and breathe into another bag. These samples are sent to a laboratory where methane and hydrogen gasses are tested. Methane levels are usually 0 to 7 parts per million (ppm). If the level between your two samples is 12 ppm or more, you are lactose intolerant. Hydrogen is normally 10 ppm, but people who are lactose intolerant often have 20 ppm after ingesting dairy. Some hydrogen breath tests only measure hydrogen. But any undigested carbohydrates (either sugars or starches) will cause more hydrogen to be released. So if you're using this test, be sure you're being tested for both methane and hydrogen. Don't have this test when you're taking antibiotics, since the test won't be accurate. Why? Because antibiotics destroy the bacteria that help break down carbohydrates.

Stool acidity test: When intestinal bacteria breaks down undigested lactose, various acids—like lactic acid—are produced. So a high amount of acid in the stool is a good indication of potential lactose intolerance. While lactose tolerance and hydrogen breath tests are more accurate, they are not completely safe for children and infants. This test is. If you suspect a child has difficulty digesting milk sugars, you can simply get their stool examined for acidity or eliminate all dairy products and see if their symptoms go away.

Acidophilus and Yogurt Might Help . . . a Little

As its name suggests, *lacto* (milk) *bacillus* (bacteria) *acidophilus* means that this friendly bacteria eats milk sugar (lactose). Acidophilus also makes lactase. So taking acidophilus supplements could help improve mild lactose intolerance, especially over time. It can also be an important part of the answer for more serious digestive problems.

But it's important for you to realize that not all dairy products cause digestive problems in lactose-intolerant people. Butter, for instance, contains no lactose. It's just a fat. Fermented dairy, like yogurt, uses up lactose during fermentation. The end product is a low-lactose food you may be able to handle. Lactaid milk, which has had some of its milk sugar removed and is low in lactose, may not cause problems.

Refined sugar and organic pure cane sugar juice, on the other hand, are sweeteners that contribute to digestive problems. If you're eating yogurt, choose one with no added sugar. Some are sweetened with fruit and fruit juice. They are fine.

SECRET #62 Sugar feeds bad bacteria and contributes to digestive problems.

When you eat foods containing a lot of sugar, you're upsetting the balance of friendly bacteria (called "probiotics") that help you digest proteins, lactose, and other substances. Beet sugar and cane sugar feed harmful, or pathogenic, bacteria like *Candida albicans.* Candida is a form of yeast that can become a fungus and sugar is its primary food.

Fructose, or fruit sugar, actually feeds the good bacteria. You can still eat limited amounts of sweet foods at times, but try to eat some that are sweetened with fruit juice. There are excellent, tasty cookies available in natural food stores that even the fussiest eater can enjoy. Try some made by Pamela's. While they're a bit high in fats (limit yourself to one or two), they taste like bakery cookies.

In the past, people have been told to avoid eating protein with starches or sugars to improve their digestion. And this can help, because your body will digest fats and proteins before starches and sugars. But this way of eating means you can never eat a sandwich again and it simply isn't practical. I believe it's better to improve a weak digestive system than to support the weakness without strengthening it. You can take a burden off your digestive system by waiting an hour or more after a protein meal to eat anything sweet.

If Your Symptoms Persist, See Your Doctor

Occasionally, digestive problems are a sign of a more serious condition. Be smart. If these suggestions I've given you do not resolve your symptoms, it's best to seek out professional advice. Always check with your physician if you have problems that don't clear up quickly. Any condition is easier to correct when it's addressed early than when it has become chronic.

If your doctor gives you a clean bill of health and you're still uncomfortable, you may have an overgrowth of *Candida albicans* or intestinal parasites. Then again, you could have an inflammatory disease called irritable bowel syndrome (IBS). For more information on treating IBS, see Chapter 13.

CHAPTER 12

This Hidden Epidemic
May Be Keeping You Sick

Approximately twenty years ago, a yeast and fungal overgrowth became the disease of the year. Just about every healthcare practitioner I knew used a series of questions from a respected allergist to determine whether or not their difficult patients could have it. More often than not their conclusion was "yes."

Don't be surprised.

It is estimated that 90 percent of Americans have either a minor or major overgrowth of this yeast, called *Candida albicans*. This condition often prevents them from clearing up a wide number of health problems. You may know that antibiotics can trigger a candida overgrowth. But so can some other little-known causes.

SECRET #63 Your genetics and progesterone levels can cause a candida overgrowth.

Antibiotics: When you take large amounts of antibiotics, or use them over a long period of time, they kill off the friendly bacteria that keep candida levels low along with the bad bacteria. The result is too much candida (bad bacteria) and not enough good bacteria (probiotics) to keep them in check. If you've taken antibiotics for more than two months at any time in your life without replenishing the friendly bacteria, it's very possible you could have a yeast problem.

Sugar: Sugar is candida's primary food. Refined carbohydrates, like white flour, also feed this yeast. Eat only small quantities of unrefined carbohydrates. And avoid refined sugar (and honey) entirely.

Progesterone: Fluctuating hormone levels can trigger candida growth. A study published in the early 1990s found an association between high levels of progesterone and high candida levels. So if you're taking progesterone—even the natural kind—and you're not feeling well, this could be the reason. Ask your doctor to check your progesterone level and make sure it's not too high.

Genetics: You may have a little-known genetic predisposition that allows candida to flourish. Here's how: Your immune system contains a protein that attaches itself to the sugars on candida cells. Then, cells that destroy bacteria and cell debris wipe out the yeast.

Usually, only 10 percent of all women have low levels of this candida-lowering protein. But I spoke with Steven S. Witkin, Ph.D., a professor of immunology at Cornell University. He said a whopping 62 percent of women with recurrent vulvo-vaginal candidiasis have low concentrations of this protective protein in their vagina due to genetics. Are you one of them? Now you can find out.

SECRET #64 This little-known test can detect a genetic propensity for candida.

A simple test is now available through Dr. Witkin. It's designed to find a particular genetic abnormality that causes a lower production of a protein that fights candida infections in the vagina. If you don't have enough of this protein, called mannose-binding lectin, you have a genetic predisposition for candida. The test is simple. You simply brush the inside of your cheek with the cotton swab that's provided in the kit and mail it in.

The test costs around $150 and you don't need a doctor to order it. All results are sent to doctors, so let yours know to expect it if you decide on your own to be tested. For more information, you or your doctor can contact Dr. Witkin's team. If you have a genetic tendency for low levels of this protein, you'll have to work harder to control your candida than other women. But I promise you it can be done.

SECRET #65 Candida is easier to control when it's a yeast overgrowth than when it becomes a fungal infection.

The first symptoms of an intestinal candida overgrowth are digestive problems. Left untreated, candida can progress to a fungal infection. In this advanced stage it can lead to chronic fatigue, migraines, weight gain, sore throats, foggy thinking, chemical sensitivities, and more.

Candida is a hidden epidemic that has been misunderstood from day one. And yet, it could easily be the source of your digestive problems. It's important to understand that you will never "get rid" of candida. It's one of more than three hundred bacteria that coexist in our digestive and vaginal tracts, keeping one another in balance. You can, however, reduce the quantity of pathogenic, or "bad" bacteria, like candida.

Candida begins in the digestive tract as a yeast. When it grows out of control, it is able to change from a yeast into a fungus, much like a caterpillar changes into a butterfly. As a yeast it is encapsulated in your intestines, unable to push its way through the intestinal lining. It causes digestive problems in this form. But as a fungus, its long, rootlike structures can break through your intestines, get into your bloodstream, and cause allergies and other problems. This is called systemic candida, and is most often found in people with severe, chronic health problems.

You may be familiar with candida as being a cottage-cheese-like vaginal discharge accompanied by itching and irritation. This form of overgrowth often comes from taking antibiotics that kill off the friendly intestinal and vaginal bacteria, which keep the yeast from overmultiplying. It is also common in women with diabetes. Vaginal candida is rarely a long-term problem. It can often be controlled with vaginal suppositories or antifungal medications, both natural and allopathic, along with temporarily eliminating its favorite food.

It takes time and a concerted effort to reduce an intestinal overgrowth of candida. Diet, probiotics, and antifungal supplements or medications are all necessary components of an anticandida program. When it becomes a fungal infection, pharmaceutical antifungals may help shorten recovery time. In addition, as the fungal form breaks through the intestinal lining, it damages this lining and can lead to intestinal permeability or "leaky gut syndrome." I'll talk about this in the next chapter. For now, just know that the more advanced your candida overgrowth, the longer it takes to get it under control. This is why it's so important to begin controlling it when it is limited to your intestines.

SECRET #66 The only way to control candida is to stop eating sugar.

Candida lives on refined sugars and other sugars that are quickly absorbed. The most important single action you can take is to starve this yeast. Eliminate all white sugar, brown sugar, pure cane sugar juice, corn syrup, molasses, honey, and alcohol. Limit your sweets to one piece of fruit a day (no juices). This isn't a permanent diet—just one you need to follow until you lower your candida colonies. Unless you totally eliminate sugar for at least three weeks—maybe more—you won't be able to get your candida under control. You may need to avoid sugar for a lot longer. Some of my patients had to stop eating sugar for six months.

I wish I could tell you differently, but I can't. And there's no way around it. It doesn't matter what else you do if you continue to eat foods with sugar. All the antifungals in the world won't help you. You can't kill off a yeast while you're feeding it and expect to get better. You simply have to starve it.

This means eating a diet higher in protein (fish, chicken, tofu, beans) and lower in all sugars and starches. A diet high in carbohydrates, such as starchy vegetables (potatoes and corn), grains, pasta, bread, fruit and fruit juice, and refined sugars is not a healthy diet for someone who has an overgrowth of any yeast or fungus. Concentrate on eating lots of vegetables and protein with small amounts of complex carbohydrates and fruit.

If your candida has progressed to a fungal infection, it has most likely suppressed your immune system. In this case, you'll also want to boost your immunity by eliminating any foods to which you are allergic or sensitive. These may be "good" foods that impair your immune system. It just means they're not good for you at this time. If you get sleepy after eating corn products (tortillas, corn chips, polenta), eliminate corn from your diet temporarily. If chicken makes you feel mentally foggy or tired, don't eat chicken for now. You're better off with a limited diet that allows you to get better than with eating a wide variety of foods that prevent you from healing. However, you probably don't have to avoid eating fermented foods or foods containing yeast.

SECRET #67 Most people with candida do not need to avoid yeast or fermented foods.

I know this is the opposite of what you've been taught. But avoiding yeast is the biggest misunderstanding connected with candida. Let me tell you how and where it originated, and why it may be safe for you to eat tofu, mushrooms, and salad dressings with vinegar.

Candida first came to our attention in the early 1980s from two doctors who specialized in treating people with severe allergies: Drs. Orian Truss and William Crook. Their patients—who had systemic candida—were put on extremely restrictive diets: nothing with yeast in it (this eliminated most breads and baked goods, as well as foods with vinegar), no sugar of any kind, no wheat or dairy, and almost no carbohydrates. Few people could stay on this diet long enough to effect changes.

What few people understood was why Drs. Truss and Crook devised such a restrictive and difficult-to-follow diet. It came out of their specialty as allergists. In their individual practices, Dr. Truss and Dr. Crook noticed that their allergy patients with chronic illnesses seemed to remain sick because of an untreated overgrowth of candida.

Remember now, these were allergy patients. They were people who had allergies severe enough for them to seek out experts in the field. And these two eminent doctors found that if their patients stopped feeding the yeast and took antifungal medications, they still didn't get better because their allergies had suppressed their immune system. Their bodies couldn't establish enough friendly bacteria to keep the disease-causing bacteria under control. So Drs. Truss and Crook took their allergy patients off the foods that most frequently provoke allergic reactions: molds and fungi (like mushrooms, vinegar, and foods with yeast), dairy products, wheat, and other common alergenic foods.

At the same time, they reduced their intake of carbohydrates and eliminated sugar, because these foods feed candida. They also put their patients on antifungal medications like nystatin and Nizoral. Patients who tried alternative medicine were put on another antifungal like garlic or caprylic acid. But many of these medical and alternative treatments didn't work because *Candida albicans* is a wily critter. Try to kill it and it mutates. By the late 1980s, there were hundreds of species of candida, and many were resistant to the antiyeast and antifungal medications.

Alternative health practitioners heard about Drs. Truss and Crook's work with candida, and began diagnosing this overgrowth in almost all of their patients. They used some of the same protocol. Instead of prescription drugs, they used garlic, caprylic acid, or other "natural" antifungals. Some patients got better, many more didn't. Instead, they grew more discouraged and more frustrated.

What was missing?

According to Hyla Cass, M.D., author of *8 Weeks to Vibrant Health,* "Everyone who has a chronic illness should look for a candida overgrowth. Some illnesses like chronic fatigue and fibromyalgia are not really caused by candida, but they're related to it. When you clear up candida, the immune system gets stronger and chronically ill patients feel better."

The diets most people were put on to control candida were often unnecessarily restrictive, causing people to "cheat" and feed their yeast, rather than kill it off. And not many practitioners addressed the issue of probiotics—friendly bacteria—that naturally keep candida from flourishing.

How to get tested

For some people, just knowing that candida may be contributing to an ongoing illness is enough. Others may want a laboratory test that says, "Yes, this is a problem for you." Genova Diagnostics does a Comprehensive Digestive Stool Analysis that's extremely accurate. This panel is a combination of eighteen tests that identify bacterial and yeast overgrowths and even show the treatments, both allopathic and natural, that will work for your specific overgrowth problem.

If you have taken nystatin, Nizoral, Diflucan, or other antifungals and still have your original problems, your candida overgrowth may be one that responds to garlic or caprylic acid instead. And, of course, the reverse is true as well. You may need pharmaceuticals to control your candida. Garlic may just not work against your particular strain.

Your doctor can contact Genova Diagnostics for the necessary information and kits. This comprehensive analysis, which evaluates digestion, absorption, intestinal functions, and microbial flora, as well as giving therapeutic information on what will correct these imbalances, costs around $200. Ask your doctor to get the prepaid customer price for you. If you pay when you send in your sample, and do your own insurance form filing, the price can be considerably lower.

Candida-Fighting Supplements

If you know or suspect you have a candida overgrowth, begin by cleaning up your diet. Then choose from the following supplements. You need at least one antifungal, a good probiotic, and something to boost your immune system.

SECRET #68 Herbal antifungals are often as effective as prescription drugs.

Antifungals: After a sugar-free, low-carb diet, prescription or herbal antifungals are the next line of defense to eliminate a yeast overgrowth. If your condition is severe and long-standing, you may need a prescription drug like Diflucan or Nizoral. Otherwise, you may get good results from a non-prescription herbal supplement. Here are some herbs you may want to try. Most can be found in health-food stores.

Caprylic acid: This is a fatty acid found in coconut oil that works in the intestinal tract. It is similar in effectiveness to nystatin, a pharmaceutical that can adversely affect liver function. The main difference is that caprylic acid is very safe to use.

Citricidal and other citrus seed extracts: In addition to being effective as antifungals in the digestive tract, citrus seed extracts also kill off parasites, like *Giardia* and *Blastocystis hominis.* If you take this supplement an hour before or after meals you can avoid any upset stomach it might otherwise cause.

Flax oil and fish oils: These oils contain essential fatty acids, which boost the immune system. They are also mild antifungals.

Garlic and onions: Both are natural antibiotics and antifungals that have been used for centuries to counteract candida. You can use deodorized garlic oil capsules if you want to avoid garlic breath.

Tanalbit is a non-prescription intestinal antiseptic used by many healthcare practitioners instead of nystatin and caprylic acid. It is made from natural tannins (resins found in tea) and zinc.

Probiotics are friendly bacteria that keep candida colonies in check. If you have too much candida, you have too little *L. acidophilus*, *B. bifidus*, and other good bacteria. Not all probiotics are the same. Get the strongest formula you can find and afford. More information on probiotics, and several excellent products, may be found in Chapter 2.

SECRET #69 High candida = low immunity.

Immune-boosting nutrients allow your immune system to fight off all infections and even a candida overgrowth. If you have candida, your immune system is most likely functioning less than optimally. When you add one or more nutrients with immune-boosting abilities, you shorten your recovery time.

Medicinal mushrooms: I frequently suggest that my patients with candida or chronic illnesses take medicinal mushrooms to support their immune systems. Dr. Crook might not agree, but Janet Zand, acupuncturist, author, founder of McZand Herbals, and longtime friend, would. When I asked Janet about using medicinal mushrooms for people with a yeast overgrowth, she said she's seen people with candida and chronic fatigue benefit *tremendously* from using them. I also found that my candida patients responded well to medicinal mushrooms—even though they're a form of fungus. See Chapter 3 for more detailed information.

Herbs that have been found to support the immune system include echinacea, garlic, ginseng, and Eleutherococcus (formerly known as Siberian ginseng). Some of these are adaptogens, as well. They help regulate the immune system. Chapter 21 explains adaptogens and identifies more of them.

Drug therapy: If you decide to use pharmaceutical medications, be sure your form of candida will respond to the drug you're taking. Not all candida is *Candida albicans*. Nor does *Candida albicans* always respond to the same medication. This yeast is tricky. It mutates quickly. If you're prescribed Nizoral, you need to know that this drug could be toxic to your liver. So if you take it, get a liver function blood test every three months. Ask your physician to rotate your drugs frequently to prevent drug resistance. If possible, include natural antifungals as well as pharmaceuticals.

Dr. Crook used pharmaceuticals with his patients. Other doctors, like Hyla Cass, M.D., coauthor with Dr. Crook of *The Yeast Connection and Women's Health,* use herbal antifungals successfully. Ask your health provider to help you design an antifungal plan.

You can't cure a chronic illness like a candida overgrowth until you identify and treat all of its underlying causes. At most, you'll be fighting an uphill battle just to keep from getting worse. The good news is you can get better! The steps I listed here are sure to defeat an overgrowth in candida and possibly resolve other chronic illnesses. I've seen it happen and you can, too!

SECRET #70 Candida may be unresponsive if you have leaky gut syndrome.

If you've done everything possible to control your candida overgrowth and still are unable to get well, there may be an underlying problem you haven't addressed. It's called intestinal permeability, also known as leaky gut syndrome. After the intestinal yeast form of candida turns into a fungus, it can damage your intestinal lining. As the fungal form of candida works its way across the intestinal mucosa it makes larger holes in the intestinal walls. This allows either particles of food or bacteria to "leak" across this barrier.

Food allergies also enlarge the lining of the intestines, making it more vulnerable to harmful particles. Leaky gut syndrome will not get better by itself or with a simple change in diet and antifungals. It can be diagnosed by laboratory tests and treated by doctors familiar with it. In the following chapter I'll explain what you can do to identify and correct leaky gut syndrome. Unchecked, it can progress to autoimmune and bowel problems. Please read it carefully, and if necessary, tackle leaky gut syndrome before beginning an anti-candida regimen. Otherwise, a leaky gut syndrome can thwart your candida eradication efforts.

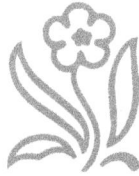

CHAPTER 13

Four Hard-to-Detect Causes and Cures of Digestive Problems

C andida isn't the only problem that causes gas, bloating, diarrhea, and other discomfort. There are four other causes of digestive complaints that many doctors either overlook or don't know how to treat naturally. They are intestinal permeability (leaky gut syndrome), irritable bowel syndrome (IBS), parasites, and *H. pylori.*

Still, if you have digestive distress, it makes sense to begin by treating yourself for an overgrowth of *Candida albicans.* It's a common enough problem for you to address before looking for more complex conditions. An anti-candida program should improve your digestion, whether or not you have other problems as well.

Years ago, I met monthly with a group of medical doctors who looked at nutritional solutions for difficult-to-detect health problems. Each month we met for three hours to discuss one illness. But it took three months of meetings—nine hours—to complete our discussion of candida. After all those hours of intense debate, input, and case histories, the conclusion this group of doctors came to was that whether or not a person has candida, allergies, or other digestive problems, an anti-candida program had a tremendous amount of value and improved symptoms.

Still, you may need to look further.

For more than fifty years, doctors and folk healers alike have said that good health begins in the colon. Now we're finding out they were right. Not only are the intestines the tubing through which nutrients are absorbed into our bloodstream, but they are designed to allow only those particles we need for cellular health to get through while keeping out larger particles that could lead to disease. When the intestinal lining becomes damaged, the result can be a more complex problem.

1. Intestinal Permeability (Leaky Gut)

SECRET #71 Your digestive distress and chronic health problems could be due to a "leaky gut."

Food allergies, candida overgrowth, and parasites (like *Giardia*) all contribute to increased permeability of the gut lining. This condition is known as intestinal permeability, or leaky gut syndrome. What this means is that the spaces between the cells in the lining of the intestines get more porous. Although these spaces are microscopic, they still become larger than they should be. These larger spaces allow undigested food particles, toxins, and bacteria to "leak" through the intestines (the "gut").

The first symptom of leaky gut is often intestinal discomfort. But it can include a myriad of complaints from food and chemical sensitivities to autoimmune diseases, headaches, inflammation, joint pain, and constipation alternating with diarrhea, gas, bloating, or cramping. Over a period of time, leaky gut can lead to irritable bowel syndrome (IBS), Crohn's disease, arthritis, or celiac disease (a sensitivity to gluten, a sticky substance found in wheat and many other grains).

Leaky gut syndrome will never correct itself or just go away. You need to work your way through a well-designed program that first identifies this problem and its causes, and then helps repair the lining of your intestines. If you've been experiencing some of the above symptoms and can't find their cause, you may want to explore the possibility of intestinal permeability.

With intestinal permeability, particles that should stay in your intestines leak through its lining. There are cells in your bloodstream that protect you from unwanted particles of any kind. When they identify a food particle, they attack it by manufacturing antibodies that are designed to destroy this foreign invader. But when these cells make antibodies to eliminate food particles, the antibodies can attach themselves to any organ in the body. This, in turn, can trigger a variety of diseases. Arthritis is one such disease. It can be caused when these antibodies attach themselves to joint tissues, producing substances that result in inflammation, swelling, and pain.

SECRET #72 Your anti-inflammatory medications could be causing more inflammation.

Not all inflammation comes from antibodies. Some come from taking anti-inflammatory drugs. That's right. One of the most common causes of leaky gut syndrome is from taking non-prescription, over-the-counter medications called nonsteroidal anti-inflammatory drugs (NSAIDs) like Motrin, Aleve, Advil, and aspirin. There are dozens of prescription NSAIDs as well. Although they are called anti-inflammatory drugs, NSAIDs actually inflame the intestinal lining, causing the spaces in the gut to widen. Some of these prescription NSAIDs have been taken off the market due to an increase in heart attacks and stroke. Ask your pharmacist if any of your drugs are NSAIDs. If so, look for safer alternatives. A number of them can be found in Part 5.

SECRET #73 Any intestinal irritation can lead to leaky gut syndrome.

Anything that continuously irritates your intestines, such as candida, caffeine, alcohol, and partially digested food particles, can lead to a leaky gut. This includes a number of irritating prescription drugs in addition to NSAIDs, like chemotherapy drugs. When chemotherapy drugs cause leaky gut, it can lead to malnutrition in cancer patients.

Leaky gut can contribute to serious illnesses, and serious illnesses can contribute to leaky gut syndrome. In fact, any condition that increases bowel inflammation contributes to a leaky gut. This includes Crohn's disease, celiac disease, inflammatory joint disease, food allergies, and alcoholism. What's more, just getting older contributes to a lack of integrity in the intestinal walls that can lead to intestinal permeability.

Dysbiosis, an imbalance between good and bad intestinal bacteria, also contributes to intestinal permeability through an inflammatory process. As I said earlier, an overgrowth of candida can cause inflammation in the gut lining. So can an overgrowth of other organisms like *Giardia* and *H. pylori.* Take probiotics to help correct this imbalance (see Chapter 2).

Diagnosing Leaky Gut Syndrome

There aren't many laboratories that diagnose this condition. The best one I know of is Genova Daignostics. They have an Intestinal Permeability Assessment test that measures the ability of two sugar molecules, mannitol and lactulose, to permeate the intestinal walls. Low levels of these sugar molecules in urine indicate there is a malabsorption problem. High levels indicate intestinal permeability. This test is highly predictive of leaky gut syndrome. This test is available only through doctors.

SECRET #74 There are natural solutions to intestinal permeability.

A number of substances can be used to reduce inflammation and the size of the intestinal wall openings. Some of them help heal the intestines as well.

Glutamine, an amino acid, is the most widely used supplement to treat intestinal permeability. It is the principal fuel used in the small intestines. Glutamine both prevents and reverses damage to the intestinal lining. It decreases bacterial overgrowth, as well. In a double-blind study conducted back in 1957, 92 percent of ulcer patients had completely healed their ulcers after taking 1.6 grams of glutamine a day for a month. Glutamine is sold in health-food stores in 500 milligrams (mg) capsules. Be sure any glutamine you buy is labeled "pharmaceutical grade" and consider taking one capsule on an empty stomach three times a day for a month or two.

Quercetin is a bioflavonoid from plants that reduces permeability caused by food allergies. It can be found in health-food stores alone, or combined with vitamin C.

Ginkgo biloba is an herb best known for its ability to improve memory through increased circulation. But it also protects the intestinal lining. If you are taking ginkgo for memory, 40 mg three times daily is the usual recommended amount. This same amount can also help repair your intestines.

Gamma-linolenic acid (GLA) is a fatty acid found in borage seed oil that prevents and treats intestinal lining inflammation. It protects against inflammatory damage from alcohol and aspirin, as well as from chemotherapy and radiation. Either GLA or borage seed oil capsules is an excellent addition to any basic supplement regime.

Probiotics: Flooding the intestines with good-quality *Lactobacillus acidophilus* and other lactobacilli such as *bifido* and *bulgaricus* is essential to establishing the proper ratio of good to bad bacteria. See Chapter 2 for more detailed information.

Digestive enzymes and hydrochloric acid. If you're not digesting your food, large particles are passing through your intestines contributing to inflammation, permeability, and food sensitivities. Consider taking two pancreatic enzyme tablets or capsules with each meal, and talk with your health provider about the advisability of including hydrochloric acid, as well. I've said it before, but it bears repeating here. Enzymes and hydrochloric acid should never be taken by anyone with an ulcer. If you're not sure, check with your doctor before using these products.

2. Irritable Bowel Syndrome (IBS)

SECRET #75 Your lifestyle may be causing your digestive problems.

If you're one of the many people who reach for an antacid whenever you get stomach pains or bloating, I've got news for you. You may not have intestinal permeability or simple indigestion. Most important, you may not need an antacid at all, even if an antacid makes you feel better temporarily. You could be among the 15 to 20 percent of Americans who suffer from irritable bowel syndrome (IBS), an abnormal functioning of the large intestines. Other IBS symptoms include diarrhea, constipation, nausea, and a disinterest in food. And while IBS is rarely life threatening it, can be extremely uncomfortable and draining. Before you reach for any medication, find out what you've got.

IBS is commonly triggered by stress and food sensitivities. This is a good thing. It puts it more in your control than in your doctor's. Other more serious colon problems like colitis and Crohn's disease are forms of chronic relapsing inflammatory bowel disease, and may require medication as well as lifestyle changes. These more serious illnesses may be genetic or could be caused by an autoimmune problem. Don't confuse them with IBS, which can respond well to stress management and dietary changes.

Begin by having an examination from your doctor and rule out the more serious problems like colon cancer, colitis, and Crohn's disease. Then, if you are told you have IBS, prepare to change your life before reaching for a medication that may only control symptoms. Ask your doctor or other healthcare practitioner to monitor you as you make some lifestyle changes.

Have you been under stress for three months or longer? Studies show that digestive disturbances occurring after prolonged stressful periods of our lives are usually symptoms of IBS. Not a lot of stress in your life? Then it's time to look to your diet.

IBS can be caused by food allergies or food sensitivities, which cause an irritation to the intestinal lining—and this can eventually lead to intestinal permeability. Try avoiding a food or foods completely for two to four weeks, and then reintroducing them into your diet one at a time. This will let you know whether or not a particular substance is causing your digestive complaints without having to get expensive tests.

SECRET #76 Irritable bowel is more common in sensitive people.

"Don't be so sensitive," my mother told me repeatedly when I was growing up. But I didn't know how. I have always been sensitive to emotional tensions, noise, colors . . . you name it. Being sensitive can work for or against you. It has allowed me to understand all kinds of people easily. And it's given me a sensitive stomach. I've learned not to eat when I'm upset and to use regular stress-reduction techniques.

IBS is an excellent example of the connection between your mind and your body. Almost all IBS patients complain of anxiety, depression, sleep disturbances, and anger. The more severe these emotions, the more severe—and frequent—their physiological symptoms become.

These physiological symptoms, in turn, contribute to psychological symptoms. For example, diarrhea contributes to malabsorption, a condition where important nutrients that are needed to alleviate anxiety, depression, and stress are not absorbed.

Stress and diarrhea cause magnesium (a mineral needed for emotional balance) to be excreted in higher quantities than usual. Since magnesium can contribute to loose stools, it cannot be adequately replenished when you already have diarrhea! To get your IBS under control, you need to first break this cycle.

SECRET #77 Your solution to IBS may be mind-body medicine, not traditional medicine.

When you focus your attention on a word, phrase, or sound, you slow down your heart rate, breathing, and metabolism. This phenomenon is what Dr. Herbert Benson, a professor at Harvard University, called the "relaxation response." Regular use of any relaxation technique lowers blood pressure, reduces chronic pain, alleviates insomnia and anxiety, and can eliminate mild to moderate depression. It also helps IBS. When you relax your mind and body, your body can more easily heal itself. Prayer and meditation are two examples of relaxation techniques.

Spirituality is a belief in a higher power and higher purpose, and spirituality heals. Recognizing that we need to move beyond our own self-absorbed concerns can help us feel connected to all life. It also allows us to relax, and our bodies to heal. Part of this concept includes accepting that all of us have limitations.

An important step in healing your IBS is to accept your body and its limitations while you look for solutions to your problem. Acceptance is not the same as resignation. Don't give up. Instead, be watchful and open to various solutions. As you become calmer and allow your stress to lessen, your body can begin healing.

Stressors are anything, positive or negative, that upset your body's balance. Skiing or a vacation is a positive stressor. A death or illness in the family is a negative stress. Both affect our health. Our reactions—both psychological (like anxiety) and biological (like diarrhea)—become our stress response.

How often should you pray or meditate? I tell my patients, "Do it every day you eat." They think I'm joking, but I'm not. Daily stress reduction is as important as food.

It may be that your IBS isn't caused by stress, but its symptoms are more likely to be present when you're under stress. This is because stress often leads to poor digestion. When you're anxious, your body doesn't make enough digestive enzymes and acids to break down the foods you eat. This leaves partially digested foods to ferment and cause IBS symptoms. Any technique or tool that breaks your stress cycle can calm down your intestines and help you feel better.

One method that has been documented as giving great results with IBS-associated stress reduction is hypnotherapy. In a study of thirty-three patients with IBS, two-thirds got relief within one and one-half months of weekly hypnotherapy treatments. Group treatments worked as well as individual ones, and the benefits lasted for three weeks after the treatments ended.

If you want to try hypnotherapy, look for a licensed psychotherapist who also practices hypnotherapy technique. This person is better able to evaluate the origins of your stresses and how they are impacting your life. A trained therapist can be a strong support for you as you make changes. You may need more than a layperson that has studied hypnotherapy. Ask to have a tape made for you that you can play at home each evening. This way your treatment can continue past your hypnotherapy sessions. Other methods of stress reduction include biofeedback, meditation, or relaxation exercises. Look to your diet for the next step if they're not enough.

SECRET #78 You may need to make major dietary changes to control your IBS.

The bottom-line is—you have to make whatever changes are necessary for your body to heal. Not just what's easy or convenient. If you have a food allergy, you need to eliminate that food forever. If you have a food sensitivity, you may be able to eat small amounts of it eventually with no problems.

Food allergies always cause a negative reaction; food sensitivities cause problems periodically. Any food can trigger IBS, but some are more commonly associated with it than others. The foods most commonly associated with it are wheat, corn, dairy, coffee, tea, and citrus. If you crave any of these, look out. Craving a certain food is often a sign that it is contributing to your problem. Many people have sensitivities to more than one of these foods. If you eat wheat, corn, or dairy daily, stop eating one or all of them—100 percent—for two full weeks. Read all labels carefully and ask questions when you're eating out.

Some prepared foods, like veggie burgers, for instance, often contain wheat or flour (made from wheat). Cornstarch, corn oil, and high-fructose corn syrup all come from corn. And to completely avoid dairy products, shop for foods marked "vegan" in health-food stores. Vegans are vegetarians who don't eat eggs or dairy.

The more processed the foods you eat, the more likely you are to find some of these ingredients lurking in them, so simplify your diet for a few weeks and eat whole foods. Rice is rarely a problem for people with IBS. Use it as your primary starch. You can find rice crackers, rice cereals, rice bread and even rice noodles either in health-food stores or in Asian markets.

Instead of dairy, use rice milk or soymilk with your cereal, beverages, and cooking. A number of delicious frozen desserts that resemble ice cream include: Sweet Nothings (their non-dairy fudge bars are remarkable!), Rice Dream, It's Soy Delicious, and Ice Bean. Avoid those with a lot of sugar. Sugar can upset the intestinal flora and cause diarrhea.

SECRET #79 You must stop eating this before you can control your IBS.

Sugar is your greatest enemy. It is the single substance that has been responsible for IBS in the majority of my patients. The fastest way to reverse your irritable bowel syndrome is to stop eating anything with refined sugar. Use small amounts of fruit-juice sweetened foods instead. Beware of the unrefined, organic, pure cane sugar juice found in a lot of "health foods" these days. I haven't seen enough studies to convince me that it's safe.

Sugar contributes to inflammation. Inflammation leads to candida, IBS, and intestinal permeability. A healthy gut is sugar free. For information on sugar substitutes—the good and the bad—see Chapter 16.

Three Helpful Supplements

There are three supplements that are key to re-establishing balance in your intestines: fiber, probiotics, and peppermint oil.

Fiber: If you're constipated, increase your fiber by eating more whole grains and vegetables. Adding more fiber increases your need for water, so drink water throughout the day. Half a glass an hour, whenever possible, is ideal, and better than drinking two or three glasses at a time, which can cause bloating.

If for some reason you can't get enough fiber from your diet, consider psyllium seed. Psyllium seed comes from the *Plantago ovata* plant. Sometimes the seeds are used, and sometimes the husks. Both are mucilaginous, which means that when you put them in water they absorb a lot of water and form a gel, softening and bulking up solid wastes. The mucilaginous effect of psyllium soothes the intestines. This is one form of fiber that doesn't cause irritation.

Psyllium is particularly resistant to fermentation, so it's not likely to cause gas.

Psyllium seed has one benefit over the husk. It contains more fiber and breaks down more slowly, producing large amounts of butyric acid. Butyric acid has an added benefit. It prevents the development of cancer cells and appears to protect against colon cancer.

Psyllium is a naturally occurring bulking agent with no side effects—unless you have a rare allergy to the plant. It is most effective when taken in 10–30 gram doses a day for several months. Begin using the lowest amount in divided doses. Whether you have constipation, diarrhea, or intestinal inflammation, psyllium seed may be an effective and inexpensive remedy. Because it contains no artificial sweeteners, sugar, or potentially harmful chemicals, it's safer than other over-the-counter bulking agents with sugar or artificial sweeteners, such as Metamucil.

Probiotics: Add a good quality probiotic to your diet for at least two or three months. (See Chapter 2 for more information.)

Peppermint oil relaxes the smooth muscles in the intestines and prevents the cramping some people get with irritable bowel syndrome. Only use enteric-coated peppermint oil capsules to ensure that the oil gets into your intestines. Enzymatic Therapy has such a product available through most health-food stores. Peppermint oil works by blocking the intestines' ability to utilize calcium. Calcium causes muscles to cramp; magnesium and peppermint oil cause muscles to relax. The first step you take might be to remove major sources of calcium from your diet (dairy products) and supplements.

3. Parasites

SECRET #80 **Even good tests can fail to diagnose parasites.**

Some of the trickiest sources of intestinal problems to identify are parasites. They're common, but extremely difficult to diagnose. I know.

For six weeks several years ago, I was bloated and had gas, diarrhea, and cramping. At first, I thought it was food poisoning. Then, as the symptoms worsened and diminished at the same times every day with no resolution, I began to look at other possibilities. I had a stool test for parasites from a very reputable laboratory come back negative. In utter frustration, I contacted my friend, nutritionist Ann Louise Gittleman, M.S., C.N.S., author of the excellent book on parasites, *Guess What Came to Dinner?*

"It sounds like parasites to me," she said after listening to my complaints. "They don't always show up on stool tests. In fact, 30 percent of stool tests come back with false negative results. I'd be happy to send you some of the anti-parasite medications I've developed if you'd like to try them," she offered. At that point, I was weak and tired and grateful to try these products. My symptoms stopped three days after starting her herbal formulas and I continued taking them for the full course of treatment. I've remained symptom free ever since.

Even the best laboratories specializing in parasite identification may fail to find them. Still, begin with tests to try to identify which parasites you have. Then, if your results are negative, like mine were, and you still believe you have parasites, go on and treat them with good-quality products.

Testing for parasites is a lengthy, difficult process and the cost reflects this (from $145–$250). But if you can get a good identification, it's worth it since different parasites respond best to specific treatments. A purged stool test using a number of stool samples is most frequently used. Follow the lab's instructions to the letter to get the best samples for them.

SECRET #81 You can't avoid parasites. You come into contact with them every day.

Intestinal parasites are more common in this country than you or your doctors may think. They're also extremely debilitating. Parasites sap your strength, compromise your health, lower your immunity, and can keep you housebound. More importantly, they often mimic other diseases such as irritable bowel, chronic fatigue, Crohn's disease, fibromyalgia, leaky gut syndrome, gallbladder problems, and ulcerative colitis. They can include symptoms such as depression, joint pains, and the inability to lose or gain weight. If you're suffering with any of these conditions and are not getting better in spite of your treatment, you may have parasites.

Parasites act like other illnesses for a variety of reasons. One is that they can break down cells faster than the cells can regenerate. When the cells in your intestines are destroyed and not replaced, you can get, or appear to have, a variety of digestive diseases. Parasites produce harmful toxins, irritate sensitive tissues causing inflammation and joint pain, and suppress the immune system.

The problem with diagnosing parasites is that few doctors are taught parasitology in medical school. Some may think of parasites if their patient recently returned from a trip to a third-world country. But many cases, like mine, are picked up right at home, because they're everywhere.

There are more than 130 varieties of parasites from microscopic protozoa like *Giardia* to long tapeworms. It's common to pick them up when traveling overseas, whether from the drinking water, eating raw fruits or vegetables, or just washing your contact lenses in tap water. You can also get them in this country from drinking or swimming in contaminated water. Chlorinated pools and hot tubs are not necessarily safe, because chlorine doesn't destroy *Giardia* and *Cryptosporidium,* two very common microscopic parasites.

If you have a pet dog or cat, you can get parasites from their fleas or from just cleaning up after them. Imported produce can carry parasites. So can organic fruits and vegetables. Raw and undercooked meats and fish, from rare beef and pork to sushi and smoked salmon, are all possible sources. Years ago, when I was a fan of sushi (raw fish with rice) and ate it at various Japanese restaurants with regularity, I asked a doctor friend whether he saw many cases of liver fluke, a difficult-to-treat parasite, in people who ate raw fish. To my surprise, he had. I stopped eating sushi then and there.

Parasites can hide within your body causing no problems unless they're disturbed. *Giardia,* for example—the parasite I had—lives in the duodenum, causing no symptoms. I apparently dislodged them during a cleansing program. Once in my intestines, they wreaked their havoc. If you haven't been exposed to parasites recently, they still could be the source of your health problem.

Most doctors believe that symptoms from parasites occur within three days of exposure. But Ann Louise, with more than twenty years of clinical experience, disagrees. She has found people who were exposed to parasites six months to a year before any troublesome symptoms began. And their symptoms were not necessarily the classic signs of abdominal pain, gas, and diarrhea.

A doctor well versed in parasitology may be able to design a course of treatment for you based on your symptoms and possible exposure to particular organisms. A lack of stomach acid (a natural barrier to parasites) and a lack of beneficial bacteria (to fight them off) are two indicators that parasites may be present.

Parasite Treatment

Flagyl (metronidazole) is the most prescribed medication for bacterial and parasite infections, but its side effects include diarrhea, abdominal cramps, incontinence, vaginal dryness, and liver damage—not much better than the parasite itself. I suggest you try herbal formulas first.

Most of the antiparasite herbal formulas on the market are based on those originally developed by Ann Louise Gittleman and sold through Uni Key Health Systems: the Verma System (for intestinal worms) and the Para System (for microscopic parasites). Each system contains a tincture and capsules. These are what I used. If you know you have worms, get the Verma System; if you're sure it's *Giardia, Cryptosporidium,* or another microscopic organism, use the Para System.

If you're not sure, or if you're traveling abroad and want good protection, take the Verma Key capsules and Para Plus tincture one week before you leave through two weeks after your trip. These products are antibacterial, antiviral, anti-yeast, and antiparasitic.

Chronic illnesses are often non-responsive because their underlying cause is not being targeted. Intestinal parasites are, in my opinion, one of the biggest reasons why people remain chronically sick.

4. Ulcers

SECRET #82 This easy-to-eradicate bacteria can be causing your ulcers.

Twenty years ago, a woman came to me with ulcers. She had tried stress reduction, a bland diet, and antacids. They hadn't helped her at all. Now her doctor wanted to give her a prescription for drugs that either blocked hydrochloric acid or had anti-inflammatory properties. The medications would allow her stomach to heal and repair itself. However, they didn't address the cause of her inflammation and pain. So she turned to me.

I remembered having read about an Australian doctor, Barry Marshall, who found that a particular bacterium, *Helicobacter pylori* (*H. pylori*) was present in almost everyone who had either gastritis or ulcers. When the bacterium was treated, the ulcers went away and didn't come back.

SECRET #83 A common over-the-counter medication could heal your ulcers.

Sure enough, a simple blood test through her doctor revealed that this woman had an overgrowth of *H. pylori*. At that time, most physicians treated this overgrowth with antibiotics. But my patient wanted to avoid the side effects from taking antibiotics, so I searched for another alternative and found one that had no side effects. It's still being used today. It's called bismuth. You know it as the active ingredient in Pepto-Bismol.

The FDA had already approved the form of bismuth in Pepto-Bismol to treat peptic ulcers, and her physician agreed to monitor her progress. Whether she had a peptic ulcer (chronic inflammation) or gastric ulcer (burning the stomach's lining with harsh gastric juices), *H. pylori* turned out to be the underlying cause of her pain. Once her *H. pylori* was under control, her pain and her ulcers disappeared.

Don't self-medicate with bismuth, however. When doctors use bismuth to treat *H. pylori*, they most frequently combine it with two or more different antibiotics. I prefer to only use antibiotics when there are no other solutions. If you want to use bismuth with or without antibiotics, you need a doctor to monitor you and make sure it works.

Get Tested for *H. pylori*

Don't assume that if you have ulcers you have *H. pylori*. If you have ulcers, or suspect you have them, the first thing to do is to see your doctor and get a diagnosis. A simple blood test or breath test can determine if you have a bacterium overgrowth.

Probiotics are always helpful when you have an overgrowth of any type of bad bacteria including *H. pylori*. In study after study, patients with *H. pylori* recovered more quickly when they took acidophilus or other friendly bacteria. This was true whether or not their treatment included antibiotics. See Chapter 2 for more information.

NSAIDs: Another cause of ulcers are NSAIDs, nonsteroidal anti-inflammatory drugs. When you take these common medications like aspirin, Advil, Celebrex, and Vioxx on a regular basis—not just occasionally—you run the risk of developing a peptic ulcer. In fact, you're more likely to get ulcers from NSAIDs than from *H. pylori*!

NSAIDs can cause excessive bleeding, kidney problems, and fluid retention. In fact, an article in the *New England Journal of Medicine* found that as many people die from ulcers caused by NSAIDs as from cervical cancer. Ulcers caused by NSAIDs need treatment that soothes and helps repair the stomach's mucous lining. Fortunately, many NSAIDs are now off the market due to even more serious side effects.

SECRET #84 Brown rice can cause ulcers.

When I first heard this astonishing claim, I didn't believe it. But the information came from a colleague of mine—author and nutritionist Betty Kamen, PhD. And like me, Betty does her homework. The truth appears to be that brown rice can cause ulcers and other intestinal problems in a small number of people. If you have these conditions and you eat a lot of brown rice, your problem may be connected with this popular grain.

Brown rice naturally contains oil along with a lot of lipase, the enzyme that breaks down fats. In fact, it has more lipase than other grains, and this is where the problem begins. When brown rice is milled and the outer husk is taken off, the fragile cells that separate the lipase from the rice oil are bruised and the enzyme begins to break down the rice oil. In a very short period of time, the oil becomes rancid.

While studies show that freshly milled brown rice, or rice bran, are protective against duodenal ulcers, stored brown rice and brown rice products have the opposite effect. Interestingly, the ulcer-inducing effects of rancid brown rice oil found in just about all brown rice products can be reversed by antioxidants like vitamin E and cysteine, an amino acid. Both are found in a number of multivitamins, such as Vitality Plus. If you're taking cysteine and vitamin E daily and eating brown rice occasionally, you *may* be fine.

If, however, you have ulcers and gastrointestinal problems, you may want to consider not eating brown rice and see if your symptoms improve.

SECRET #85 Licorice root is one of the most effective herbs to heal ulcers.

There are a number of medications used for ulcers. Fortunately, there are also more natural remedies that work. Of all herbs, DGL made from licorice root has been used and studied the most for ulcers.

DGL is deglycyrrhized licorice (*Glycyrrhiza glabra*). It is a form of licorice root that helps heal your stomach lining. It is not licorice candy. Licorice root has been used therapeutically for thousands of years in both Eastern and Western medicine. It is used in orthodox medicine to treat ulcers. Dosage, according to the *Expanded*

Commission E Monographs (the gold standard of herbal information) is to chew two to four DGL tablets before each meal. Don't take it for more than four to six weeks except under the supervision of your doctor. If you're taking any medications, check with your pharmacist before taking DGL. Some other drugs, when taken with DGL, can cause a loss of potassium.

There are other plant-based ulcer remedies, from aloe vera gel (one teaspoon after meals for up to two months) to fresh cabbage juice (drink one cup every three to four hours and expect to have gas). Personally, I'd use DGL or the newest ulcer remedy, zinc-carnosine.

HELP YOUR TREATMENT OF CHOICE WORK FASTER BY AVOIDING THESE SUBSTANCES:

- alcohol
- aspirin
- coffee (even decaf)
- refined sugar
- tea

SECRET #86 **This natural formula kills *H. pylori*, soothes stomach tissues, and stops inflammation.**

Some ulcer remedies, such as bismuth, kill *H. pylori*. Others have anti-inflammatory activity. Still others soothe damaged mucous membranes. A newly formulated combination of zinc (a mineral) and carnosine (an amino acid) does all of these. It is another example of a combination that outperforms either nutrient alone.

I first heard about zinc-carnosine, a formula developed in a laboratory, from Dr. Georges M. Halpern, a medical doctor who has written an excellent book, *Ulcer Free! Nature's Safe & Effective Remedy for Ulcers*. There are a number of studies on the use of zinc-carnosine for gastric ulcers. I would use it for mild to moderate conditions without hesitation. But I think that any severe condition should be both evaluated and monitored by your doctor. Here's what this combination does:

It's an antioxidant. Zinc-carnosine destroys hydrogen peroxide, a free radical that's produced in the stomach. But hydrogen peroxide also damages the stomach lining. Zinc-carnosine reduces this damage.

It's an anti-inflammatory and inflammation is painful. In addition to reducing inflammation in general, one study found it reduced inflammation caused specifically by aspirin.

It inhibits H. pylori. Zinc-carnosine creates an environment that appears to keep *H. pylori* from growing by strengthening your stomach lining.

Zinc-carnosine is more than a good Band-Aid. It seems to address the major causes of ulcers. Because it works at the source of your pain, it takes a while to work. Give it a two-month trial, and don't be surprised if you start to feel better much sooner.

Studies indicate several doses for zinc-carnosine. To end my own confusion and to eliminate yours, I contacted Dr. Halpern directly. Based on all the studies he reviewed in writing his book, he recommends taking 37.5 mg twice a day. You can get this formula from GNC stores under the name of PepZin GI. A one-month supply costs around $20—less if it's on sale.

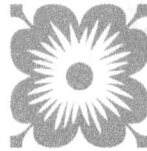

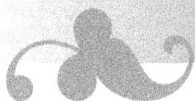

PART 3

LOSE WEIGHT and LOOK YOUNGER

Let me begin by saying there's nothing wrong with aging. But like anything, we can do it well . . . or we can do it poorly. We may not be able to stop the clock, but we can certainly slow it down and look and feel our best. And we can take steps to prevent premature aging.

Pain, illness, depression, and fatigue all contribute to how young or old we look and feel. I'll discuss them in the following chapters. For now, let's see what you can do that will affect your appearance and vitality.

Excess weight and dry, wrinkled skin make you look older than your years. We can do something about them, and this section is filled with tips to help you look your best.

Many women gain weight and begin to age in their forties and fifties when hormone levels begin to shift. No matter what doctors tell you, estrogen therapy (natural and synthetic) contributes to weight gain. It's much more difficult to lose weight if you've been on hormone replacement therapy (HRT) than if you haven't. Still, it's possible.

Your skin, on the other hand, responds to HRT. Estrogen keeps skin from thinning and wrinkling. Moist skin looks younger than dry skin. There are solutions that can revitalize your skin even if you're not on hormone therapy.

What's the best diet for losing weight and keeping it off? Is it high protein? Low fat? Are there really good carbs and good fats that are safe to eat? And why isn't willpower enough to avoid foods with empty calories?

Everyone's looking for the perfect weight-loss program—one that can help take weight off and keep it off. Obviously, if there were one such program, everyone would be doing it and we'd all know just what to do. But each of us is different emotionally, and our bodies are different physiologically. There's no one simple answer for everyone. But there are answers. There are ways to lose weight and have younger-looking skin. Let me show you.

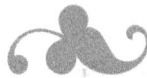

CHAPTER 14

Beyond Willpower—
Weight-Loss Secrets
That Really Work

Do you overeat or eat foods with empty calories because food cravings get the best of you? Do you struggle to control your cravings and constantly fail? If so, I've got great news for you. I discovered ways to stop these cravings and they have nothing to do with willpower.

It's easier to lose weight and get healthier when you're not being ruled by your cravings. It's easier to create new eating patterns and stick to them when chips or chocolate are out of your mind. Frankly, the reason so many people fail at adopting healthier eating habits is that they're relying on willpower. What most women don't realize is that by emphasizing self-control, all of us, including doctors and diet gurus, are overlooking an entire aspect of weight management. There are physiological reasons for various food cravings. Until you address them, you'll never be free from them.

SECRET #87 **Weight loss is not about willpower. It's about cravings.**

Sticking to any diet isn't a matter of discipline and willpower. It's about craving certain foods. In 1989, I wrote a book called *Overcoming the Legacy of Overeating*. It was the first book that addressed both the emotional and physical reasons for our food choices. This book was revolutionary because it explained why so many people fail to stay on a healthy diet. You can't simply look at the emotional reasons for overeating or choosing to eat certain foods. You need to address the physiological ones as well.

Many psychologists and registered dieticians (R.D.s) still concentrate on behavioral modification techniques and understanding psychological needs to control weight. But there's more to overeating—or eating foods that are counterproductive to your health and weight goals—than your emotions. And you probably know by now that it's not a matter of self-control.

I've found that both physiological needs and nutritional deficiencies can trigger bingeing. You may crave a food because it contains a high amount of an essential nutrient that your body desperately needs. Or because a particular food will raise your low blood sugar. You may crave a particular food because you have a sensitivity to it and by eating it you can avoid withdrawal symptoms. Willpower won't help any of these.

Before you can be free from your cravings, you need to address both the emotional and physiological reasons for your cravings. Trust me. You have both.

SECRET #88 Craving chocolate is a sign of a magnesium deficiency.

Are you a chocoholic? I was. As a child, I stole money from my parents to buy chocolate. I spent most of my allowance on chocolate. And I ate most of the candy my father gave to my mother on special occasions. I couldn't help myself.

It wasn't until I was in my thirties that I discovered why I craved chocolate. That was when I met Dr. Guy Abraham, a doctor working with nutritional solutions to PMS. He had found that a deficiency of magnesium and vitamin B$_6$ contributed to many PMS symptoms. As an aside, he mentioned that chocolate was highest in magnesium of all foods.

A lightbulb went off inside my head. Did he mean that women who craved chocolate would lose their craving if they took more magnesium? If so, this was astonishing news!

I decided to investigate for myself.

I increased my intake of magnesium in my diet and supplements. Sure enough, my chocolate cravings disappeared after a few months.

Next, I increased magnesium in my patients who craved chocolate. Their cravings left, as well. I still like the taste of chocolate and eat it occasionally. But I can also pass it by—and frequently do. In fact, yesterday I gave away a bar of excellent quality chocolate to a friend instead of keeping it for myself. It was easy. I really didn't care whether or not I ate it.

Craving chocolate can be a sign of a calcium/magnesium imbalance. It could mean that you're getting too much calcium and not enough magnesium. Most women need 500–600 milligrams (mg) a day *each* of supplemental calcium and magnesium. The rest we get from a healthy diet. But most of us are being told by doctors and healthcare practitioners to take 1,500 mg of calcium and half as much magnesium. This isn't enough magnesium and our chocolate craving tells us so.

Magnesium is an extremely important mineral that is often overshadowed by its partner, calcium. Magnesium helps muscles relax. It helps carry calcium into bones. And while magnesium is abundant in nuts, seeds, and legumes (beans), it is excreted in higher-than-usual quantities when you're under stress. This is why so many women crave chocolate before menstruation, a time when magnesium levels are lower from physiological stress. When magnesium is increased, chocolate cravings decrease.

Too much calcium and not enough magnesium can lead to brittle bones and heart disease. See Parts 7 and 8 for more detailed information on the consequences of a high-calcium, low-magnesium intake. For now, if you're a chocoholic you may want to decrease your calcium to 500 mg a day in your supplements, limit dairy products, and increase your magnesium supplement to bowel tolerance (comfortably loose stools).

SECRET #89 You may crave sugar because you have a yeast overgrowth.

Craving any food that turns into sugar quickly can be either due to an overgrowth of the yeast *Candida albicans* or a blood sugar imbalance.

Sugar is candida's food. Like all living things, this tiny yeast fights hard to stay alive. When it's starving, it will do whatever it can to trick or beg you to give it food. But eating sweets and refined carbohydrates and starches just perpetuates an overgrowth and another craving cycle. If you have too much candida, you have to starve it, kill it with antifungals, and increase your colonies of yeast-fighting friendly bacteria with probiotics. Take a look at any other symptoms you may have and see if candida might be at the root of your problems. If so, you will need to reduce candida colonies before you can eliminate your sugar craving. See Chapter 12 for more information.

Craving carbohydrates can also be a sign of low blood sugar. All foods eventually turn into sugar. Refined carbohydrates (sugar, white flour) turn into sugar quickly. Protein turns into sugar more slowly, but its energy lasts far longer. If you don't eat enough protein, your body may be crying out for immediate energy from sugar or refined starches. A sugary donut or energy bar will rapidly lift your blood sugar. But it will also drop it quickly, causing another sugar craving. To stop this craving, eat protein at each meal and eat every four to five hours.

Some people have a sensitive response to insulin. If your body produces more insulin than it needs, or if it produces it inappropriately, you'll crave sugar, refined carbohydrates, fruit juice, or alcohol. Or you may crave starches that turn into sugar quickly, such as potatoes, corn, bread, and potato chips. If so, the first step to take is to eliminate refined sugars and carbohydrates. Then you can add supplemental chromium (500 mg twice a day for two months) to your increased protein and frequent meals to help regulate your blood sugar. Studies show it's worked well for many people.

SECRET #90 **You may not be craving just any fats, but particular fats.**

One reason many people eat a high-fat diet is because fats fill them up and leave them feeling satisfied. Others just can't eat enough fats. These people may be misinterpreting their body's cry for a particular kind of fat: essential fatty acids (EFAs).

Essential fatty acids are fats your body needs and can't make. Your brain and reproductive system need them throughout your life. They can help your memory, heart, PMS, and hot flashes, to name just a few. The foods highest in EFAs are fatty wild fish (farmed fish are low in EFAs), flax oil, soy, and walnuts. Add them to your daily diet or begin taking two or more essential fatty acid capsules a day. Watch your craving for fats decline. A variety of EFAs will give you the balance your body needs. For more information on the effect EFAs have on your heart, see Chapter 40.

Some EFAs are best taken in supplement form, like borage oil, evening primrose oil, and fish oils. It doesn't matter whether you get your EFAs from food, supplements, or both. If you don't get enough of them, your body may crave fatty foods. Any fatty foods. And eating too much of the wrong fats can be harmful.

You need a balance of fats, but many people get too many animal fats and not enough EFAs. As you increase your EFAs, decrease your consumption of animal fats and cooking or salad oils. See Chapter 40 for more information.

EFAs can help you lose weight. They actually create heat and help your body burn calories faster. As you move away from some of the other fats found in desserts and dairy, and substitute them for more fish, walnuts, and vegetable oils, you'll lose weight without even trying.

SECRET #91 **Craving salt can be a sign that you're under a lot of stress.**

Your adrenal glands, which handle all kinds of stress, need a little sodium to function. When you're stressed and these tiny glands are working overtime, you may crave salty foods.

There's nothing wrong with eating a little salt, but eating too much of it can raise your blood pressure and cause water retention. Sugar causes water retention also, by the way. If you alternate eating salty foods with sweet foods, you may be adding an extra five pounds or more in water weight.

Instead of reaching for salted nuts or chips when you crave salt, recognize that you're stressed. Then take steps to reduce the stress. Drink more water, meditate a few minutes each day, and get a little extra sleep. Eat healthy foods. Pamper yourself a little. And watch your salt cravings lessen.

SECRET #92 Craving certain foods can be a sign of a food sensitivity.

Have you ever been hooked on coffee and then suddenly stopped drinking it? Then you know what it's like to experience a withdrawal. Coffee withdrawal often comes in the form of a headache and foggy thinking, but there are other withdrawal symptoms like depression, anger, and food cravings.

Years ago, I met a woman who had a lot of health problems. She ate eggs every day for breakfast, and ate chicken most days for either lunch or dinner. In fact, she confessed to me that she felt terrible if she didn't. Her mind became fuzzy, she was tired, and she became depressed. A lightbulb went off as I listened to her describe her diet. I was sure she had a sensitivity to chicken and eggs.

Time proved me right. She didn't begin to get better until she stopped eating them. It took a long time for her to be convinced that this was even a possible problem. Once she stopped eating the foods to which she was sensitive, her cravings and her health problems improved. She also lost weight, because food sensitivities can cause your body to retain fluids.

We often crave foods to which we're allergic or sensitive, setting off a never-ending bingeing cycle. And the culprit can be almost any food. You can have a sensitivity to coffee, sugar, alcohol, or to healthy foods such as corn, chicken, or bananas. Here's how I help my patients decide which foods may be contributing to their cravings.

Make believe you're going to spend two weeks on an island. It's a true paradise, complete with your favorite friends and your own private chef. The chef asks you, "Which three foods do you want me to be sure to include as I pack for this trip?" If you have a food sensitivity, you will find you're sensitive to one or more of these foods.

To eliminate your craving, it's essential that you avoid every trace of the food or ingredient for two weeks. At the end of that time, you should be free from the craving. Test the food you've eliminated. If you have any negative reactions, stop eating that food for three months and try it again. If there's improvement, ease back into it. Just don't eat it daily, and keep its quantities low.

SECRET #93 You could have a "craving brain" that causes you to overeat.

If you crave food even when you're not hungry, your brain has become addicted to certain foods. We all have an intellectual brain and a biological brain. You may "know" what to eat, but if your biological brain—controlled by food, safety, and intimacy—is in charge, you'll have an uncontrollable urge to eat.

Your biological brain is controlled by neurotransmitters like dopamine, serotonin, GABA, and endorphins. These neurotransmitters can malfunction, causing food cravings. You can take medications to correct these imbalances, or try natural therapies instead. For instance, regular exercise can help your brain make needed endorphins. Magnesium and vitamin B_6 help it make serotonin. You can lower excessive dopamine levels by reducing stress. And GABA can be enhanced with herbs like hops and valerian root.

SECRET #94 Don't eat until you're full. Stop when you're not hungry.

I never knew what it felt like to be hungry when I was growing up. Although our family never had much money, food was always plentiful. It was a reward, punishment, friend, and my mother's way of sharing her love. Like many people, I ate even when I wasn't hungry, and I didn't stop until I was too full to take another bite. Consequently, I was never able to lose my excess weight.

This pattern isn't unusual. Many people eat until their stomach is full and they feel pressure. But this is more food than they need. They eat so often that they never experience hunger. There's nothing wrong with feeling hunger. It's not your enemy. It's just a signal that your body needs food. Wait until you hear this signal before you eat. And stop eating when the hunger goes away, not when the pressure in your stomach is already uncomfortable.

It takes twenty minutes for a message to travel from your stomach to your brain telling you that you're no longer hungry. One way to eat less is to eat only when you're hungry and stop as soon as you feel "not hungry." There are a lot of calories between "not hungry" and "full"! After twenty minutes, eat a little more if you're still hungry.

In time, you'll get a better idea of how much food it takes to eliminate your hunger. Then you can take smaller portions, always knowing that if you want more you can have it.

Exercise belongs in every weight-loss program. It's no secret, but it's such an essential part of your weight-loss and antiaging program that I have to mention it here. Regular exercise helps you keep your muscle tone and balance. They, in turn, help prevent falls and their consequences. Exercise increases your circulation that helps your heart and brain. And, of course, exercise helps you lose weight.

It's obvious. Eating more calories than you burn results in weight gain. Find some activity you enjoy doing—walking briskly through the mall, walking or biking with a friend, or gardening (weeding and digging can burn up plenty of calories). If you like going to a gym or working with a personal trainer, that's fine. Do it. If not, there are plenty of other ways to be active. But you're not going to lose the weight you want and stay healthy without regular exercise. Four to five times a week, for half an hour or more, is ideal. But forget perfection. Just begin today. And I don't mean tomorrow!

SECRET #95 These five supplements can help you lose weight.

Some weight-loss supplements are designed to speed up your metabolism and burn calories faster. Many, like ephedra and guarana, are high in stimulants and not safe for everyone. Other supplements help restore your body's balance by removing sugar cravings and depression. Out of the myriad of weight-loss supplements on the market, I've chosen five that can help you lose weight through different actions. Choose one or two that best seem to fit your needs.

Chromium: Do you crave sugar? If so, your chromium levels may be low. This mineral helps regulate blood sugar. It also helps your body burn carbohydrates rather than store them in fat tissues. Chromium has been found to help diabetics and people with low blood sugar (hypoglycemia). The dose used in various studies is 200 micrograms (mcg) two or three times a day. If you crave sugar, you may want to take extra chromium in addition to your multivitamin/mineral. Don't forget to count the amount of chromium in your multi toward the daily total.

Bulking agents: Consider taking a supplement that will fill you up before you eat to reduce your calorie intake. Glucomannan and apple pectin are two high-fiber substances added to some weight-loss formulas for this purpose. You could also mix a tablespoon or two of ground psyllium seed or oat bran in a little water and drink it before your meal. Or simply add more vegetables to your diet. The fiber in these supplements also helps reduce cholesterol levels.

Starch blocker: There's now a substance made from white kidney beans and other natural ingredients that prevents from 60 to 70 percent of the starches you eat from being absorbed. You will get all the vitamins and minerals from these starches without absorbing all of their calories. As a result, it increases your stools and will occasionally give some people a bit of gas. This is a small price to pay for the ability to eat starches without wearing them tomorrow. The starch-blocker ingredient is called Phase 2, or Phaseolin. You can find some products with Phase 2 in health-food stores and in the Resources section at the end of this book.

Antidepressant: It's difficult to eat properly and get into an exercise program if you're feeling depressed. 5-HTP (5-Hydroxytryptophan) is a precursor to the amino acid tryptophan found in health-food stores. It helps regulate moods by helping your body produce serotonin, a "feel good" hormone, in your brain. Since low-level depression is often a cause for overeating—and for not exercising—this supplement could address some reasons for your excess weight. 5-HTP also helps regulate your appetite. Taking 50–100 mg, three times a day, appears to be sufficient. St. John's wort is an herb used for depression. If you're not taking any medications, it may be safe for you. But studies have shown this herb interferes with the absorption of numerous drugs, so check with your doctor before taking this supplement.

Green tea: Many weight-loss supplements on the market contain caffeine because it's an effective product for weight loss. But some of these supplements are associated with serious side effects including hypertension, tightness in the chest, and even death. Green tea or green tea extract has less caffeine than other caffeine substances. It also has the advantage of increasing thermogenesis, which helps you burn calories faster. In addition, green tea is high in beneficial antioxidants. Unlike coffee and black tea, green tea is less likely to keep you awake at night or make you feel anxious. Supplements with green tea extract are low in caffeine. You can find them in health-food stores and in the Resources section at the end of this book.

Bottom-line

In more than twenty-four years of clinical practice, I've found that a permanent weight-loss program consists of the following key components:

- Addressing both the physical and emotional reasons for overeating or choosing problem foods like sugar and fatty foods.
- Eating the proper amount of the right foods.
- Exercising at least four times a week for thirty minutes or longer.
- Using safe supplements to increase your metabolism and reduce hunger.

CHAPTER 15

High Protein? High Carb? Your Best Diet May Surprise You

These days it's difficult to know which diet you should follow to lose weight and stay healthy. Should you go on one of the popular high-protein, low-carbohydrate diets? Or should you try one of the high-carbohydrate, low-protein programs that used to be in favor? What about a vegetarian, vegan, or raw-foods diet? There are too many options, and the arguments for each diet are persuasive.

If you want to lose weight, and both look and feel your best, you need to begin with a healthy diet filled with vitamins, minerals, and other nutrients. Your best diet will help you reach your ideal weight. And it will provide you with the nutrients you need to be and stay healthy.

SECRET #96 Your best diet depends on your metabolism.

Some people have a fast metabolism and burn calories quickly. They tend to feel and look their best when they eat a diet containing more complex carbohydrates. Hint: Usually they are, or were, thin. Other people have a slower metabolism and burn calories slowly. These people, who tend to be heavy, feel and look best when they eat more protein and fewer carbohydrates of any kind. Either way, getting sufficient protein is vital. So is eating good-quality foods—foods rich in vitamins, minerals, and essential fats, and low in toxins. Your best diet should be high enough in protein and very low in toxins.

You might think that because I'm a vegetarian, I'm biased against meat-based diets. Actually, I'm biased against unhealthy diets. It's tough to be a healthy vegetarian and get enough

> Among modern hunter-gatherers, the percentages of total protein and fat have been found to vary from 36 to 97 percent, with total carbohydrates varying from 3 to 64 percent—and the people at both "extremes" are equally disease-free.
>
> JONATHAN V. WRIGHT, M.D.

111

protein. It's not much easier to be a healthy carnivore and eat good-quality protein that's not laced with toxins.

SECRET #97 This sensitivity explains why many people do poorly on a high-carbohydrate diet.

It has many names: carbohydrate sensitivity, insulin resistance, Syndrome X, or hyperinsulinemia. They all mean that when you eat a lot of refined starches or sugars, your blood sugar quickly rises too high and your body doesn't secrete insulin appropriately. Instead of using these foods for energy, your body stores the calories in fat tissues. Carbohydrate sensitivity causes weight gain, raises your cholesterol, and contributes to diabetes.

What causes this carbohydrate sensitivity? Yo-yo dieting, not exercising, a diet high in refined carbohydrates (sugar, white flour, white rice, etc.), alcohol abuse, and smoking. About 25 percent of all Americans and 75 percent of overweight people have insulin resistance. Dr. Robert Atkins developed his high-protein diet to correct this problem.

SECRET #98 Dr. Atkins had a good point . . . but he left something out.

Robert Atkins was a medical doctor who used nutrition in his practice for more than forty years. He noticed a common problem in many patients that affected their health and weight: fluctuating blood-sugar levels. His solution was simple. Avoid refined carbohydrates and greatly increase both animal protein and unprocessed fats to stabilize blood sugar. Eat more vegetables high in antioxidants to counteract the damage from free radicals that occurs in a diet high in rancid and processed fats.

To meet the needs of his overweight patients, Dr. Atkins developed a radical weight-loss program emphasizing animal protein and eliminating carbohydrates, even those that were unrefined. His patients lost weight and their glucose levels stabilized. However, his original diet left something out—food quality. The proteins he suggested were high in pesticides, hormones, and other toxins that are stored in the fat tissues of meat, chicken, dairy, and fish. Eventually, they could contribute to chronic illnesses. And a long-term diet high in animal protein naturally contains fats that increase inflammation, a condition that leads to many chronic illnesses.

While Dr. Atkins insisted that eating a lot of meat won't raise your cholesterol, my brother's cholesterol skyrocketed on this diet—and he ate lots of veggies like a good boy. He's not alone in this response. If you eat a high animal-protein diet for more than a few months, get your cholesterol checked. My greatest quarrel with the Atkins weight-loss diet is that until recently it didn't emphasize food quality.

This omission was huge. Although later dietary modifications included information on better quality food, I'll bet that the majority of people who are on the Atkins diet never heard anything about the importance of eating organic.

While Dr. Atkins was shouting the praises of his high-protein diet for weight loss, nutritionist Ann Louise Gittleman began teaching the importance of eating a healthy diet with an emphasis on protein sufficiency. Her book *The Fat Flush Plan* was the first in a series of "Fat Flush" books that explains in detail how and where to find healthy foods and still get enough protein. For instance, a diet high in essential fats (EFAs) is a healthy diet. Animal fats don't contain EFAs. You need to eat a lot of fish to get more EFAs, and these fish need to be free from common contaminants like pesticides and mercury. A diet high in the fats found in meats is less healthy because animal fats contribute to increased inflammation and contain a lot of toxins. EFAs are found in many plant foods like flaxseeds and walnuts. A healthy diet should include getting some EFAs daily.

SECRET #99 You can remove many pesticides with Clorox.

A good weight-loss program should go beyond losing weight. It should help you retain or improve your health. There are many convincing studies that link toxins to chronic diseases. Some pesticides act like synthetic estrogen, raising your risk for breast cancer. Other pesticides are known carcinogens and neurotoxins. Many of these contaminants, including heavy metals, are stored in your liver. As they increase, they can affect your health. Your best answer is to buy organically grown foods whenever you can find and afford them. Still, there's no way we can completely avoid toxins. But there is a way to remove some of them from your produce.

Wash any non-organic foods in a Clorox bath. That's right, Clorox. I wrote about this technique in my first book, *The Nutrition Detective* (now out of print) in 1985. It originated with naturopath Hazel Parcells in the 1950s and has been used ever since by practitioners of integrative health.

Use one-half teaspoon of Clorox for each gallon of water, and place your fruits and vegetables in this solution. Use a fresh Clorox bath with each batch of food. The length of time each type of food needs to soak is as follows:

- Frozen, leafy vegetables, or thin-skin fruits—15 minutes

- Thick-skin fruits and root vegetables—20 minutes

- Thick-skin squash—25 minutes

Take the fruits and vegetables out of the solution and soak them in clean water for fifteen minutes. They will have no aftertaste, and many people report that they stay fresher longer when this method is used. If you have any immune problem, use this wash for organic fruits and vegetables to kill any parasites and bacteria. You can also find vegetable washes that remove pesticides in health-food stores.

SECRET #100 A one-day fast can help you lose weight quickly.

Ann Louise Gittleman has gone beyond *The Fat Flush Plan.* She has written a revolutionary new book with a plan that can help you lose three to eight pounds while you detoxify. This plan is detailed in *The Fast Track One-Day Detox Diet.* It consists of a seven-day diet to strengthen your body in preparation for a one-day fast. The fast, itself, alkalinizes your body and helps your liver and colon get rid of toxins. It's followed by a three-day diet to help you ease back into a more normal— and more consciously healthy—diet.

Get ready for the one-day fast by eating a diet with plenty of vegetables to support your liver and to begin unclogging a sluggish colon. Then you're ready for the one-day fast that consists of a drink made from specific spices and juices.

For three days after your fast, you'll be adding supplements to enhance your digestion. This prevents your colon from getting blocked, and allows the nutrients in your foods to break down into small enough particles to be absorbed into your cells. The "Fast Track" diet isn't the only detox diet there is. But it is the one that makes the most sense to me. And it can help you lose weight quickly and safely.

SECRET #101 No matter which diet you choose, you're probably not eating enough protein.

The issue isn't whether or not you should be eating a predominately protein or carbohydrate diet. It's whether or not any diet is giving you enough protein. I was initially surprised to learn that an adult woman needs about 60 grams of protein a day—20 mg at each meal. This is a lot if you're a vegetarian, or if you're a meat-eater who has cereal or toast for breakfast. After all, a breakfast of two eggs has only 12 grams of protein. But when you increase your protein to this level, you may find, as I did, that you have increased energy and strength. This increased stamina can help you increase your exercise program and lose more weight, increase your muscle tone, improve your circulation, and support your health and vitality.

Since many contaminants are stored in fat cells, the fats in meats are storage bins for health-destroying toxins. However, meats (including chicken and fish) are much higher in protein than soy and other legumes.

Like the old gray mare, the quality of protein just "ain't what it used to be." Once, clean and lean, it's now fatty and laced with pesticides, antibiotics, hormones, mercury, and other toxic substances. Wild game contains 3.9 percent fat. Today's beef and pork is 25 to 35 percent fat.

PROTEINS IN COMMON FOODS	
Beef (4 oz lean ground)	28 grams
Chicken (3.5 oz lean)	30 grams
Egg (1)	6 grams
Garbanzo/Kidney beans ($\frac{1}{2}$ cup)	7 grams
Peanut butter (2 Tbsp)	7.7–9 grams
Protein powder (1 Tbsp, rice)	12 grams
Soybeans ($\frac{1}{2}$ cup dry roasted)	34 grams
Soybeans ($\frac{1}{2}$ cup boiled edamame)	11 grams
Tofu (3 oz)	6–7 grams
Tuna (3 oz water packed)	25 grams
Veggie Burger (Amy's/Gardenburger)	12–15 grams

If you eat meat, buy grass-fed rather than the widely available grain-fed animals whenever possible. They're lower in saturated fat and higher in essential fats (omega-3 and conjugated linolenic acid, or CLA). If you eat grain-fed meats, add more essential fats to your diet like fish oil and flax oil. Dozens of sources for grass-fed beef can be found in The Fat Flush Plan.

Eating most chicken isn't any better than eating grain-fed meat. In fact, I think it's worse. Commercially raised chickens are overcrowded, diseased, and given high amounts of antibiotics and growth-stimulating hormones. Studies show that 30 percent of them have salmonella contamination, while more than 60 percent have *Campylobacter*, a bacteria found in fecal material.

You can avoid these problems if you buy free-range chickens. They're healthier and lower in total fat with 100 percent more essential fats (EFAs). Free-range eggs contain 400 percent more EFAs than ordinary eggs. Omega-3-enriched eggs have even more. Two eggs a day provide good, quality protein without elevating cholesterol.

Most oceans, lakes, and streams are polluted. Still, wild rather than farmed fish are your best choice for animal protein. Much farmed fish is overcrowded and low in EFAs. Choose smaller fish. They contain fewer pesticides and less mercury than larger varieties. If you're taking fish-oil supplements, make sure they're free from both mercury and pesticides.

Soy is a healthy low-fat protein you can safely eat once a day. Choose organic or non-GMO (genetically modified) soy. We don't know the safety of genetically modified foods. They're not safe enough to be sold in Europe, but safe enough for U.S. corporations to sell them to you. Until we know they're safe, eat only non-GMO soy products. Soy contains healthy plant estrogens that get into our estrogen receptors and block the uptake of harmful estrogens. The safety of soy has been greatly debated. I still think it's a healthy protein in moderation.

Legumes, or beans, are high in both protein and unrefined carbohydrates. To slow down their conversion from starch to sugar, add healthy fats, such as one teaspoon of olive oil or flaxseed oil, to them so they turn into sugar more slowly.

Bottom-line

Get enough protein. Eat more carbs if you're thin and burn energy faster. Eat fewer carbs if you have a weight problem. Most important, concentrate on the quality of all the foods you eat.

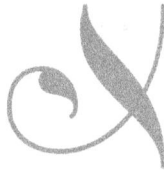

CHAPTER 16

Good Carbs, Bad Carbs

If you were to listen to everyone hawking low-carb foods, you'd believe that all carbohydrates were alike. This is far from the truth. And if you're on a strict high-protein, very low-carbohydrate diet, I have important news for you: You may be throwing the baby out with the bathwater and doing more harm than good. A diet too low in carbohydrates isn't healthy.

SECRET #102 A low-carb diet can be dangerous.

Starches and sugars are your body's main source of energy. You need them to fuel your muscles. In fact, your brain needs 130 grams of carbohydrates a day just to function properly! A carbohydrate-free diet, or a diet that's too low in carbs, can be both dangerous and too low in nutrients.

A low-carb diet has to be high in something. That something is protein. And as I've said before, a lot of animal protein is high in harmful fats and pesticides. Or it's high in soy, a low-carb vegetable protein. Now, I don't think there's anything wrong with eating soy. But not three times a day!

A low-carb diet is low in plant-based nutrients like antioxidants. It tends to be low in potassium, a mineral found in abundance in fruits as well as vegetables. And it lacks the fiber we need for a healthy digestive tract.

If you're on a high-protein diet, you still need carbohydrates. The good ones.

Some carbohydrates support your health while others drag it down. Too many of the bad carbohydrates raise your triglycerides and make your blood thicker, putting you at risk for heart disease. They also contribute to carbohydrate cravings and diabetes. The trick is to eat enough good carbs and very few bad ones. It's a balancing act, but not too difficult once you understand the concept. So just which carbs are good and which are bad? And why?

SECRET #103 Some carbs cause insulin resistance. Some don't.

When you eat any carbohydrate—either a sugar or a starch—your pancreas releases insulin to help your body utilize it. When you eat a lot of carbohydrates, especially those that are refined and low in fiber, you run the risk of having high amounts of insulin that remain in your blood.

Over time, your body may stop using insulin properly. This is called insulin resistance or Syndrome X. It often leads to diabetes, heart disease, obesity, hypertension, and blood clots. Good carbs are digested more slowly. They rarely lead to insulin resistance when you eat them in moderation. In fact, they tend to stabilize your blood sugar.

Good carbs are whole foods from plants that contain both sugars or starches and fiber. They include beans, whole grains, starchy vegetables, and fruit. Substitute some of them for saturated (animal) fats and they can lower your cholesterol. Their fiber content also keeps your blood sugar level.

Bad carbs are processed starches and sugars. They include sugar, honey, and refined grains like white flour and white rice. They are absorbed quickly and can trigger an insulin response, causing your blood sugar to drop suddenly.

SECRET #104 The health food industry is promoting bad carbs.

I'm disgusted with the health-food industry. There are no regulations about which foods are healthy and which are being sold just to make a buck. Unfortunately, there are a growing number of those in the second category. Health-food stores are filling up their shelves with junk foods. I'm disheartened with the amount of foods they're selling that contain bad carbs.

The following are a few to watch out for and avoid:

- *White rice:* It's not unusual to find organic white basmati rice in health-food stores. Think it's a good carb? It's not! White rice has been stripped of its nutritious hull that contains important fiber along with B vitamins and magnesium. Eat it along with vegetables and protein and it isn't so bad. But I don't consider any white rice a "good carb." It's low in nutrients and turns to sugar too quickly.

- *Unenriched or enriched wheat flour:* This is white flour, plain and simple. "Unenriched" wheat flour means the food contains white flour stripped of nutrients with none put back. Enriched flour is no better. Neither the fiber nor many of the nutrients that were removed are replaced. You may find white flour in organic breads, crackers, and cookies, but "organic" doesn't necessarily mean "nutritious." Treat refined flour like white rice—okay in very small quantities, but with little nutritive value.

- *Spinach and tomato pastas:* Just because they look dark doesn't mean they're unrefined. Most spinach and tomato pastas are made from white flour dyed a darker color from the added vegetables. Vegetable juices just make white pasta look healthier than it is.

- *Pure cane sugar juice:* I know a lot of cane sugar juice is organic and that's great for the environment. But this form of sugar acts the same as plain old sugar. It contains a minimal amount of nutrients, feeds candida and cancer cells, and causes insulin reactions just like white sugar.

Five years ago, a nutritionally minded doctor put out a line of instant cereals. I noticed that they contained organic pure cane sugar juice. "What's the difference between this sweetener and refined sugar?" I asked him. "Nothing," he answered. "I use it because people like the way it tastes."

- *Fructose and high-fructose corn syrup:* These sweeteners don't raise blood sugar levels very much, but they raise total cholesterol levels and harmful LDL cholesterol. Worst of all, they contribute to a sluggish immune system. Fructose may be the single substance that's causing an increase in diabetes. It's found in soft drinks and many fruit drinks.

- *Honey and maple syrup:* These sugars trigger an insulin response, contribute to inflammation, and can lower your immunity. Just because they're natural does not mean they're healthy. If you want a safe sweetener without any calories that won't affect insulin levels, stick to stevia, a powder made from the leaves of the *Stevia* plant that's available in health-food stores. I'll talk about it in more detail in the next chapter.

SECRET #105 Sugar alcohols are bad carbs.

No, you haven't died and gone to heaven.

Yes, it's too good to be true.

Low-carb foods are suddenly pouring into supermarkets and health-food stores tempting you at every step. All at once it looks like there are brownies, cookies, protein bars, ice cream, shakes, and other foods with low "net carbs" you can eat safely in almost any quantity. But before you rush out to buy them—or restock your pantry—there are some things you should know about the sweeteners in these foods that could change your mind.

Low-carb sweets contain higher amounts of sugar alcohols than other sweeteners. Sugar alcohols originate from plants such as fruits and berries, so they seem safe and natural. You've heard some of their names before: mannitol, sorbitol, and xylitol are the most common ones. But chances are you don't know much about them. Let me tell you the truth the food manufacturers don't want you to know. Basically, although manufacturers say that the sugars in these foods don't count, the calories in sugar alcohols, counted as net carbs, do count. These sugars don't taste like sugar. They can have unpleasant side effects. And we don't know the effects from eating a lot of them over time.

SECRET #106 Net carbs do count and are not lower in calories than other sugars.

Carbohydrates from sugar alcohols turn into glucose more slowly than sugar and don't affect blood sugar levels in the same way. So manufacturers subtract the sugar alcohols from the total grams of carbohydrates. The sugars that are left are called "net carbs." The idea is to give the impression that these low-carb foods are lower in calories because the grams of sugar alcohols "don't count."

Rubbish!

These carbs do count, all right. And the American Diabetes Association agrees with me. They raise blood glucose levels—a danger to diabetics—and have a significant amount of calories. Your weight is affected by the amount of calories you eat and the amount of energy you expend. Read labels and compare the calories in low-carb versus regular foods. They're often either close or the same.

Don't be fooled. A product may say "sugar-free" and be high in sugar alcohols. Technically, sugar alcohols aren't sugar. Sneaky, isn't it?

If you limit your carbohydrates as part of a weight-loss program, net carbs are deceptive. A low-carb energy bar with two net carbs does not have eight calories from carbohydrates. The 25 grams of total carbohydrates it contains, when sugar alcohols are included, means that 100 of its calories come from carbs. Count all the carbs and all the calories.

SECRET #107 Sugar alcohols don't taste just like sugar.

I sent for samples of some low-carb protein bars that were advertised as "Rated #1 in Taste!" They didn't impress me in the least. They tasted dry, sweet, and cool. Although they were chocolate, they had very little chocolate flavor. Just a cool, sweet, mealy feeling in my mouth.

When I compared this low-carb bar with a Luna bar (another popular protein bar), there was little difference in total carbohydrates and calories. But there was a huge difference in taste. The Luna bar tasted much better with strong flavors and more moisture. Other low-carb protein bars and cookies I tasted were dry and mealy, as well. I was confused about why until I struck up a conversation at my gym with a local baker.

She had been using the sugar alcohol xylitol in some baked goods. "When I add xylitol crystals to my brownie batter, it causes the melted butter to get stiff quickly. The batter is very cold when I touch it, and the brownies taste much drier than those made with sugar, even though they have a lot of butter. It's weird," she said.

Sugar alcohols tend to dry out low-carb products that are not naturally moist.

You can tell whether or not a protein bar is high in sugar alcohols without even reading the label. Pick one up. If the package feels cold to the touch, the bar is probably high in sugar alcohols. Although sugar alcohols are alcohols derived from sugar molecules, they taste artificial to me. For the extra 5 grams of carb between a low-carb bar and a Luna bar—just 20 calories—I'll have a Luna bar, thank you.

SECRET #108 Sugar alcohols cause digestive problems.

Remember the potato chips that contained Olestra, a fat blocker that caused loose stools? Well, sugar alcohols have the same effect. If you eat enough of them, you could become bloated, gassy, and have diarrhea.

Mannitol is the most likely form of sugar alcohol to cause bloating and diarrhea because it remains in the intestines for a long time. However, sorbitol and xylitol can also cause these side effects. Taking between 30 and 50 grams of sorbitol or xylitol, or 20 grams of mannitol, commonly causes a laxative effect. This may seem like a lot, but if you binge on sweets, it translates to two or three low-carb energy bars. And you could have side effects with lower amounts.

One protein bar I ate had 17 grams of sugar alcohols. It caused gas and bloating for hours. Like many products, the label didn't indicate which sugar alcohols it contained.

Sugar alcohols derived from sugar remain in the intestines longer than other sugars, so they're most likely feeding bad bacteria. Could eating a lot of foods high in sugar alcohols feed candida? We don't know. Why take the risk?

SECRET #109 There aren't enough studies on sugar alcohols to convince me of their safety.

We really don't know what effect eating large quantities of sugar alcohols over a long period of time will have on our health. Dr. Walter Willett, professor of epidemiology and nutrition at Harvard University, cautions, "There haven't been adequate studies of sugar alcohols or glycerin when they're consumed in the large amounts contained in the new low-carb processed foods." The amount of sugar alcohols naturally found in a bowl of blueberries or in an ear of corn is negligible compared with the amount in a single serving of a low-carb dessert.

Dr. Willett notes that researchers have found a slight increased risk for colon cancer in people who ate a lot of prunes. Prunes are naturally high in sorbitol, which may be why they act as a laxative. It's possible that the sorbitol in prunes is contributing to increased colon cancer. We just don't know.

Be smart. If you're going to eat any foods with sugar alcohols, eat them only occasionally and in small portions until we know more about their safety.

SECRET #110 Good carbs include whole foods.

Good carbs come from whole foods. Get 90 percent of your carbohydrates from beans, brown rice, corn tortillas, polenta, and starchy vegetables. Eat small amounts of them along with protein and vegetables rather than one large carbohydrate meal.

Some good carbs, such as potatoes, have gotten a bad rap because they're high on the glycemic index. This means they turn into sugar quickly. But Nancy Appleton, Ph.D., author of *Lick the Sugar Habit,* is furious about this.

"The glycemic index is a hoax," she told me. "If you eat any one of these foods alone that's high on the glycemic index, it will raise your blood glucose. But if you eat them with protein and fat, it won't. That's the way we should eat!"

Don't be afraid or reluctant to eat some carbohydrates with your meals if they are unprocessed and are eaten with plenty of vegetables, protein, and a little fat. Just make them the good carbs, and keep your portions small.

SECRET #111 This sweetener with no calories has been used in Japan for decades and is safe.

One afternoon about twenty years ago, I got a phone call I'll never forget. A man who had listened to my radio show for years was calling me all the way from Japan. "There's a sweetener that's being used all over Japan that doesn't affect diabetics," he said, excitedly. "I don't know what it is, but if I send you some of it can you get the label translated? I know a lot of people in the United States would want to use it and you've always done a lot of research on products. I'm diabetic, and I can use this sweetener without any changes in my blood sugar!"

I asked the Japanese parents of one of my friends to translate the labels for me. The common ingredient in all the products he sent to me was called "stevia." I began studying then, when there was little information about it. So while some of you may not be familiar with stevia, I am. And I'm still impressed. In my opinion, there are no sugar-free sweeteners as good or safe as stevia.

Stevia rebaudiana is a South American shrub. Its leaves contain natural sweeteners called stevioside and rebaudioside that are 250 times sweeter than table sugar. Stevia has no calories, doesn't cause dental caries, won't kill off beneficial bacteria in your colon, causes no allergic reactions, and won't raise your blood sugar.

So why haven't you heard much about it? Ask the folks at the Food and Drug Administration (FDA) who appear to be protecting the sugar industry more than your blood sugar and waistline. Stevia is an unapproved food additive, they say. No one has convinced them that it's safe, although numerous toxicology reports say it is.

Apparently, the FDA became concerned after reading a 1968 study on rats that hasn't been duplicated, and that one of its researchers says does not necessarily even apply to humans. It found that stevia could act as a contraceptive—after the rats drank the equivalent of $2\frac{1}{2}$ quarts of stevia-liquid, containing parts of the plant we don't ingest, in half an hour! Isn't it nice to be protected by the FDA? Still, you can buy stevia in any health-food store. It's approved as a dietary supplement, but can't be promoted as a sweetener unless you live in Brazil or Japan, where stevia is an approved food additive and sugar substitute.

SECRET #112 You can use this sweetener to lose weight and to control blood sugar.

Probably the most valuable use for stevia is to replace sugar in your diet. There's a rise in both obesity and type 2 diabetes, and sugar-sweetened sodas are one of the biggest culprits. In fact, a Harvard study found that women who drink one or more sugary drinks a day have an 80 percent increased risk of diabetes over women who rarely drink sodas with sugar. Some of my patients took a small packet of powdered stevia and made a week's worth of sweet lemonade with it.

For many years, stevia extracts have been used to treat diabetes in Paraguay and Brazil. This herb is being used successfully to fight diabetes, obesity, hypertension, fatigue, depression, infections, and sweet cravings. Several studies on rats with type 2 diabetes strongly suggest that stevia could become a new anti-diabetic drug because it stimulates insulin secretion and lowers blood sugar.

But what about those of us with normal blood sugar? Stevia extract increases glucose tolerance. Used in very high quantities—an unlikely occurrence—it can lower blood sugar in people with hypoglycemia. Basically, it looks like stevia is not only an acceptable sweetener, but a valuable one as well. Too bad there's no way to patent it and to raise its price.

In Japan, the largest consumer of stevia in the world, the leaves and extracts are used in soy sauce, confections, soft drinks, pickles, and just about anything else that needs sweetening. In fact, Coca-Cola sweetens their drinks with stevia in Japan and other countries. In my opinion, it's an excellent option for anyone who wants to lose weight and still occasionally eat sweet foods.

You won't find commercially made foods with stevia in this country yet, but it's easy enough to use this sweetener. Here are a few tips to get you started.

You can find stevia powder or liquid in your health-food store. Use the smallest amount necessary. If you get a bitter aftertaste, you've used too much. One-quarter teaspoon of the powder equals about half a cup of sugar. The powder is convenient to use for baked goods. But if you're sweetening a drink, like lemonade, coffee, or tea, add a few drops of an extract. You can make an extract by mixing one teaspoon of stevia powder into three tablespoons of pure water. Put it in a dropper bottle, refrigerate, and shake well before using.

If you're looking for recipes using stevia, I have several suggestions. *The Stevia Cookbook,* by Ray Sahelian, M.D., and Donna Gates, is packed with recipes for breakfast crepes, salad dressings, sweet and sour entrees, and desserts. It also has a lot of background information on stevia. If you're more interested in desserts, *Stevia Dessert Cookbook* by Kristen Younger has tasty recipes. It includes a section on adapting recipes for vegans, gluten-free diets, and people with lactose intolerance.

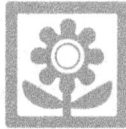

CHAPTER 17

A Saturated Fat That's Healthy and Promotes Weight Loss

Like so many things, fats are separated into several categories: the good ones and the bad ones. As I've said, some of the healthiest fats are essential fatty acids (EFAs). They are important for good heart health, a healthy reproductive system, good memory, and a host of other conditions. You can find more about them in Chapter 40.

Of the less healthy fats, trans-fatty acids are the ones you should avoid completely.

SECRET #113 The worst fats are not found in nature. They're man-made.

No wonder they're bad for you.

Trans fats are made in a laboratory. You can't find them anywhere in nature. So it's no surprise that your body doesn't know what to do with them.

To make trans fats, hydrogen gas is forced into a vegetable oil and bonded to fat molecules. This turns the oil into a solid substance that is used in baked goods, crackers, and other processed foods. When you read a label and it says "hydrogenated oils," or "partially-hydrogenated oils," this is what's in the food you're holding. Crisco and most margarines are made from hydrogenated trans fats. Dr. Walter Willett, a professor at the Harvard School of Public Health, calls trans fats " . . . probably the most toxic fats ever known." There is no amount of trans fat that is safe to eat. It is, however, safe to eat some saturated fats. Just not large amounts of them. And not to the exclusion of more beneficial fats like EFAs.

SECRET #114 Not all saturated fats are harmful.

Most saturated fats are semi-solid and come from animal products, but not all of them act alike. The most harmful saturated fats are those found in meat. They are made up of long-chain fatty acids. A small amount of these saturated fats won't hurt most people, but large quantities are difficult to digest and can raise "bad" cholesterol (LDL) while lowering "good" cholesterol (HDL). You want the opposite effect for a healthy heart. If you eat dairy products or meat once a day, you're probably not getting too many saturated fats. But if you eat these foods at every meal, you may be putting your health at risk. Since everyone's body is a little different, it's not possible to tell you exactly how much saturated fat is safe for you. A diet that includes fish and soy protein, both of which contain EFAs, will give you a healthier mix of fats than one that relies entirely on animal products.

In general, fats are difficult to digest. They burn slowly, and collect in tissues and arteries when you overeat them. However, some plant-based oils are made from medium-chain fatty acids. The molecules in these oils are one-third to one-half the size of molecules in other oils. They are more water soluble—easier to digest—and burn quickly. Two of these oils are palm kernel oil and coconut oil. They don't contribute to heart disease. That's right. The fats you've been told to avoid are both healthy. Of the two of them, coconut oil is easiest to find, although palm kernel oil is gaining in popularity.

SECRET #115 Coconut oil is a healthy saturated fat.

"I'd really like to have the vegetable curry with coconut milk," my friend Patricia said, looking over the menu at our favorite Thai restaurant, "but I know coconut milk is not good for me. And besides, it's fattening."

She was wrong on both counts. If one of my best friends was uninformed about the benefits—not the harmfulness—of coconut products, you may be, too.

Undoubtedly, you've heard that coconut oil is a saturated fat that's bad for your heart. This statement is simply erroneous. Coconut milk, meat, and oil have gotten an undeservedly bad reputation. There's never been any reason to avoid coconut products. This is just another myth perpetuated by makers of polyunsaturated fats (cooking oils) who found they could profit from this piece of misinformation. Once again, vested interest groups reared their ugly, profit-motivated heads at the expense of your health.

Coconut oil is not only safe, it's a valuable addition to your diet. It contains fatty acids that fight bacterial and viral infections, as well as fungi like *Candida albicans*.

Saturated fats from plants have a different chemical makeup than saturated fats from meats and dairy. Coconut oil, for instance, contains lauric and caprylic acids, fatty acids that are antifungal, antimicrobial, and antiviral. These are not found in meat or dairy fats.

When a fat is saturated, it means that it doesn't oxidize (spoil) quickly. Oxidation leads to the formation of harmful free radicals. This is why saturated tropical oils like coconut, palm, and palm kernel used to be added to baked goods and other processed foods. They don't spoil as quickly as other oils. Now hydrogenated or partially hydrogenated oils like shortening and margarine that create toxic trans fats and contribute to free-radical production have replaced much of these tropical oils in our food supply.

SECRET #116 Manufacturers of hydrogenated oils perpetuated the rumor that coconut oil is harmful.

In the late 1950s, a researcher in Minnesota announced that hydrogenated vegetable fats cause heart disease. The food oil industry insisted that any health problems were not caused by hydrogenation. After all, they made hydrogenated oils. Instead, they claimed that the saturated fats contained in these hydrogenated oils were harmful. What bunk! We all know that the less processed any oil (or food), the healthier it is.

Around this same time, a Philadelphia researcher announced that polyunsaturated fats lower cholesterol without explaining just how this occurred. It happens because polyunsaturated fats drive cholesterol out of the bloodstream and into the liver and arteries—just where you don't want them. Increasing cholesterol in your arteries is a terrible idea. Still, this little fact was ignored and polyunsaturated fats were perceived to be healthy.

The oil industry jumped on this single researcher's statement and convinced us to eat more polyunsaturated fats and fewer saturated fats. Polyunsaturated fats include oils containing omega-3 fats (found primarily in flax, fish, and walnuts) and omega-6 fats (found in corn, safflower, and soy). The omega-3 fats are particularly healthful EFAs. But we're now seeing that eating a diet high in other polyunsaturated fats—the omega-6 oils—is not as healthy as we once thought. Coconut oil is not only safe, it's also beneficial and can help you lose weight.

SECRET #117 Coconut oil is easy to digest and burns like a carbohydrate.

Both animal fats and tropical vegetable oils contain saturated fats. But the fats in coconut oil, as well as palm and palm kernel oils, are medium-chain triglycerides (MCTs), not long-chain fats. As explained previously, this means the fat contains smaller molecules than those found in other oils. The longer the chain of molecules in an oil, the more difficult it is to digest and the longer it takes to burn. Most oils burn like large, moist logs and don't always get completely burned. What isn't burned is stored in fat cells and can become rancid. MCTs burn like dry wood chips and are used up rapidly. In fact, this fat is easy to digest and burns as fast as a carbohydrate!

Because its molecules are small, it is less viscous—or thinner—than other oils. It absorbs other flavors, like garlic, with more intensity than other oils, as well. In addition, it has no cholesterol and doesn't raise blood cholesterol levels. Coconut oil has been used for years for premature babies with underdeveloped digestive systems. Ordinarily, these babies would have starved for lack of sufficient calories. But coconut oil with its smaller molecules doesn't need to be broken down by their digestive system. It goes directly to the liver where it burns like a carbohydrate, giving preemies life-saving fuel.

This thinner viscosity means you can use less oil in a recipe. This translates into fewer calories. If you eat the same amount of fat as before but replace some of the fats with coconut oil, you can lose weight effortlessly. Also, less fat will get stored in your fat cells. If the fats in your diet give you gas—which is a sign of poor fat digestion—coconut oil probably won't.

SECRET #118 Coconut oil contains fats that fight fungal infections.

Many doctors of integrative medicine use two fatty acids found in coconut oil to fight an overgrowth of *Candida albicans*. These are caprylic acid and lauric acid. Lauric acid converts into monolaurin in the small intestines, and it's monolaurin that has strong beneficial activities.

Caprylic acid: Years ago, I found that when I gave patients with an overgrowth of candida a supplement containing caprylic acid, their fungal infection began to improve. I used caprylic acid for years with great success as an antifungal agent. Although there is much less caprylic acid in coconut oil than in capsules, coconut oil should help control intestinal candida. If you want to try caprylic acid to lessen your candida, look for caprylic-acid supplements in your health-food store. (Take 1–2 grams, three times a day with meals for three months.)

Lauric acid: Lauric acid is a fat that is found in higher quantities in coconut than in any other food. In fact, nearly 50 percent of the fat in coconut oil is comprised of lauric acid. When you eat coconut oil, this acid is broken down into other fatty acids. One of them, monolaurin, has strong antimicrobial activity.

Monolaurin is one reason why breast milk enhances the immune systems in babies. You see, lauric acid is one of the main fats in breast milk. It is thought that the lauric acid, and the monolaurin it converts into, is responsible for protecting an infant's intestinal tract from viruses, bacteria, and fungal infections. Coconut oil, also high in lauric acid, can help protect you from bacteria and viruses as well.

Studies have shown that monolaurin inactivates candida and bacteria like *Listeria*, *Staphylococcus*, and *Streptococcus*, herpes simplex, Cytomegalovirus, flu, and measles. When coconut products, especially the oil, are added to your diet, you're maintaining very low levels of potent antibacterial/antiviral substances, which fight disease early.

SECRET #119 Coconut oil is available in several forms and flavors.

Coconut oil is readily available in canned coconut milk. Look for it in your grocery store, health-food store, or Asian market. I use it to make soups creamier and add it to vegetable curries. Since coconut oil is beneficial and helps you lose weight, you can use the full-fat variety without feeling guilty.

All coconut products contain at least a little oil. When you add desiccated (dried) coconut to your cereal, muffins, breakfast smoothie, or pancakes, you're getting a little of this safe fat.

Popcorn made with vegetable oils, and biscuits made with shortening, are examples of fats with larger molecules that taste greasy in your mouth. Coconut oil doesn't. And because it really is less viscous—thinner—it carries flavor better than thicker oils, so a little goes a very long way. If you add a few drops of hazelnut extract to a bottle of ThinOil, you can have a lot of flavor in your salad dressing and use much less of the oil than if you use a commercial salad dressing, olive oil, or vinegar. I used to spray butter-flavored ThinOil on my popcorn. Delicious! And I've used the oil for baking (use about one-third less oil than the recipe calls for), for sautéing, and in salad dressings.

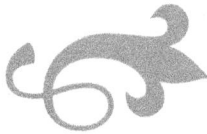

CHAPTER 18

Skin-Care Secrets for Young-Looking Skin

From our thirties to our eighties, we spend millions of dollars every year to have moist, wrinkle-free skin.

Some amount of wrinkling can be genetic. But dry, flaky, irritated, blemished skin is often caused by poor nutrition—both inside and out. Your skin is an organ, and like all organs, it needs antioxidants, good fats, and minerals. A healthy diet, good-quality supplements, and the right kind of skin-care products all contribute to youthful-looking skin.

One of your skin's functions is to help eliminate toxins. If you don't get rid of them through your kidneys, colon, and lungs, they tend to come out through your skin. This is why exercise and a good diet are essential for healthy skin. They help the other paths of elimination to work better.

When I begin working with a new patient, I take a comprehensive health history. It includes the question, "Do you have any skin problems?" While I'm looking for any skin diseases, such as acne or rosacea, they most often tell me, "I have very dry skin."

SECRET #120 Winter is the worst season for young-looking skin.

Your skin would like you to live in a tropical rainforest. It wants to be shielded from the sun's damaging UV rays. It wants to be in a moist environment. It doesn't want to be exposed to winter's drying heat from your furnace or cold, dry winter winds, either. It would like you to reach up and pick a piece of tropical fruit high in antioxidants and smear it all over your arms, legs, and face. But you don't need to live in a rainforest or rub yourself with an avocado or mango to have young, supple skin.

Our skin changes and needs increased care after menopause. That's when lowered estrogen levels cause some of the fat in our face to decrease. Our face begins to sag and we get more wrinkles. Collagen shrinks and our skin gets thinner. It loses some of its elasticity and has less oil.

Of all the seasons, your skin dislikes winter the most. The combination of dry skin, heated rooms and cold, outdoor weather makes it even more important to take good care of your skin at all times. You can keep your skin from aging and repair some of the damage by winterizing it no matter what the season. I don't mean slathering on moisturizers because your skin doesn't like too much moisturizer. Begin by stopping the damage.

SECRET #121 Three things to avoid that age your skin.

Soap: I never liked the feeling of soap on my face. Now I know why. Soap is drying and can inflame sensitive skin, and my skin is both dry and sensitive. Anything that dries your skin ages it. Using the right kind of cleanser is the first step in winterizing your skin.

Choosing a facial cleanser can be confusing, especially since the most popular brands touted by dermatologists, Cetaphil and Eucerin, contain sodium lauryl sulfate, a substance that can also dry and inflame sensitive skin! Cold-cream type cleansers can clog your pores and leave a film on your skin. This prevents moisturizers from penetrating.

Drying Ingredients: Acetone, alcohol, benzoyl peroxide, camphor, citrus, eucalyptus, menthol, and mint all dry the skin. Some of them may be "natural" and smell good, but they have drying effects nevertheless. Make sure that the products you use are free from these substances. If you happen to like soaking in a bath with citrus or eucalyptus oils, make sure you moisturize your skin afterwards. And don't stay in hot water too long.

Hot Water: Long, hot showers or baths, and sitting in a hot tub, dry your skin. Either avoid soaking in hot water for very long, or be sure to moisturize your skin well afterwards. But before you moisturize, be sure to remove the dead cells on your skin's surface.

SECRET #122 Only use the right kind of cleanser.

If you have dry skin, use a water-soluble liquid cleanser without sodium lauryl sulfate. It will clean your skin and remove makeup without being greasy or irritating. Buy a cleanser in a pump bottle. This prevents bacterial contamination from dirty hands and bathroom air found on soap.

If you have oily skin, use only facial cleansers with alcohol-free toners. Alcohol is drying, but it could dry your skin too much and backfire on you, causing more oil to be secreted.

After cleansing, exfoliate and then moisturize your skin.

SECRET #123 Prepare your skin before you moisturize.

Exfoliating removes dead cells from your skin and leaves it ready for moisturizing.

If you don't remove dead cells, you're just mixing them up with lotion. This can clog your pores.

Not all exfoliants are alike. Some are gentle on your skin while others are harsh. Alcohol-based exfoliants are effective by burning off dead cells, but they're also irritating. Fruit acids, like alpha hydroxy acid (AHA), are good exfoliants if your skin is oily, but can be harsh if you have dry, sensitive skin.

SECRET #124 These effective exfoliants cost little or nothing.

To avoid damaging sensitive skin, you may want to use a facial scrub to exfoliate only once a week. The rest of the week you can get rid of dead cells at no cost. Simply scrub your face gently each day with a washcloth and warm water. The washcloth will exfoliate your face, arms, and legs without damaging your skin. Or make an inexpensive exfoliant by mixing a little baking soda into your liquid cleanser and rub it into your face with clean fingertips.

Avoid products with apricot kernels and walnut shells if they feel scratchy. Most do. These are often too coarse and irritating for older, thinner skin. Some gentler ingredients like jojoba meal or oats can safely remove dead surface skin without causing any damage.

To remove dead skin, dry brush your body with a loofah sponge every day. Use a softer brush for your face to avoid bruising delicate skin. After you've exfoliated, you're ready to moisturize. But not with just any lotion or cream.

SECRET #125 Use a moisturizer that nourishes and repairs your skin.

The best moisturizers are packed with antioxidants. They reduce future damage and repair some of the existing damage as well. This is why your skin would like you to rub avocado, papaya, and other tropical fruits all over it. They're high in healing antioxidants. If you think you can't afford a good moisturizer, I have good news for you. You can. Pick up a ripe avocado the next time you go to the market and gently massage some of it on your face. Allow its oils to penetrate your skin, then remove whatever remains with warm water and blot carefully. If your skin is too oily, rub a little fresh cucumber on it instead.

Canola oil, evening primrose oil, hazelnut oil, kukui nut oil, olive oil, safflower oil, soy oil, sunflower oil, and herbs such as comfrey, and calendula are soothing, effective moisturizers. Find or make products with some of these ingredients. Apply any of them to your face for half an hour, and cover it with a hot, moist towel. Rinse it off with warm water, then seal your pores with cool water.

SECRET #126 These products noticeably turned back my aging clock in one month.

Studies show that vitamins A, C, and E, and omega-3 fatty acids help protect and repair the skin when they're used topically. You can find moisturizers that contain one or more of these nutrients in beauty supply and health-food stores. Some products also include herbs that are beneficial to the skin. Dr. Janet Zand, head of Z Mei Skin Care Therapy System, knows that the better the nutrition—both inside and out—the better your skin will be. She has developed skin-care products that reflect her knowledge of nutrition and Chinese herbs I've known her for more than twenty years. In addition to her knowledge and integrity, she has the most beautiful skin I've seen. I've aged some over the past twenty years, but Janet hasn't!

Janet includes Chinese and Western herbs along with vitamins and minerals in her Z Mei products. I am mentioning her products because of the dramatic improvement I saw in my own skin after using them for one month. Whether you use Z Mei or a different brand is your choice. But get good, quality products. Since you should use sunscreen, you can choose a moisturizer with SPF 15 and combine your needs into one product. For best penetration, apply a moisturizing cream after exfoliation while your skin is still warm and damp. Only moisturize dry skin or skin that shows signs of being dry in the winter. Oily skin doesn't need more oils!

SECRET #127 Don't put products with oil on oily skin.

When the oil glands in skin, called sebaceous glands, make too much oil (or sebum), your skin becomes oily. The nice result is that your skin remains moist and you're likely to have fewer wrinkles. But too much oil can plug up your pores and cause them to stretch and break, resulting in acne. Or you can have shiny, oily patches that are unsightly areas for dirt to collect.

If you use a moisturizer, use very small amounts of one that is oil free. In fact, all of your cosmetics should be free from oil. Here are a few natural products you can use for cleansing:

- Gently rub your skin with apple-cider vinegar and water (1:1 ratio).

- Cleanse your face with a strong, cool, sage tea. Make it ahead of time and store it in your refrigerator.

- Rub a slice of raw potato on your face and rinse with cool water.

- Add three drops of any of the following essential oils (found in natural-food stores) to your favorite cleanser or shampoo: lemon, orange, peppermint, rosemary, tea tree, jasmine, or geranium.

Also consider your diet. Are you eating plenty of whole grains, nuts, seeds, beans, and yeast, which are high in vitamin B$_2$ (riboflavin)? A vitamin B$_2$ deficiency can contribute to oily skin. Next, look at the skin-care products you're using. Finally, don't forget the importance of a nutrient-dense diet.

SECRET #128 These dietary tips will improve your skin.

Dry or oily, your skin needs to get sufficient quantities of the right kind of oils from your diet. A low-fat or no-fat diet will age your skin. Essential fatty acids (EFAs), such as the omega-3 and omega-6 fats found in flax oil, raw walnuts, fatty fish, evening primrose and borage seed oils do more than help control weight and support your immune system. They keep your skin healthy and moist. If you're not eating enough foods high in EFAs every day, or taking them in supplements, you may be contributing to your dry skin. Don't rely on applying oils topically. Take one teaspoon of flax oil, or two capsules of flax, borage, or evening primrose oil, twice a day. Add two to four capsules of fish oil daily, except on days when you eat oily fish, like salmon.

Your skin needs vitamin A to repair and make healthy skin. Supplement your diet with 15,000–25,000 mg of carotenoids—or 5,000–10,000 international units (IU) of vitamin A in your multivitamin. Make sure you get enough vitamin C, which is needed to make the skin protein collagen. Take 1,000–2,000 mg a day and eat potatoes, citrus, and bell peppers, all high in this vitamin.

"Internally and externally, skin degeneration is caused by a lack of good oils and trace minerals," Janet Zand told me. "But you need to take them orally as well as use them topically," she said. "And you need to not only take them, but digest them. Often, I suggest that older women take enzymes along with fish oils for best absorption."

It's not enough to apply nutrients topically. You need to include them in your diet every day. Vitamin A and its carotenoids improve wrinkles and rough skin. Yellow, orange, and green vegetables, egg yolks, and fish oils contain carotenoids, used to make vitamin A. Include several good portions of these foods every day. Vitamin C, in vegetables and citrus, helps stabilize collagen. And vitamin E, in oils, nuts, and seeds, moisturizes and softens the skin. Be sure to include a good-quality vitamin/mineral supplement to ensure that you're getting enough nutrients.

SECRET #129 The best thing for your skin costs nothing.

Caffeine dehydrates you and dries out your skin. Water and herb teas have the opposite effect. This is why the number-one remedy for dry skin is to drink enough water or other liquids, without caffeine, throughout the day. Drinking water isn't a

---

problem for the majority of women I counsel. Going to the bathroom frequently is. But there's no way around it. If you don't drink enough water or other liquids, your skin will not be as moist and supple as if you do.

Extremely dry or excessively oily skin can lead to skin problems. Diet, environmental pollution, and soaps compound them. With so many skin-care products available, it's easy to choose the wrong kind for your particular type of skin. When you know which ingredients will minimize overly dry or very oily skin, you can often find inexpensive products that work well. If you happen to have dermatitis, I've found a simple solution that could calm down inflamed tissues.

SECRET #130 This common beverage can get rid of dermatitis.

"Itis" means "inflammation," so dermatitis means that you have a skin inflammation. Chapter 38 will give you a lot of information on treating inflammatory conditions, but you may not even need them.

Chances are that if you have itchy, inflamed skin that doesn't clear up, you're already using topical or oral treatments to suppress the inflammation and itching. This form of dermatitis often runs in families of people with sensitive skin or various allergies.

Make sure that the skin-care products you're using are not irritating or causing an allergic reaction. Parabens, a preservative found in many products, can cause inflammation if you're sensitive to them.

In addition to using cortisone creams, antibiotics, antihistamines, and ultraviolet-light treatments to reduce inflammation, I may have found a simple and inexpensive solution for you—drinking tea.

A group of Japanese researchers noticed that when animals with allergic skin conditions were either given green, black, or oolong teas, their dermatitis improved. So they decided to test the teas on humans. Their results are encouraging.

Each person in the study drank one cup of oolong tea (steeped for five minutes) after each meal over a six-month period. Almost 50 percent of them had a moderate improvement in their skin lesions after just one month. At the end of the study, half the participants still were moderately improved and a few had significant improvement.

Since the animal studies used green, black, and oolong teas, you can choose any of these to drink regularly. All are high in polyphenols—chemicals that reduce allergic reactions. The cost for this little experiment is just pennies a day. But don't stop using your medications and switch over to tea. First, see whether or not your skin improves after drinking three cups a day of the world's most popular beverage. If it does, then speak with your doctor about reducing your medications. You may even find you can eliminate them.

SECRET #131 You can get rid of cellulite.

When I was in my thirties, I had "cottage cheese" thighs. Little clumps of unsightly fat covered my buttocks and thighs. At that time, I was a professional masseuse in Southern California. I discovered that my condition was not unusual, although it seemed to progress with age. Lots of women had pitting and bulging, especially in their thighs and buttocks. In fact, other masseuses I knew concentrated in giving "cellulite massages" to actresses and other women who wanted smoother skin at any cost.

I never heard any men complain of cellulite, and never noticed that they had it, and for good reason. For the most part, they don't. Cellulite is a condition where the tissue that lies just below a woman's skin (called subcutaneous tissue) is structurally different from a man's. Between 90 and 98 percent of people with cellulite are women. And a good number of women would look and feel younger with less cellulite. Is there any way to get rid of it? Very possibly.

The Difference Between Men's Skin and Women's Skin

First, it's important to understand why cellulite occurs in women and not in men. All skin begins with the epidermis—the covering. Beneath the epidermis lies a layer of connective tissue called the corium. Below the corium is subcutaneous tissue.

In women, the skin's subcutaneous tissue has large standing fat-cell chambers separated by walls of connective tissue. These fat chambers are attached to the corium.

Men's skin has thicker, stronger corium. Their subcutaneous tissue is thinner with criss-crossed connective tissue walls that don't allow fat to accumulate. This difference assures men of having smoother skin at all ages. How unfair!

As our skin ages and our estrogen levels decline, it becomes thinner and looser on all levels. The connective tissue walls between our large fat-cell chambers get thinner. This allows the chambers to balloon out, and lets fat cells migrate into the corium. So if you didn't have cellulite when you were younger, you probably will as you get older. Unless you decide to do something about it.

SECRET #132 These three steps can reduce cellulite.

Diet, exercise, and massage all help get rid of cellulite. Diet and exercise help by reducing the size of your fat-cell chambers. Keep animal protein and animal fats in your diet low. The one exception is good-quality fish. Eat more raw nuts and beans. Drink water throughout the day to flush out unwanted toxins and reduce your food intake if you want to lose weight.

If you want to get rid of cellulite and are overweight, it's important for you to lose some of that excess weight. Weight loss takes pressure off the connective tissue structures. Exercise improves your circulation that, in turn, strengthens the connective tissue structures. Stronger structures mean that your fat chambers can't bulge as much. It also means that fewer fat cells can migrate toward the surface of your skin.

A slow, steady weight loss allows your skin and connective tissues to gradually improve their strength and tone. Rapid weight loss, on the other hand, accelerates the negative changes and worsens your cellulite. As tempting as it may be to lose weight quickly, concentrate on losing two to four pounds a week.

Massage improves your circulation and moves blood and lymph through your body more quickly. Some cellulite is caused by protein masses that are not being eliminated through the lymphatic system. This is why some massage therapists use a lymphatic drainage massage with their clients who have cellulite.

SECRET #133 You can easily drain your lymphatics at home by yourself.

Gently jump on a rebounder trampoline to get your lymphatic system pumping. If you don't have a trampoline, jump lightly on the balls of your feet for a few minutes. Then lie on the floor with your legs raised up on a wall or chair and gently massage the crease between your legs and belly. This opens up the deep lymph nodes where the protein masses tend to accumulate.

Use a dry bath brush or dry loofah sponge and lightly brush your skin in the direction of your heart. You can massage this area in the same direction with your hands if you don't have a bath brush or sponge. Do this for a few minutes each day.

SECRET #134 Two herbs can help reduce your cellulite.

Gotu kola (Centella asiatica) reduced cellulite in 80 percent of the people who tested it. It appears to improve the integrity and strength of connective tissues. The participants took a gotu kola extract containing 30 mg of triterpenes (asiatic acid and asiaticoside) three times a day.

Horse chestnut extract (Aesculus hippocastanum) contains an active ingredient called escin that reduces swelling and has anti-inflammatory effects. You can take horse chestnut extract containing 10–20 mg of escin three times a day, or apply a salve with 0.5–1.5% escin topically.

Both gotu kola and horse chestnut extracts have been used successfully for varicose veins as well as for cellulite. For this reason, you may want to consider combining equal amounts of each extract and taking $1/_2$ teaspoon three times a day.

SECRET #135 Coffee reduces cellulite. But don't drink it.

When you use caffeine topically, it can reduce cellulite more effectively than if you drink it. Look for a salve or ointment with 0.5–1.5% *Cola vera* extract (14% caffeine). Apply it morning and night to the areas where you have the most cellulite.

FOUR STAGES OF CELLULITE

Stage 0 is where the skin is smooth when you stand or lie down and doesn't pit or bulge when you pinch it. Forget it. You won't have this type of skin unless you're slender and in your twenties. Let's move on to a more realistic stage.

Stage 1 is when your skin looks smooth when you're standing or lying down, but when you pinch it you get the pitting and bulging. If you can get to this stage, you're doing well.

Stage 2 is when you look just fine lying down but you get the pitting and bulging when you stand. This stage is not unusual for women over forty or for women who are obese.

Stage 3 is when you have cottage cheese thighs and buttocks all the time. Standing, lying down, and sitting. If you're past menopause, you know what I'm talking about.

SECRET #136 There's a connection between cellulite and varicose veins.

Both cellulite and varicose veins are conditions where connective tissues have become weaker from age. Both can be corrected by reducing fat in the subcutaneous layer of your skin through diet and exercise. Even if your cellulite doesn't bother you, it makes sense to take steps to avoid or reduce varicose veins. If your buttocks and thighs look smoother and younger as a result, that's an extra benefit.

Can you really get rid of your cellulite? I did, without even trying. I was concentrating on increasing my exercise, eating more fresh fruits and vegetables, and eating fewer junk foods. Each week I exchanged a massage with a friend who was also a masseuse. One day she commented, "Your cellulite is gone." Yes, I have a little cellulite now, but not much at all. In my late sixties, I can still wear shorts without feeling embarrassed.

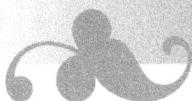

PART 4

RELIEVE FATIGUE
and REDUCE STRESS

When you look and feel tired, you look and feel older than your years . . . no matter what your age may be. Fatigue can come from a number of sources, including blood-sugar imbalances, physical exertion, too little sleep, pain, chronic fatigue syndrome, depression, and stress.

Of all of them, stress seems to be the one that's hardest to get and keep under control. And yet when you do, the effects can be immediate. Instead of looking worn out, you look vital. Instead of wishing you could go to sleep, you feel refreshed.

The world—and our lives—has never been so stressful. As soon as we relax, something else happens. There's no way to escape it. Stress is everywhere. It's stressful to live in a polluted environment with bad air and water. It's stressful to drive on roads filled with angry drivers and to breathe toxic exhaust fumes. It's stressful just to make a living. And we add to our stress when we try to find time to reduce it with regular exercise, and preparing healthy food. But hang in there. While you're looking for ways to simplify your life—and I truly hope you are—I've discovered a number of simple solutions you can use to reduce your stress and fatigue. I'll guarantee you haven't heard or tried all of them.

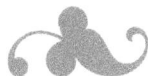

CHAPTER 19

Hormones Can Cause or Reduce Stress

Stress is anything—positive or negative—that makes more demands on you than you can meet. This includes vacations, eating junk foods or skipping meals, being too hot or cold, illness, insufficient sleep, and emotional tension. Holidays add more emotional and financial stress. And many hormones add to your trouble. But there are substances, including some hormones, that can help.

All stressors have something in common. They trigger a physiological response that causes your adrenal glands—tiny glands that sit on top of your kidneys—to pump out more adrenal hormones. When your body identifies a stressor, your brain releases hormones that tell your adrenals to jump into action and produce hormones to help you meet the challenge before you.

Your body doesn't know the difference between various types of stressors. It keeps pumping adrenal hormones in response to any and all of them. The result is too much cortisol and too little DHEA, a hormonal imbalance that can lead to health problems. This is a bigger problem than you may realize.

SECRET #137 The cortisol response is more damaging than the "fight-or-flight" response.

There are two types of stress responses. One is the "fight-or-flight" response, which is controlled by epinephrine and norepinephrine. These hormones give you the extra strength and agility you need to run to safety, such as when you're being chased by someone with a knife or escaping a rampaging tiger. But too much of these hormones can cause fear and anxiety, leading to more stress. The end result is that your adrenal glands become exhausted.

The other stress response is triggered by cortisol, a hormone that results in a big push of energy. But this extra energy comes with a high price tag. It raises your blood sugar to give you the ability to burn more energy (sugar) and increases insulin sensitivity. This can lead to anything from sudden fatigue to diabetes. Some stressors that increase cortisol levels include heat, cold, pain, radiation, obesity, disease, overexertion, and worrisome events in our lives. In other words, almost everything. Now you're in a cycle of stress that's difficult to break. Stress makes cortisol, and cortisol causes other stressors.

You may not be able to change the stressors in your life, but you can change your response to them.

SECRET #138 Morning meditation and exercise reduce cortisol.

Our cortisol levels tend to be highest in the morning. If you're stressed, morning is the best time for you to use two stress-reducing techniques: meditation and exercise. But don't push yourself and overexercise. This perpetuates your stress cycle. Walking, swimming, biking, low-impact aerobics, gardening, and dancing are easier on your adrenal glands than running. If you're too tired to exercise, don't do much. Listen to your body and take a ten-minute walk instead of a longer more strenuous workout. Mild to moderate exercise from four to six times a week will help lower your cortisol. And it takes only ten to thirty minutes of prayer or meditation to help break the stress cycle.

SECRET #139 Stress can affect your memory.

You may remember times when you were under tremendous stress and couldn't think clearly. This is a temporary response. But when too much cortisol is secreted and too little is eliminated, it can destroy your brain cells, increase the aging process, lead to insomnia, and lower your immune system. Once more, cortisol increases stress. Chronically high cortisol levels are associated with a greater deterioration of the hippocampus, a part of the brain that is associated with memory. Reducing cortisol levels by reducing stress is the most important thing you can do to improve your mind.

SECRET #140 Stress ages you.

Do you have more weight around your stomach than you had in the past? Does your blood sugar fluctuate? Do you have a loss of memory, depression, muscle weakness and wasting, low blood pressure, allergies, flu and bronchitis, or thin skin? Do you fly off the handle at the slightest provocation? These are not only signs of aging; they come from years of chronic stress and excess cortisol resulting in adrenal fatigue.

"Cortisol is a killer," Dr. Uzzi Reiss, gynecologist and author, told me. He said that people with high cortisol levels have a lower life expectancy than people with normal levels. This is why he counsels every patient to deal with stress before they begin any hormone program. Whether you are using estrogen replacement therapy

(ERT) or not, you need to find ways to reduce your cortisol levels. It can prolong your memory and your life. One way to get cortisol levels under control is to take DHEA.

RELAX—AND SAVE YOUR PROGESTERONE!

Your adrenal glands are designed to produce their hormones as needed—not constantly. When exhausted adrenal glands can't make enough stress-relieving hormones, your body makes them out of progesterone, resulting in even less progesterone than naturally occurs with aging! Before taking progesterone, it's important to reduce your response to stress.

SECRET #141 Balance cortisol with this anti-stress hormone.

DHEA (dehydroepiandrosterone) is a steroid hormone made from cholesterol by your adrenal glands. Structurally, DHEA is similar to other steroid hormones, such as estrogen, progesterone, and testosterone. In fact, DHEA can be converted into both estrogen and testosterone, boosting estrogen and testosterone levels. But DHEA is more than a reservoir for these hormones.

It's a popular anti-stress androgen hormone that has a number of beneficial actions. It helps regulate various hormones and enzymes. And animal studies indicate it can help prevent diseases like cancer, lupus, rheumatoid arthritis, Alzheimer's disease, heart disease, and chronic fatigue. DHEA supports the immune system and is considered to be anti-carcinogenic. It also helps prevent osteoporosis by slowing down bone loss and increasing the formation of new bone.

Does this sound like a miracle? Read on. DHEA may slow down aging and increase your libido. Because it is abundant in brain tissue and has been found to increase neurons in laboratory tests with nerve-cell tissue cultures, DHEA can support your brain function as you age.

Does this mean you should rush out to your nearest health-food store and buy this over-the-counter hormone? I don't advise it.

SECRET #142 Too much DHEA can cause problems.

DHEA can be converted into other hormones, including testosterone. When you take too much it can cause the same side effects as testosterone, such as facial hair. Self-medicating with any hormones isn't as safe as you may have been told. Author Hyla Cass, M.D., says, "It's a delicate balance, this hormonal dance." Our bodies handle hormones differently. For instance, in some women, DHEA remains as DHEA. But in others, it's converted to testosterone or estrogen. This is why it's so important to be monitored by a physician.

Dr. Reiss, author of *Natural Hormone Balance for Women,* echoes this concern. Studies using DHEA have been too short and have used doses much too high. Many of his patients who take DHEA can take only 5 milligrams (mg) without having side effects. Too much can damage your adrenal glands.

Last year, my doctor suggested I increase my DHEA from 5 mg to 10 mg, but a follow-up lab test revealed that the extra 5 mg had begun to shut down my adrenal glands. I'm now taking just 5 mg a day. A small amount of supplemental DHEA can support your adrenals, but self-medicating with any hormone is tricky.

To determine whether or not you need this hormone, have your doctor do a DHEA-sulfate blood test. Discuss a slow method of gradually increasing your levels if you're deficient. The amount of DHEA you need may vary considerably from 5 to 50 mg a day. However, many doctors are finding that from 5 to 15 mg is sufficient. Check with your doctor first and be sure to take the right amount—not too much, not too little. Remember, taking too much DHEA too quickly can give you undesirable side effects. The many studies done with DHEA conclude that it sometimes works and it sometimes doesn't.

SECRET #143 Not all DHEA supplements are good quality.

You want any hormones you're taking to be of the highest quality. Some DHEA is better quality than others. Also, DHEA may not be effective because it may not contain the amount it says on the label. The head of a natural compounding pharmacy told me that many DHEA products sold in natural-food stores that claim to contain 25–50 mg of the hormone contain only 5–10 mg. "At least people aren't hurting themselves," he said.

Many doctors prefer DHEA made by natural compounding pharmacies or sold through nutritional supplement companies that primarily sell to healthcare practitioners. For more information on where to get quality DHEA, see the Resources section at the end of this book.

SECRET #144 Mexican yam supplements don't work as well as DHEA.

Mexican wild yam is a precursor to DHEA. In theory, this means that it can help make DHEA. But don't count on this if you're over fifty. Your body's ability to convert precursors into DHEA decreases with age, so this natural product isn't likely to have much, if any, of an effect on your hormone levels.

Still, some women swear by wild yam supplements. Why is this? Their increased feelings of well-being most likely come from a stimulant effect in the product. If that's what you want, then there's nothing wrong with taking the supplements. But the only way we know to raise DHEA levels is to take DHEA. Not a precursor.

STRESS CONTRIBUTES TO . . .

- Bone loss
- Depression and mood swings
- Digestive disturbances from gas to Crohn's disease
- Immune problems like colds, flu, and cancer
- Insomnia
- Low libido
- Muscle wasting
- Slow wound healing and thinning skin
- Water retention and weight gain

From *Tired of Being Tired*, Jesse Lynn Hanley, M.D., and Nancy Deville (Berkley Trade, 2002)

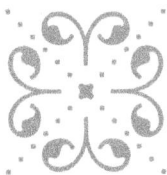

CHAPTER 20

Treat Trauma and Stress with Flower Essences

Jillian was hysterical. Between long bouts of crying, I was able to understand why. Her beloved dog, Thor, had run full steam into a recently washed sliding-glass door and had died in her arms from the injuries. I told her I'd be over in a few minutes, picked up one of my favorite remedies I keep handy for emergencies, and drove to her home.

SECRET #145 This formula made from flowers can instantly reduce trauma.

When I arrived, Jillian was sitting with her best friend and was crying so hard she could barely speak. I told her to open her mouth, placed four drops of the Rescue Remedy flower essence formula tincture in it, and waited. Within a few minutes, she had calmed down enough to talk.

While I was with Jillian, I gave her additional drops of Rescue Remedy whenever her voice started to sound hysterical. She calmed down each time. Flower essences provided her with the relief she needed at this very difficult time.

Rescue Remedy is one of a number of formulas made from five particular flower essences that has been used for decades for trauma. It works equally on people and animals. It's sold under two names: Rescue Remedy and Five Flower Formula. Each contains the same flower essences prepared in the same manner. I keep a small vial of either formula in my purse and in my medicine chest. I won't travel without it. I've found these flower essences invaluable for emergencies on camping trips and vacations when people were injured or traumatized.

SECRET #146 Flower essences are an effective component of mind/body medicine.

In the 1930s, English pathologist and bacteriologist Edward Bach discovered that small quantities of water infused with specific plant essences could affect emotional health. He categorized the plant essences according to particular personality traits.

Bach was so fascinated with the effects that these essences had that he stopped making vaccines for physicians. He spent the rest of his life learning about the healing properties of flowers and how they affected various moods. It was this combination of mind/body medicine that resulted in the thirty-eight individual flower essences known today as the Bach Flower Remedies.

Dr. Bach spent hours examining the habits and characteristics of flowers and trees and came to the conclusion that plants and flowers had different vibrations, and that diseases could not co-exist with some of them. While many plants had medicinal qualities, Bach found only a few healed the emotions. He noticed that physical healing was accelerated when a person's outlook became positive and peaceful. By restoring the emotions to harmony and balance, the body could heal itself more rapidly.

I've been using Dr. Bach's essences for forty years on friends, patients, and myself. I find an immediate effect as soon as I place the drops in my mouth, although some people find it takes a little longer.

SECRET #147 These five essences are used in Rescue Remedy and Five Flower Formula.

There are thirty-eight different flower essences in the Bach flower repertory and numerous combinations you can make from them. Any of the books on Edward Bach will give you the information to make your own formulas. However, you may find that the combination that's sold under the names Rescue Remedy or Five Flower Formula are all you need to help reduce stress.

Star of Bethlehem: This essence is particularly useful for shock and trauma. Some examples include hearing about the death of a loved one, or the fear that comes after narrowly escaping an accident. You can also use this flower essence to comfort someone who refuses to be consoled.

Rock Rose: It's used for terror and panic. This essence is useful in emergencies even when the situation appears to be hopeless. Use it for accidents, sudden illnesses, or whenever anyone is feeling terrified.

Impatiens: Best for physical and mental tension and irritability. As its name implies, this essence can help reduce feelings of impatience.

Cherry Plum: This essence is helpful for people who have a fear of losing control. Useful when you feel overwhelmed, heading for a nervous breakdown, or are afraid you'll do something you'll later regret.

Clematis: For a tendency to pass out from stress. This essence helps when you feel detached from reality, are daydreaming, or feel indifferent.

The combination can be used for any and all of the above situations. There are some people who claim that flower essences work only if you believe they will. How, then, can you explain their effectiveness with animals?

SECRET #148 Flower essences work well with animals.

My parrot, Pancho, and I lived in Los Angeles when a big earthquake shook the house for several long and terrifying minutes. I heard Pancho's wings flapping wildly as she flew off her perch. When the shaking stopped, I put her in her cage. Her eyes were wide open with fear, and Pancho climbed around and around inside her cage. I used to be a veterinary assistant and knew that fear could kill a bird, so I reached for my bottle of Rescue Remedy.

I managed to get a drop of it into her beak. She became calm and rested on her perch almost immediately. Pancho still wasn't looking completely normal, but she was greatly improved and the terror in her eyes was gone. I put another drop of the tincture in her water dish and soon she was back to normal.

If you have a pet that is experiencing anxiety, put one or two drops of this remedy in its mouth or water dish. If you have an injured pet that's in shock, this is an appropriate remedy. Use it if you're transporting your pet by car or plane, especially if the animal tends to get motion sickness.

SECRET #149 Just two to four drops of this formula can ease trauma.

I usually put two to four drops of Rescue Remedy in a little water and hold it in my mouth for a few seconds before swallowing it. Or I place a drop or two under my tongue. Some people recommend you place four drops of the tincture in a small glass of water, juice, or cup of tea and sip it slowly, drinking it within fifteen minutes. If necessary, repeat. It's safe to take more. You just don't need more.

You can also buy a spray bottle of Rescue Remedy. This is an excellent way to get the formula in the mouth of pets and infants.

You can use a cream containing these flower essences. Rub a small amount on the inside of the wrists, the neck, or ankle—any place with thin skin will do—and the effect is the same as with the drops.

Most health-food stores sell either Rescue Remedy or Five Flower Formula. These combinations of flower essences are not to be used instead of emergency treatment, but for those times when emergency treatment is unavailable or someone is in a cycle of stress they're unable to break. It's simply wonderful for life's little emotional emergencies.

CHAPTER 21

How Adaptogens Can Relieve Your Stress, Fatigue, and Trauma

Stress pushes your body and emotions out of balance. It speeds up some functions and slows down others. You need plenty of vitamins, minerals, and amino acids to keep feeding your cells. But when you're under stress, you need to normalize your body to allow it to heal and restore itself. Adaptogens are some of the best supplements you can take for this purpose.

Adaptogens are substances—usually herbs or mushrooms—that help regulate and balance your body by normalizing its physiological functions. By doing so, they increase your resistance to harmful physical, chemical, and biological stressors. For this reason they are often called "antiaging" herbs.

Few people know that there's a mineral with adaptogenic qualities as well. This mineral may be an important key to improving women's health. It regulates the thyroid, protects against breast cancer, and can help our hormones work better.

Read on. The subject of adaptogens is fascinating, and their ability to keep you healthy may surprise you.

Plant-based Adaptogens

Two of my favorite adaptogens from the plant kingdom are *Rhodiola rosea* and *Cordyceps* mushroom. I talk at length about *Cordyceps* in Chapter 3. Now let me tell you about *Rhodiola*. It may be your best choice for support when you're under a lot of stress.

SECRET #150 **This herb has a history of relieving stress.**

The ancient Greeks knew about this stress-relieving herb thanks to physician Dioscorides, who included it in his giant book on herbal medicine 2,000 years ago. From there, word of its value quickly spread throughout Europe and Asia, where it's been used ever since for many health conditions. Yet chances are you haven't heard of it.

The Vikings used it to give themselves greater strength and endurance.

It was used to prevent altitude sickness and fatigue, and to promote longevity.

It was considered to be the most effective of all herbs for colds and flu during harsh Arctic winters when respiratory problems were often fatal.

More recently, the Russians gave it to their astronauts and professional athletes to relieve fatigue and enhance their performance.

I'm talking about a root that grows high in the mountains of Europe and Asia called *Rhodiola rosea* (*R. rosea*). It was so prized that Russian families carefully guarded its locations for centuries. They harvested the root in secret and smuggled it down the mountains where they traded it for rare foods and wines. Chinese emperors sent messengers to Russia to bring back this prized herb.

R. rosea was then studied at length by Russian botanist G.V. Krylov in the mid-1900s. He found it protects against physical and emotional stress, toxins, and cold weather. Nearly 200 papers and studies over the past thirty years support effectiveness in a wide variety of conditions. It increases energy, alleviates depression, helps with weight loss, relieves mental fatigue, protects the heart during stress, and improves the function of the thyroid, thymus, and adrenal glands. Its ability to restore balance to organs and glands gives it a prominent place among adaptogens.

SECRET #151 *Rhodiola* excels in reducing the effects of physical stress and stress-related mental fatigue.

When it comes to stress, few people are under more physical and mental stress than professional athletes and doctors. *R. rosea* dramatically increased the endurance, performance, and mental clarity in a group of master-level competitive skiers. It also shortened their recovery time.

Who are more stressed and tired than medical doctors who are on night duty in hospitals? A group of them were given 170 mg of *R. rosea* extract just once a day for two weeks. This one-time daily dose resulted in a significant reduction in fatigue compared with doctors who took a placebo.

But what about ordinary people like you and me?

A fifty-year-old computer analyst suffered from extreme fatigue. Any of us who work at computers know from experience how stiff and tired you can get sitting in front of a monitor day in and day out. This woman's doctor gave her 50 mg of *R. rosea* extract to take in her morning tea and her fatigue disappeared within a few days! That's less than one-third the amount that the doctors took.

If you know anyone who has ever had chemotherapy, you know it often leads to depletion and exhaustion. Take the case of a sixty-two-year-old woman with breast cancer. She was forced to stop her chemotherapy treatment because of fatigue and a low red and white blood cell count. She took 150 mg of *R. rosea* extract twice a day. It relieved her fatigue and normalized her red and white blood cell numbers so she could continue her chemotherapy.

SECRET #152 The amount of *Rhodiola* you need to take is not critical.

High or low amounts of this herb both work. Last year, the results of a randomized, double-blind, placebo-controlled study of 161 stressed and tired cadets were published. Some of the cadets were given higher amounts of *Rhodiola* than others, but there was no difference in results between the two groups. *R. rosea* worked in smaller or larger quantities. This is good news, because it means that if you're extremely stressed, a larger dose is not necessarily more effective than a standard dose.

SECRET #153 *Rhodiola* stimulates brain chemical production.

You need sufficient serotonin, a calming chemical, to handle stress and think clearly. But stress decreases your body's production of serotonin. *R. rosea* has the unique ability to "turn on" brain chemicals, such as norepinephrine, dopamine, and serotonin, which help you think and feel better. It also inactivates those chemicals that block memory activity, which improves your memory.

SECRET #154 All *Rhodiola* is not equally effective.

The problem with *Rhodiola* supplements that are being sold today is that not all of them are effective. There are more than fifty species of *Rhodiola*. The only one that's proven effective for the conditions I've described is *Rhodiola rosea*—the species used in every one of the studies. Any *Rhodiola* product you buy should be a standardized extract and say *Rhodiola rosea* on the label.

   R. rosea is an effective adaptogen whether it's dried or in a tincture. It works well alone or in combination with other herbs. You can find standardized *Rhodiola rosea* extracts from Nature's Way and Planetary Formulas in many health-food stores. HerbPharm, one of my favorite herb companies, makes an excellent *R. rosea* extract from roots harvested in the Russian Arctic Circle—where some of the studies were done.

   The answer to stress and its side effects—memory loss and fatigue—is to reduce stress with exercise, daily meditation or prayer, more rest, a healthy diet, and specific supplements. An adaptogen like *R. rosea* is an excellent addition to any stress-reduction program. It isn't the only adaptogenic herb there is, however. Here are a few others I've found useful.

SOME KNOWN APPLICATIONS FOR *RHODIOLA ROSEA*

- Antidepressant
- Protects the heart
- Improves appetite
- Improves work performance
- Improves sleep

- Reduces mental fatigue
- Improves mental alertness
- Improves short-term memory
- Enhances weight loss
- Reduces heart palpitations

SECRET #155 Siberian ginseng is not a ginseng, but it is an adaptogen.

More than twenty years ago, I came upon a particularly potent adaptogen from Russia. It was called Siberian ginseng, but it wasn't a form of ginseng at all. It was a root used in traditional chinese medicine (TCM) for thousands of years, and researched by Russian scientists in the 1900s. This root was mislabeled for over a dozen years. Now it's called by its real name, *Eleutherococcus senticosus,* or eleuthero, for short.

Eleuthero has a wide number of applications related to stress and fatigue. It increases immune system function and keeps you from getting sick. It's a tonic, adaptogen, and anti-stress herb. One of its actions is to tranquilize the central nervous system, which can help you feel calmer. Eleuthero appears to support and boost adrenal gland function, supporting both physical and emotional stress. It improves mental performance, enhances recovery from exercise, and reduces stress.

You can find eleuthero in health-food stores both in tinctures and in capsules. I prefer a tincture with an alcohol base. When I first began researching this herb, I found evidence that the active ingredients were more potent in an alcohol extraction. You can use two to four ml (1–2 droppersful) of the extract from one to four times a day, or 100–200 mg of dried root three times daily.

SECRET #156 These are three other proven adaptogens.

Korean ginseng (*Panax ginseng*) has been used for thousands of years in China, Japan, and Korea. This species of ginseng is primarily used as a tonic and adaptogen. Like *Rhodiola*, Korean ginseng improves the memory. It has properties that reduce physical and chemical stressors.

In Eastern medicine, ginseng is rarely used alone. It is usually one ingredient in an adaptogenic formula. The primary active ingredients in ginseng are called ginsenosides. A great deal of research on Korean ginseng root suggests that 200 mg of a 4% standardized extract (8 mg of ginsenosides) is an effective daily dose. However, there are numerous Asian studies that suggest between 80–240 mg of ginsenosides may be needed for the desired effect.

American ginseng (*Panax quinquefolius*) is one of about six species of ginseng. Most of it is exported to Asia where it is thought to be superior in many ways to Korean ginseng. This isn't true. All ginsengs have slightly different actions. American ginseng has been used for the exhaustion and anxiety that comes from overworking. It is also a stomach tonic. American ginseng has also been used to improve one's mood from fatigue. To improve physical endurance, take 330 mg of the dried herb three times a day.

Ashwagandha (*Withania somnifera*) is an Ayurvedic herb. It is known as "Indian ginseng" because it has many of the same adaptogenic activities as Korean ginseng. It has been used for thousands of years in India where it is considered to be the strongest adaptogen of all Ayurvedic herbs. It's been used for insomnia, nervous exhaustion, and stress. In addition, it stimulates the immune system in people with low white blood counts. Dosage is from 75 to 250 mg a day.

Ashwagandha is being sold as an herb for sexual enhancement, especially for men. It's not. It's an adaptogen just like the others I've talked about. But by regulating various body functions, some people may find it enhances their sexual desire and performance.

SECRET #157 This mineral may be the ultimate adaptogen.

I talk about iodine and the thyroid in Chapter 1. And I explain its role in preventing breast cancer in Part 9. This mineral never ceases to amaze me. It plays such an integral role in regulating a number of body functions that it may, indeed, be the ultimate adaptogen. It's an essential mineral, crucial to your health, that hasn't yet been recognized for its adaptogenic effects. And I'll bet you need more of it.

Last year, I organized a seminar in Northern California for forty doctors of integrative medicine on the subject of iodine. Dr. Guy E. Abraham, a research endocrinologist from Southern California, led the presentation. Drs. David Brownstein, from Michigan, and Jorge Flechas, from North Carolina, joined him.

The physicians who attended this presentation were impressed. "If this turns out to be true in my practice, as it has with these other practitioners, I'll have to change the way I practice medicine!" said Dr. Richard Shames, co-author of *Thyroid Power.* "I'm going to try it on some of my very sick patients," another one told me. Months later, this second doctor confessed that he found that the majority of the patients he tested were iodine insufficient. When he increased their iodine supplementation, he was able to take them off some of their medications.

Iodine is best known for its role in thyroid function. But it was Dr. Abraham who discovered that if you take enough iodine—100 to 400 times the recommended dietary allowance (RDA)—it helps regulate other body functions as well. Dr. Abraham found that more than 90 percent of us are low in iodine. He's not alone in this finding. Drs. Flechas and Brownstein, who have tested for iodine and used iodine/iodide supplementation for years, are convinced that whole-body iodine insufficiency is contributing to numerous health problems from hypothyroidism to breast cancer and fibromyalgia.

SECRET #158 Fifty milligrams of iodine/iodide a day acts as an adaptogen.

If you're familiar with iodine at all, it's probably in relation to your thyroid function. But it does much more. It's used throughout the body to help normalize a number of body functions. Iodine is found in breast tissues, the ovaries and testes, parotid glands, and salivary glands.

The RDA for iodine is 0.15 mg—400 times less than the amount Dr. Abraham found was needed for iodine sufficiency. His testing showed that most people need 50 mg of iodine/iodide a day. In this amount, iodine acts as an adaptogen, regulating various body functions.

IODINE INSUFFICIENCY MAY PLAY A ROLE IN THE FOLLOWING CLINICAL DISORDERS:

• Autoimmune thyroiditis	• Hormone resistance syndromes
• Cardiac arrhythmia	• Hypertension
• Diabetes (types I and II)	• Obesity
• Fibrocystic breast disease	• Polycystic ovary syndrome
• Fibromyalgia	• Sleep apnea
• Graves' disease	• Subclinical hypothyroidism

Not just any iodine will do. Kelp and iodized salt just won't give you even close to this amount. Neither will seaweed nor fish, unless you eat enough of them every single day. As I explained in Chapter 1, which you may want to re-read now, some forms of iodine are harmful. Dr. Abraham has used a safe, stable, inorganic, non-radioactive iodine and iodide identical to Lugol's solution, a well-absorbed form of iodine that has been used for 180 years.

SECRET #159 Seven ways iodine normalizes various functions.

Here's what sufficient iodine can do for you::

1. *Normalizes hormone receptors:* Hormones have "parking spaces" called receptors that are reserved for them. These receptors need to have iodine attached to them for optimal function. Without enough iodine, your hormones won't work at their best. If you and your doctor can't explain why the hormones you're taking aren't working the way they should, insufficient iodine may be the reason.

2. *Regulates the thyroid:* Your thyroid gland needs iodine whether it's working normally, is underactive (hypothyroidism) or overactive (hyperthyroidism), or is enlarged (goiter). Enough iodine normalizes all these conditions. See Chapter 1.

3. *Reduces fibromyalgia in patients with low thyroid function:* Dr. Flechas observed some improvement in his fibromyalgia patients on iodine supplementation. This could be because of the effects of bromide on inflammation. Excess bromide displaces iodine. Dr. Abraham has reported that iodine removes bromide from the body, improving fibromyalgia symptoms.

4. *Protects your breasts:* When bromide gets into breast tissues, it displaces iodine, which is essential for breast health. Some women with fibrocystic breast disease find their cysts and tenderness disappear after iodine supplementation. Low levels of iodine have been found in numerous women who were then found to have early breast cancer. Iodine appears to protect against this cancer.

5. *Supports the adrenal glands and stress:* Your adrenal glands need sufficient iodine to function properly and respond to life's many stresses.

6. *Helps the stomach make HCl:* Low hydrochloric acid (HCl) production is frequently caused by iodine insufficiency. We need iodine to pump chloride into stomach cells (hydroCHLORIC acid). Without enough HCl, we can't digest protein or utilize calcium, magnesium, or iron efficiently. As we age, our bodies make less and less HCl. By increasing iodine, you may also be able to increase your body's natural production of HCl.

BROMIDE IN YOUR DRINKS

Mountain Dew, Fresca, and orange Gatorade all contain bromide in the form of brominated vegetable oils. While the manufacturers say the amount is negligible, Dr. Flechas has observed that drinking beverages with bromide caused low thyroid function in some of his patients.

7. *Improves immunity:* Iodine protects us from two toxic elements, fluoride and bromide, by competing with them for a place in our tissues. These toxins are in our water, non-organic foods, and some soft drinks. Bromide is even used in some asthma drugs. If you don't have enough iodine, chances are you have too much fluoride and bromide. Sufficient iodine pulls these toxins out of the body.

SECRET #160 The only way to know if you need iodine, and how much to take, is by getting an iodine-loading test.

In the past, alternative healthcare practitioners suggested painting iodine on the skin and watching how fast it disappears. When the iodine disappeared quickly, it meant you needed more. This test is not accurate. I wish it were. Get a dependable test developed by a doctor and read by a doctor. A twenty-four-hour urine test will show more accurately whether or not you need more iodine.

This test is available for $75 through Dr. Jorge Flechas (see the Resources section). You don't need to have a doctor order this test. You can get a test kit directly from Dr. Flechas. He will send your results and an interpretation to both you and your doctor. If you don't have a doctor to monitor your iodine supplementation, Dr. Flechas will do this for you. He will also see that you get Iodoral, Dr. Abraham's supplement containing both iodine and iodide.

SECRET #161 You can't get enough iodine from your diet.

The Japanese have adequate iodine, but we can't get enough from our diet unless we eat high-iodine seaweed every single day. Why? Because we're extremely deficient. We've been on a low-iodine diet all our lives and they haven't. And it's rare for anyone in this country to eat seaweed daily.

I thought I was getting enough iodine from my supplements and diet but I wanted to know for sure. I took Dr. Abraham's iodine-loading test and it indicated I was very low in iodine. I took Iodoral and noticed more mental clarity, energy, and a better complexion. These positive effects disappeared when I stopped taking it. Needless to say, I'm back on the iodine supplement. I was tested five times in the first year to see whether or not I was still deficient. Even though I could feel iodine's normalizing effects, it took one year of Iodoral to reach sufficiency. But everyone is different. You may find other benefits.

All of us need a combination of iodine and iodide, the two forms of iodine used throughout our bodies. The only supplements containing these two nutrients I know of are Iodoral and the foul-tasting Lugol's solution. See the Resources section for information on where to find Iodoral. Lugol's solution is available through many pharmacies.

Use Your Breath to Stay Sharp and Energized

You can live for days without food and go for hours without water, but stop breathing and you're gone in a matter of minutes.

Oxygen is not only essential to your life, your brain uses a full 25 percent of all the air you breathe. If you're doing mental work, not just exerting yourself physically, you need to take deep breaths to supply your cells with oxygen.

Your lungs may hold an important clue to lagging energy, because fatigue is caused by a deficiency of oxygen in the cells. This is why if you have difficulty concentrating or suffer from fatigue, the first step for you to take could be one that costs you absolutely nothing—a few deep breaths.

SECRET #162 Frequent yawning or sighing can mean you need more oxygen.

Do you breathe shallowly or yawn or sigh frequently? These may be signs that you need more oxygen.

I first became aware of the importance of deep breathing after talking with Karen. She was a therapist who constantly yawned during her clients' therapy sessions. One of them complained to me that Karen's frequent yawning was the reason she decided to look for a different therapist. This client, and apparently others as well, thought she was bored or not paying attention.

Nothing could have been further from the truth. Karen didn't even realize that she was yawning as much as she was. She insisted that she was listening intently to everything her clients said. And she was. Her body was just crying out for more oxygen. By breathing more deeply throughout the day, Karen would have felt more energized. She would have kept her clients as well.

SECRET #163 You can increase your energy with conscious breathing.

Of all your organs, your lungs are the only ones you can control with your will. Think of it. Your heart beats on its own. Your liver performs hundreds of different functions whenever they're needed. But you can consciously fill your lungs with full breaths of air for increased energy or breathe slowly to calm yourself down. Still, few of us breathe consciously. Take more control of your breath. It can directly affect your health and energy.

I discovered the effectiveness of conscious breathing one day when I was kayaking in a local bay. Suddenly, strong winds began to blow against me. Paddling became extremely difficult and I was several miles from my car. I knew it was unlikely that the wind would die down, and I was worried that I'd run out of energy before I reached shore.

My energy began to decrease and I noticed that my breathing was shallow. I was beginning to panic and was taking in very short rapid breaths. "Breathe deeply," I reminded myself. With each stroke, I either took in a breath or exhaled. Within minutes, my energy had returned. I was able to paddle without stopping even once or feeling weak during the hour-long ride back home. Oxygen—and my lungs— rescued me. Now, whenever I'm paddling, I check to make sure that I'm taking in complete breaths. I'm rarely tired even after hours of strenuous exercise.

SECRET #164 You need to become aware of your breathing patterns before you can increase your energy.

Pay attention to your breathing patterns. Do you breathe differently when you're walking, exercising, or sitting? When you're under stress or particularly happy? Before you can change your breathing patterns, you need to be aware of what you've been doing. Notice how your breath changes with different moods and activities and how these changes affect your energy.

Awareness is the key to changing any of our habits, so for the next few days pay more attention to your breathing patterns.

Begin making changes slowly. If you breathe shallowly when you walk or exercise, make a concerted effort to spend a few minutes breathing deeply. Do you sit and type at your computer for hours, barely breathing? Take frequent deep breathing breaks and open up your chest with a simple exercise.

SECRET #165 Increase your energy in five minutes with this simple exercise.

Watch your posture when you're sitting. Are you hunched over or are your shoulders back and your chest open? You can breathe more deeply and easily when your body is in an open position. To help correct the hunched over effect that comes with sitting, stand up and put your arms straight out in front of you at shoulder height. Make two fists, and tighten your arms.

Then bring your hands toward your chest with your elbows out to the sides. Point your elbows toward the ground and try to touch them behind your back. You won't be able to, of course, but you will stretch the muscles that keep your lungs (and heart) shielded, tight, and unable to function at their best. Notice how you can breathe more deeply and easily after this stretch. Pay attention to your increased energy. Repeat this exercise throughout the day.

If you would like to make more significant changes, I suggest you pick up a wonderful little book, *Ways to Better Breathing*. It contains specific, gentle experiments and exercises that will give you more information about your current breathing patterns and tell you how to modify them.

SECRET #166 It's not always smart to breathe deeply.

I lived in Los Angeles for more than thirty years. For a while, I ran on a grassy path beside a busy street every morning with a friend. We thought it was healthy. However, as we ran we took in deep breaths, breathing in the carbon monoxide from car exhausts.

YOU NEED TO BREATHE DEEPLY . . .

- when you're under stress.
- when you're exercising.
- when you need to think clearly.
- when you're tired.
- whenever you think of it.

One day it hit us. This was about the worst thing we could do for our health. We immediately changed our route and ran along the beach. The air was much cleaner. Still, there's not really any clean air in Los Angeles and other major cities, especially during the summer months when the air tends to be heavy and still. When I decided to move to Northern California, a doctor friend of mine said, "Good. You can't be healthy when you're constantly breathing bad air." He was right. I had chronic lung problems all my life. They healed a few years after my move to the country.

Here are a couple of rules for deep breathing:

- Don't breathe polluted air deeply.

- If you live in a heavily polluted area, reduce your exposure to carbon monoxide and other pollutants by exercising as early as you can in the day, and not near busy streets or industries.

SECRET #167 You can use acupressure to clear your lungs when they're congested.

Chinese medicine teaches that energy pathways for each of our organs, called meridians, have points along these meridians that affect particular functions. The lung meridian runs from your collarbone down your arm to the end of your thumb. Lung 7, one of the points along the lung meridian, can help clear congested lungs. This point can be stimulated by rubbing it (acupressure) or by placing a thin needle in it (acupuncture).

To find Lung 7, travel up your wrist along the line of your thumb for three finger widths. Lung 7 is at that point just under the bone that leads to the outside of your thumb. If this point is tender, massage it gently, but deeply, for a minute or two. Repeat this periodically throughout the day and see if it helps your lungs.

SECRET #168 There are effective herbal formulas that are specific to the lungs.

There are a number of herbal formulas that can help strengthen your lungs. My favorite one that is also useful for repairing damaged lungs is called *Usnea barbata*. I talk about it in depth in Chapter 3. Native Americans called Usnea "the lungs of the earth." The tincture form is more potent than the dried form. You can find it in health-food stores or through the Resources section.

Clear Lung Plus is an herbal lung formula that has colloidal silver added to it. The colloidal silver works best for people with bronchitis, pneumonia, and chronic coughs. I prefer using it only when Usnea isn't strong enough. Use products with colloidal silver sparingly. It is antibiotic and antibacterial, but you don't want to kill off beneficial bacteria by using it for more than a week or two.

Keep your lungs healthy and breathe deeply. You'll increase your energy, and improve your overall health at the same time.

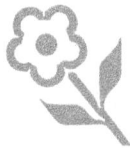

CHAPTER 22

Five Ways to
End Sudden Bouts
of Depression

S ome people are chronically depressed. They often have a chemical imbalance and either need to be on medication or should see a doctor of integrative medicine for an evaluation. Specific supplements, including the right amino acids, are natural ways to reverse some types of chronic depression. If you are depressed because of a chemical imbalance, I want you to know that there are answers. However, you're not likely to find them on your own.

I'm talking here about a different type of depression—temporary depression. It's the "down" side of life's ups and downs. All of us get depressed at times, such as when a good friend moves away or dies, or during the holidays when we're alone. We may also get depressed from lack of sunlight during dark winter months, or when we listen to the news.

I used to sit around reading escape novels and watching TV when I would get depressed. And I would eat anything with chocolate. Now I know that inactivity and sugar are sure-fire ways of turning temporary blahs into chronic depression. I've consolidated a lot of information on depression into a five-step program, because when you're depressed, you need something that's simple. If five steps are too many, just do the first one. It will help you move on to the rest.

Put a copy of these five steps on your refrigerator. Then you'll know where to look when you or your friends are feeling down and can't get up.

SECRET #169 Force yourself to take this first step. You'll feel the effects immediately.

Step One: Keep moving. Hundreds of studies show that regular exercise improves your mood as much as medication. It releases endorphins, "feel good" chemicals made in your brain, such as serotonin. The more you sit around and stew in your depression, the lower your endorphins are likely to be.

I know. The last thing you want to do when you're depressed is exercise. But it's the most important step you can take. I've been exercising regularly for more than a year, and there are days when I feel blue and don't want to do anything but take a nap. Instead, I force myself to go to the gym and get on the treadmill or exercise bike with a good book. Reading helps distract me so I can exercise longer. Within twenty to thirty minutes, I have more energy and feel better emotionally.

It may take more time or less time for you to get these effects. But once you've experienced them, you'll know just how vital exercise is to your mood and energy.

Force yourself to get out and walk. In fact, if it's still daylight, get up right now and walk for just twenty minutes. Then check off each day you exercise on your calendar. You need to exercise four or five times a week to beat depression. Daily is even better.

Both exercise and exposure to bright lights reduce depression. You can make your exercise doubly effective by exercising outdoors or in a well-lit room. This will give better results than walking on a treadmill in a dim room. Walk around your neighborhood. Drive to a lake, river, the ocean, or the mountains once a week. Being in nature and experiencing its vastness is healing, says psychotherapist Sara Harris who often combines counseling with walks. She's right. When I feel "down," I go to the river and kayak. It always lifts me out of my blahs.

SECRET #170 It's more difficult to be depressed when you're alone than with someone who cares about you.

Step Two: Don't isolate yourself. This second step is not much easier than the first one. When you feel depressed it's difficult to reach out to others. But, that's just what you need to do. When you're depressed, you're focusing inward. It's natural to immerse yourself in negative thoughts when you have nothing to distract you.

Stop making excuses. Your friends love you even when you're feeling down. They want to help you as much as you want to help them when they're in need.

Pick up the phone and make a date with a friend or friends to get together. Invite them over if you can't get out. You don't have to invite someone over for a meal. A cup of coffee or tea is enough.

Look for activities that will distract you and take your mind off your problems. Arrange to go for a walk and exercise with a friend. Ask someone to help you pick out a new pair of shoes. Reach out, even if you don't feel like it. If no one you know is available to get together, volunteer your services at a church, hospital, senior center, or non-profit organization. Offer to help out one time for just a few hours. If you like it, do it regularly. You'll meet new people and feel better being around others.

SECRET #171 Foods affect your moods differently.

Step Three: Eat healthy foods. Some foods will add to your depression. Others have the opposite effect. For instance, it's important to eat enough protein—as much as 15–20 grams with each meal. You need protein to help make mood-regulating chemicals. Protein also helps keep your blood sugar from dropping. Low blood sugar can cause fatigue and temporary depression.

Avoid any foods that trigger a low blood sugar response, such as sugar (honey, pure cane sugar juice, etc.), alcohol, fruit juices, and high quantities of refined carbohydrates (bread, crackers, white rice). Get junk foods out of the house today, or put them in tins if they must be around for other family members. When you want something sweet, eat a piece of fruit. Often, your craving for other sweets will lessen.

Eat small amounts of unrefined carbohydrates such as beans, fresh fruit, and brown rice. They help your brain release serotonin. Half a cup of a starch, such as brown rice or potatoes, or one piece of fruit, is a reasonably small amount.

Make eating good foods easy by planning in advance. Buy healthy frozen meals, especially those that are organic. Get pre-washed, pre-cut salad greens and vegetables to either eat raw or to sauté with your entree. Have some bean dip on hand to eat for a meal or as a snack with carrots and celery. Buy healthy prepared soups, either dried, frozen, or in boxes. You can find these at your health-food store or in the health food section of your supermarket.

SECRET #172 The reason St. John's wort is so effective is due to its side effect.

Step Four: Use supplements. There's been a lot of bad press surrounding St. John's wort (*Hypericum perforatum*), and much of it has been due to poor studies or poor interpretations of good studies. It's the most popular and well-studied herb for minor and moderate depression. In fact, St. John's wort has been tested head-to-head with Prozac. The bottom-line is: It often works just as well as the drug with fewer side effects.

One reason St. John's wort works is because of its side effect. It causes photosensitivity—a sensitivity to sunlight. Bright light therapy helps reduce depression. By increasing your sensitivity to light, St. John's wort magnifies the effects of normal light. It acts just as if you're being exposed to continuous light therapy.

The daily dosage of St. John's wort varies from 300–900 mg a day. Try it for at least a month. For a more thorough explanation of its actions, you'll want to read *St. John's Wort: Nature's Blues Buster* by Dr. Hyla Cass. One warning: St. John's wort can reduce the effectiveness of some medications. If you take any drugs at all, consult with your doctor or pharmacist before taking this herb.

SECRET #173 This supplement helps your body produce natural antidepressants.

Serotonin, a neurotransmitter made in your brain, is one of your body's natural antidepressants. One reason why some people are depressed is a lack of serotonin production. Here's what happens: Neurotransmitters carry messages to your brain cells. When the levels of neurotransmitters are unstable they can trigger a change in your mood. In addition to depression, low serotonin production can cause a variety of symptoms, including obsessive thinking, anxiety, violent behavior, alcohol and drug abuse, premenstrual syndrome, and increased sensitivity to pain.

SECRET #174 Why 5-HTP is a better and safer choice than SSRI drugs.

Medical doctors treat depression induced by low serotonin levels with medications called SSRIs (selective serotonin re-uptake inhibitors). These drugs increase your body's production of serotonin. A growing number of doctors and other health practitioners who use integrative medicine are now suggesting 5-HTP, a safe form of tryptophan, as an alternative. Tryptophan is an amino acid that helps your body make serotonin. If your depression is not due to a lack of serotonin, 5-HTP may not be your answer. If it is, however, you may be on your way to a more natural, safer type of serotonin-producer than SSRIs.

Prozac is the first SSRI that came on the market in 1987. Today, more than six million people in this country alone use it regularly. In fact, Prozac was considered so effective as an antidepressant that other pharmaceutical companies came out with their own SSRI medications like Zoloft and Paxil. One problem with SSRIs is the side effects they may cause. These include headaches, nausea, anxiety (just what it's supposed to treat!), insomnia, drowsiness, diarrhea, and on and on. SSRIs also cause a lack of libido. This side effect alone is enough to make you depressed!

More than a dozen studies using 5-HTP for depression have appeared since the early 1970s. These have included more than 500 people with various kinds of depression, including some seriously depressed patients. More than 50 percent of the patients were significantly improved after taking 5-HTP. In a Swiss study, 5-HTP was compared with SSRIs. Both groups improved. Slightly more people on 5-HTP improved over those taking conventional antidepressants. In addition, there were fewer side effects with people taking 5-HTP. The most common side effects were mild nausea or slight gastrointestinal discomfort, and these usually disappeared within a few days.

The dosage of 5-HTP for depression is usually 50 mg, three times a day with meals. After a few weeks, if there is not sufficient response, it can be increased to 100 mg three times daily. 5-HTP should not be taken along with Prozac or other SSRIs. Check with your doctor before taking this supplement, especially if you're on any medication for depression. A month's supply of good quality 5-HTP will cost between $25–$30.

SECRET #175 In spite of what the FDA said, tryptophan is safe.

Tryptophan is an amino acid that was taken off the market in 1985 when a batch from Japan was found to have a bacterial contamination. This contamination led to a chronic debilitating condition called eosinophilia myalgia. No one in the supplement industry I talked to was surprised. They told me that this particular manufacturing plant was less stringent in its quality control than was thought to be prudent. This was an accident waiting to happen.

The FDA managed to restrict tryptophan sales to doctors only, and the price skyrocketed. This damaged the supplement industry and made tryptophan both unaffordable and difficult to obtain for those people who found it to be helpful. I was in close contact with the company that produced a tryptophan powder that the FDA used in their tests as their level of purity. This tryptophan reversed eosinophilia myalgia. Nevertheless, tryptophan remains off the over-the-counter market.

SECRET #176 Why 5-HTP is better and safer than tryptophan for depression.

Before tryptophan can affect the neurotransmitters in your brain, it has to be converted in your body into 5-HTP. Then 5-HTP, with the help of vitamin B_6 and magnesium, converts into serotonin. When you take 5-HTP, you start out a step ahead on the process. It's a faster way of making serotonin than taking tryptophan.

Much of the 5-HTP found in health-food stores is extracted from the seeds of a plant called *Griffonia simplicifolia*. This means it's safer than tryptophan. While any product, from SSRIs and other prescription drugs to processed foods can become contaminated, bacteria are not present in large quantities in 5-HTP.

The risk for contamination in 5-HTP is very, very low no matter what you may have heard.

Several years ago, researchers at the Mayo Clinic implied that contamination in 5-HTP had, indeed, occurred. They found indications that all six samples of the 5-HTP they had tested had markers they claimed were similar in chemical structure to two contaminants once found in the batch of tryptophan from the 1980s. However, none of the contaminants in the tryptophan have ever been identified as the ones that caused eosinophilia myalgia.

The research from the Mayo Clinic was not published in a peer-reviewed journal (this is what often separates good science from possibly bad science). It was published as a letter to the editor in *Nature Medicine* journal in September 1998, a dozen years after the tryptophan contamination issue occurred.

There is no indication at present that 5-HTP has any contaminants that can cause problems. If you decide to use 5-HTP, get it from the best source possible. Preferably, from a company known to you or your healthcare provider.

SECRET #177 Aromatherapy can help you move through your depression more rapidly.

Step Five: Use fragrances to heal your emotions. Particular fragrances have specific effects. I talk about flower essences in Chapter 20, but there are highly concentrated fragrances made from plants that also affect the emotions. They're called essential oils.

Essential oils are usually used topically. Never take them internally unless you are under the care of a healthcare practitioner skilled in using them. They are powerful enough to cause side effects when they're ingested. However, you can safely rub a few drops on your wrist, put them in your bath, or add them to oil and give your hands or feet an aromatherapy massage.

Aromatherapy massage has been the subject of several studies. Perhaps the most impressive one was conducted in a hospice. All depressed patients who were given massages with added lavender oil had dramatically improved moods. If it worked for their depression, essential oils should work for yours. You can find them in all healthfood stores and in many bath accessory stores. Use only pure essential oils. Synthetic ones won't work as well. Here are a few to try.

SECRET #178 These four essential oils reduce depression.

Lavender is not just a popular and light fragrance. It's known for its ability to lift depression. It relaxes and stimulates, calms and invigorates.

Ravensera is energizing and uplifting. It helps relieve chronic depression and promotes energy and mental clarity.

Bitter orange (Citrus aurantium, or neroli) helps lift anxiety, depression, nervousness, and insomnia.

Patchouli calms the nerves, improves concentration, and lifts depression.

A Final Note: Remember that everything changes. Today's depression will turn into tomorrow's peacefulness and joy if you'll allow it. Concentrate on everything you have rather than what you don't have. Appreciate each little blessing.

CHAPTER 23

This Homeopathic Can Heal Your Grief Quickly

You know that the loss of a loved one, or any other tragedy, is difficult to handle emotionally. While the grieving process usually passes eventually, sometimes it hangs on, unchanged. In these cases, or when grief first hits, there's a simple remedy that's extremely effective. Let me show you how it helped me, and how you can expect similar results.

Two and a half months after my mother died, I still found myself bursting into tears for no apparent reason. The profound sadness that welled up inside me took me by surprise. It wouldn't leave me. It didn't lessen. So this is part of the natural grieving process, I told myself. It will eventually pass. But it didn't. It remained, unchanged, until a friend reminded me of a particular homeopathic remedy. I took a single dose of it and my intense grief vanished permanently. I'm still sad at times, of course, but I'm no longer overwhelmed with sadness and tears.

This friend, Cathie-Ann Lippman, is a psychiatrist in Los Angeles who works with integrative medicine. We occasionally consult with one another over difficult cases and her insights have been extraordinarily helpful to me. In the past, Cathie-Ann has been right on the money. This time was no exception. Her advice? Take "Ignatia 30C."

"Ignatia is a homeopathic remedy that's specifically for acute grieving," she reminded me. "Use the 30C potency and take three or four pellets. If you need to, you can repeat it once or twice daily."

SECRET #179 Energy medicine is a powerful tool for healing the body and mind.

The term homeopathy is from the Greek words "homios" (similar) and "pathos" (suffering). This means that a substance causing a negative symptom in a healthy person can help heal a sick person with the same symptom. In other words, "like cures like." Homeopathic supplements are tiny amounts of greatly diluted substances that have a subtle but often profound effect on the body. For instance, if you have poison ivy, you would take a homeopathic remedy called Rhus toxicodendron, which contains minute quantities of poison ivy. Instead of making you worse, you'd get better.

Unlike essential oils, homeopathic remedies have been "watered down" so many times that they no longer contain the substance they were made from. Instead, they have the "energy" of that substance.

The trick is to take the right remedy with the right potency at the right time. Dana Ullman, M.P.H., is a homeopath, the author of nine books on homeopathy, and a friend. Over the years he found that, "When you hit the right remedy, the results are substantial." They were for me. I took one dose of Ignatia 30C and my intense emotional reactions disappeared as if I had turned off a water faucet.

SECRET #180 How to know when Ignatia is the best remedy to help you through your grief.

Ignatia isn't the only remedy for grief. There are others. But it is the most appropriate homeopathic to use for the first stage of a new heartache. Use it when there's been a recent death or breakup, or when you move and miss your close friends.

Ignatia is effective for those times when you hold in your emotions and don't break down in front of other people. It is helpful for grief that's expressed with frequent sighing, a lump in your throat, or uncontrollable crying and extreme sadness.

If your grief is old, try Natrum muriaticum 30C instead. It's more appropriate for chronic grieving. You can take Natrum mur. either by itself or with Ignatia. Most health-food stores sell homeopathic remedies. There are many different potencies for each remedy. Generally, the 30C potency is most appropriate for new grief. Your local health-food store can usually order Ignatia if it's not in stock.

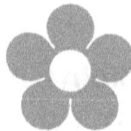

CHAPTER 24

Friendship Reduces Stress

We are social animals. Even those of us who are hermits know that we are "people who need people." There's a physiological reason for our need to form close relationships with others. In fact, friendship reduces stress. I know you've experienced it. Now I'd like to explain how and why it's so important for you to find time to spend with a good friend. I make sure I do this regularly.

Almost every week, I find time to see my friend Lydia. We don't do anything much. We have breakfast, shop, and talk about what's going on in our lives. We go to a movie or have a cup of tea. But spending time with Lydia and my other girlfriends is both nourishing and calming. All of us get more than the emotional response that comes from enjoying one another's company. Our friendships actually trigger a hormonal response that reduces stress.

SECRET #181 Women benefit more from friendships than men.

I've noticed for a long time how we women seem to have more close friends than men. We tend to talk over our problems with one another more than they do, especially during times of stress. But until recently, I didn't realize that there's a biochemical reason for this. Friendship reduces stress in women more than in men, and the reason is fascinating. It begins with our basic survival mechanism and carries over into other areas of our lives. Our friendships with other women keep us calm and healthier by stimulating the same hormones that are released during breast-feeding and labor. If anyone you know says you're wasting your time hanging out with a girlfriend, tell him (or her) that it's a natural form of hormone therapy!

SECRET #182 "Fight or flight" is a male response. "Tend and befriend" is our response.

Remember hearing about the stress mechanism known as the fight-or-flight response? It's based on the idea that when you're cornered by a saber-toothed tiger, your body produces the hormone adrenaline. Adrenaline gives you enough immediate strength to fight the tiger or enough speed to outrun it. Personally, I never identified with the description of the fight-or-flight response. There aren't many saber-toothed tigers where I live and, if there were, I'd look for a hole to crawl into and wait the tiger out much like our female ancestors did. "Fight or flight" never felt much like "me." Now I know why. It's more of a male response.

We women are our children's nurturers and protectors. We shield them from harm rather than fight our way out of dangerous situations. We band together with other women and their children, sharing resources for our mutual benefit. And we create and maintain these social groups to help us through stressful situations. Shelley E. Taylor and a group of other researchers on human behavior at the University of California, Los Angeles, calls this response "tend and befriend."

We pass these social interactions on to our children. This type of communication and caring has a direct effect on their future friendships. My parents had a close circle of friends that were their extended family. My brother and I have formed similar bonds with close friends who live near us. Now I realize this was no accident.

Children who bond to their mothers and other children during their early years have an easier time forming close relationships when they become adults. So, the depth of the friendships we have today is based upon the early attachments we formed when we were young—along with the release of a chemical that's found more in women than in men called oxytocin.

SECRET #183 Friendship activates the same calming hormone that's released during breast-feeding.

Oxytocin is a hormone with a calming effect that is released by our pituitary gland when we're stressed. It is one of the earliest hormones released during a number of different forms of stress. It stimulates the uterus to contract during labor and promotes the release of milk during breast-feeding.

Oxytocin reduces anxiety and has a mild sedative effect both during labor and nursing and at other times as well. It balances cortisol, the stress hormone produced by your adrenal glands to handle a fight-or-flight response. Cortisol is stimulating; oxytocin is calming. Studies indicate that oxytocin appears to reduce blood pressure, depression, and aggression.

Women have more oxytocin than men, and the effects of this hormone are enhanced in the presence of estrogen. In fact, estrogen's influences on oxytocin production are some of the most powerful of all estrogenic effects. Postmenopausal women on hormone therapy release more oxytocin than those who do not take estrogen. If you're not using hormone therapy and feel anxious, you can still produce oxytocin. You may just need to stimulate its production a bit more often. You can do this by spending more time with your friends. Fortunately, the effects from this hormone are long lasting, which may be why a weekly "fix" with a friend can be so satisfying.

> Oxytocin is released during stress. It reduces anxiety and stimulates social contact. Social contact, in turn, promotes the production of more oxytocin. When you're anxious, spend time with a friend.

Sadness decreases oxytocin levels, but researchers found that close friendships can help keep oxytocin high during times of sadness or distress.

Colds, flu, and chronic diseases like coronary heart disease can result from wear and tear on the sympathetic nervous system, the pituitary, and the adrenal glands. Oxytocin reduces this wear and tear, protecting you from stress-related illnesses.

SECRET #184 Massage increases oxytocin.

Touch is healing. In fact, it can produce more oxytocin. Oxytocin levels increase after a relaxing massage, so consider getting regular massages for your own stress reduction. I have one massage every month. The feeling of well-being I experience afterward goes beyond the physiological release that occurs when tense muscles relax. You can either get a full-body massage from a massage therapist or exchange a foot, hand, or shoulder massage with a friend.

Remember that sadness lowers oxytocin levels and friendship raises it. When stress strikes you, don't be a hermit, even if this is your tendency. Whether or not you want to talk over your problems or just spend quiet time with someone, it's important to call a girlfriend and up your production of oxytocin!

When someone you care about is going through difficult times, reach out and spend time with her. It will help raise her calming hormone levels when she's anxious or sad and help reduce her anxiety. If you don't know what to say, don't say anything at all. Often, Lydia and I don't talk. We just enjoy being with one another. We found that we don't need any words to help produce oxytocin. Just the presence of a friend.

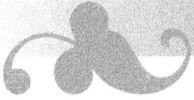

PART 5

NEW WAYS to
CONTROL YOUR PAIN

Pain-control therapy is often limited to choosing one drug or another. If one pharmaceutical isn't effective, perhaps another one will be. And when prescription and over-the-counter pain medications were found to have life-threatening side effects, pharmaceutical companies began to look at other painkillers that might not cause heart attacks and stroke. The problem is that the FDA and pharmaceutical companies continue to look in the same places for safer solutions. This is because they're looking for solutions that can be patented.

All pharmaceuticals have side effects. Some are more dangerous than others. Safe, natural solutions already exist, but there's less profit in an herb or vitamin that can't be patented. As long as we continue to fill ourselves with synthetically produced substances, some people will have uncomfortable or life-threatening side effects.

Magnesium, and the herb feverfew, can relieve the pain from migraine headaches in many people. But drug therapy is much more lucrative. Which is worse: dying of a stroke from taking a patented painkiller or having loose stools from taking too much magnesium?

There are other pain-relieving therapies that have been studied for decades and used by physicians. They still have not gained respect from the mainstream medical community. Prolotherapy is one of them. It can totally erase pain caused by loose ligaments through a series of sugar-water injections! My own knee pain vanished after a series of prolotherapy sessions. So did the tendonitis in my elbow I'd had for more than a year.

There are many safe, effective therapies that can reduce or eliminate your chronic pain. Not all of them will work for you. My hope is that you'll find some new information in this section that can lead you to a more comfortable pain-free life. Through my research and my experience with patients, I know it's often possible.

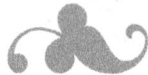

CHAPTER 25

Sugar-Water Injections Could Save You from Chronic Pain and Surgery

If you have chronic pain, chances are you've tried many therapies including anti-inflammatory drugs, nutrients, physical therapy, and self-help techniques like massage, exercise, and stretching. Sometimes it seems like there's no permanent answer.

I think the reason for this is because pain is often treated with a Band-Aid approach. What I mean is that many therapies work by blocking pain receptors or increasing circulation. However, they don't address the bottom-line cause of the pain. As the Health Detective, I'm always looking for the underlying reason behind any problem. And unstable ligaments that lead to inflammation often cause chronic pain. These weak ligaments can be strengthened, and when this happens pain decreases or disappears.

SECRET #185 Your pain may be in your ligaments, not in your muscles.

Muscles and ligaments are different structures. Muscles are large, strong tissues with a good blood supply, while ligaments are smaller tissues with a poor blood supply. Muscles heal quickly because they get plenty of blood. Ligaments heal slowly and incompletely because they have a decreased blood supply.

Aging doesn't help. As years go by, and as we reduce our mobility by not exercising enough, our ligaments get weaker and more lax. Weak ligaments are more easily injured. You might not think that there's a way to strengthen and tighten weak and damaged ligaments and stop chronic pain, but there is. It's a technique called prolotherapy.

SECRET #186 Prolotherapy works by correcting the cause of pain.

Prolotherapy works by strengthening weak, relaxed ligaments that cause joints to loosen. The muscles around weak ligaments contract to help stabilize the joint. This causes pain from tight muscles. You can't just relax these muscles with heat and massage. Even a good blood supply to your muscles isn't enough. You need to strengthen the ligaments to stop the muscles from contracting. Since many ligaments have been injured for long periods of time, when these ligaments are treated, people who have had pain for many years can be cured. *Prolotherapy gives lasting relief because it corrects the cause of the pain.*

SECRET #187 Prolotherapy has been used successfully for fifty years.

Prolotherapy isn't new. It was originally called sclerotherapy and developed in the 1950s by H. I. Biegeleisen to treat varicose veins. But the Father of Prolotherapy, George S. Hackett, M.D., wrote a book on the subject in 1955 and used prolotherapy extensively to rid more than 10,000 patients of chronic pain during his career.

Prolotherapy is not yet a mainstream approach although it should be. Fewer than 1,500 physicians are using it in this country. It is well thought of by respected doctors like former Surgeon General C. Everett Koop, M.D. Dr. Koop has never been considered to be on the cutting edge of complementary medicine, yet he has come out in support of prolotherapy as an excellent method of eliminating pain.

Dr. Thomas Dorman first introduced me to the concept of prolotherapy more than a dozen years ago. He was a physician I met at a nutrition seminar in Southern California. Dr. Dorman explained that he specialized in a technique called prolotherapy. It turns out that he not only researched this technique, he wrote the textbook for other doctors!

Dr. Dorman used prolotherapy for years on seniors with osteoarthritis. Prolotherapy improved their range of motion and decreased their pain. He began using it when he was an internist. In 1987, Dr. Dorman published the results of a double-blind study on prolotherapy and low back pain. He conducted the study with rheumatologist Robert Klein, M.D., in Santa Barbara, California, on more than eighty patients who had at least ten years of pain. Of the people who were given prolotherapy treatments, 88 percent of them experienced moderate to marked improvement.

And he's even found a great number of other conditions for which this technique is appropriate. Prolotherapy can help osteoarthritis, knee pain, back pain, neck pain, fibromyalgia, old whiplash injuries, carpal tunnel syndrome, degenerated or herniated discs, sports injuries, sciatic pain, TMJ (jaw) pain, and partially torn tendons, ligaments, and cartilage.

SECRET #188 You may not need prolotherapy. You may just need to drink more water.

Still, while some people think of prolotherapy as being a miracle, it's not appropriate for everyone. For instance, if your pain is coming from rheumatoid arthritis (RA), prolotherapy is not likely to help. RA is not caused by loose or damaged ligaments.

Often, dehydration causes joint pain, which progresses to stiffness. Before you go hunting for a doctor who uses prolotherapy, first make sure you're drinking enough water!

SECRET #189 Prolotherapy causes an inflammation that rebuilds and strengthens ligaments.

It sounds crazy, but prolotherapy works by injecting an irritant solution into areas where ligaments are weak or damaged—at the place where ligaments and tendons attach to the bone. The solution is made from sugar water, saltwater, or a vitamin C solution. What happens next is an example of how the body heals itself, and is why I think prolotherapy is such a clever concept. It actually tricks your body into making stronger, healthier ligaments.

The solution that's injected into the weakened ligament causes a low-grade inflammation. The cells that are part of your immune system (called macrophages) then move in to remove the irritant solution and any ligament debris. The job of macrophages is to act as scavengers and remove old cells and cellular debris. When the macrophages are finished cleaning up damaged ligaments, cells called fibroblasts that produce collagen and elasticin rebuild the ligaments. The new ligament that is rebuilt as a result of these injections is stronger than the original one—sometimes as much as 40 percent stronger! What's more, the treatments lead to a faster regrowth of cartilage. This means that you're left with stronger, more stable connective tissue and less pain both now and in the future.

Don't think that all of this happens in one quick treatment. It doesn't. You might need only four to six treatments to get rid of your chronic pain, or you might need more than ten. A doctor who uses this technique can probably give you a good idea of whether or not prolotherapy is appropriate for you and, after an initial treatment or two, approximately how many sessions you will need. The good news is that scientific studies on prolotherapy indicate that it cures chronic pain in 92 percent of cases for which it has been deemed appropriate. What's so nice about this technique is that it can't hurt you to try it. As Dr. Koop says, "How could placing a little sugar water at the junction of a ligament with a bone be harmful to a patient?"

SECRET #190 Prolotherapy corrects other painful knee problems.

As we age, we all have some signs of wear and tear in our knees. Arthroscopy removes bits of torn cartilage caused by arthritis, injury, or infection, and trims torn structures in the knee. A surgeon can undoubtedly find and remove some debris in a painful knee. There are times when arthroscopic surgery is the perfect solution to knee pain. But if your pain comes from a knee that isn't tracking properly, it won't solve anything. That's what I found for myself.

One morning, I kneeled down to look under my bed. "Ouch!!" I had a sharp pain on the outside of my left knee. I touched the spot and it was tender. Apparently, I had bumped my knee without paying much attention to it. I expected the pain would get better in a few days, but it didn't.

Two months later, my knee was still extremely painful if I knelt on it. So I paid a visit to my favorite doctor, Terri Turner, D.O. Dr. Turner is an osteopath, and osteopaths are medical doctors who are skilled in manipulating bones and muscles when they're misaligned. I knew she'd do more than give me a prescription for a pain pill, and I was right.

After my exam, she announced, "Your knee's not tracking properly. If you don't do anything, the pain will gradually increase." Most doctors would then recommend arthroscopic surgery.

Instead, Dr. Turner adjusted my knee. In fact, she adjusted it three times. But the adjustments didn't hold because the ligaments that keep the knee in place were loose. To compensate for flabby ligaments, the muscles around them tightened, causing pain.

Dr. Turner's solution to strengthen my weak ligaments was prolotherapy.

Let me share my experience of prolotherapy with you so you'll know what to expect if you have some treatments. It hurts!

Prolotherapy treatments are painful, even with pain-killing lidocaine added to the solution. It's not unbearable, but it's darn uncomfortable. After being injected with the solution, the area may become hot and sore for a day or two. This is a result of the inflammation. Ice packs help reduce this temporary pain, but you can't take aspirin, Advil, or Motrin. They are anti-inflammatory medications and this is one time when you *want* inflammation. If you're taking anti-inflammatory herbs, nutrients, or medications, it's important to stop taking them temporarily.

The number of prolotherapy treatments needed to strengthen loose ligaments varies. In my case, I had four injections for the inside ligament of my knee, and two for the outside ligament. After the first two treatments, I was surprised to find that there was very little pain or discomfort.

Would I do prolotherapy again? In a heartbeat. Especially if it means avoiding surgery. Prolotherapy didn't just remove my pain. It corrected the problem!

SECRET #191 Prolotherapy works for pain in other parts of your body.

Prolotherapy has been used to successfully eliminate chronic back pain, shoulder pain, carpal tunnel syndrome, migraines, chronic neck pain, sports injuries, arthritis, and fibromyalgia. If you have chronic pain that's caused by loose ligaments or tendons, consider prolotherapy. If you don't know whether or not loose or damaged ligaments are causing your chronic pain, get an evaluation from a doctor skilled in this technique. You can find them through organizations listed in the Resources section at the end of this book.

SECRET #192 The cost for prolotherapy treatments varies considerably.

How much does all of this cost? It depends on the doctor you see and how many sessions you need. A single treatment can range from $90 to $200. Even if you need ten treatments, the total cost is considerably less than the $5,000 or more needed for back or neck surgery. Some insurance policies cover prolotherapy treatments. Medicare does. If, like me, you can find a doctor who uses prolotherapy who accepts Medicare, your treatments won't cost you a penny. And prolotherapy treatments save insurance companies thousands of dollars over the years. Most of all, they can get rid of your chronic pain.

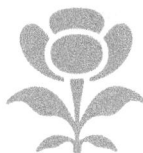

CHAPTER 26

Say Goodbye
to Migraines

Anyone who has experienced the pain of a migraine knows how disabling it can be. These vise-like headaches can come without warning and may be accompanied by sensitivity to bright lights, nausea, anxiety, and disturbed thinking. They can last for hours or days, upsetting your life and the lives of people around you.

Migraines affect up to 30 percent of women, twice as many as men. Traditionally, migraines are treated with various pharmaceuticals from ibuprofen and antihistamines to stronger drugs such as Inderal and Imitrex. These medications tend to have unpleasant side effects. There's no one cause for migraines, so you may need to be a bit of a detective to figure out what causes your headaches and which solution might be best for you. The beauty of integrative medicine is that it offers multiple views of any condition.

SECRET #193 Here's what you can do to prevent a full-blown migraine.

Pay attention to early warning signs. Up to 60 percent of people with migraines get a warning up to a day before the headache begins. It's called a prodrome, and its symptoms include depression, food cravings, fatigue, yawning, and urinary retention. Be aware of how you feel prior to a migraine. If you have a migraine prodrome, you can begin treatment before you have a full-blown migraine. You may even prevent its onset, especially if you can identify its source. So put on your detective hat and start unraveling the mystery of migraines. When you find one or more possible causes, match them to the appropriate solutions.

SECRET #194 Weak ligaments and unstable blood vessels can cause migraines.

Weak ligaments in the neck: Dr. Ross Hauser, physician and author of numerous books on prolotherapy says, "Prolotherapy is the best curative treatment for migraine headaches." He finds the most common cause to be weak ligaments in the neck. If you get a pain or tightness in your neck just before a migraine begins, it's an indication that your headache might be from weak ligaments and is likely to respond very well to prolotherapy.

Unstable blood vessels: Migraines can be caused by an abnormality in blood vessel constriction and dilation due to unstable blood vessels. In this case, large blood vessels become dilated (widened) while smaller blood vessels constrict. This prevents normal blood flow and causes pain.

Serotonin: Platelets and small blood vessels store serotonin (a "feel good" chemical made in the brain), which helps blood vessels relax and constrict. Some people with migraines have platelets that clump together more than normal and release excessive amounts of serotonin. As serotonin levels increase, migraines occur. Often, a mitral valve prolapse is present as well. Known as a leaky heart valve, this condition can damage platelets, continuing the circle of pain.

SECRET #195 Too much, or too little, serotonin can cause migraines.

Migraines may be caused by too much or too little serotonin. The drug Imitrex and monamine oxidase (MAO) inhibitors increase serotonin production and are suggested for migraines that occur from too little serotonin. But there's a safer and more natural treatment: 5-HTP, a natural serotonin precursor. It can give you similar results without side effects. You can find this supplement in natural-food stores.

Vitamin B_6 is also needed to help produce serotonin. Be sure to get enough of both 5-HTP and B_6. I suggest 25 mg of vitamin B_6 along with 100–200 milligrams (mg) of 5-HTP three times a day. Using these nutrients for two or three months may prevent your migraines from recurring.

SECRET #196 Substance P causes food-related migraines.

Stress: Chronic stress triggers the production of a pain-producing substance by nerve cells called "substance P." Substance P dilates blood vessels and releases allergic compounds like histamines. Both food allergies and chronic stress may be implicated in this type of migraine. This explains why some people get migraines when they're under stress and eat a particular food. At other times, they may eat the same food yet not be under enough stress to cause a migraine.

Food sensitivities: Any food can cause a migraine, but some foods are more closely associated with them. Foods high in chemicals called amines, including phenylethylamine (in chocolate and aged cheeses) and tyramine (in red wine, beer, dairy, nuts, citrus, and beans), commonly trigger migraines. I know it's inconvenient to eliminate so many foods. But a study in the *Lancet* found that 93 percent of people with migraines improved when they stopped eating these trigger foods. So it's highly likely you could benefit from an elimination diet!

SECRET #197 A sensitivity to any food can cause migraines.

Whether you're sensitive to foods high in amines or some other foods, one or more of them could be the source of your problem. A migraine-provoking food could be something you eat in a large quantity, such as a glass of milk or some yogurt, or in small amounts like the dairy in a ranch-style salad dressing. Food reactions are difficult to identify because an allergic reaction like a migraine doesn't always occur right after you eat. It can take as long as seventy-two hours.

Keep a food diary and look for any patterns between particular foods and headaches. If you suspect one, eliminate that food in all forms for at least three months. Then test it by eating it alone. If you have no reaction, you can try eating it again in small amounts. Don't eat it more than once or twice a week, however. You don't want that sensitivity to come back. In addition to amines listed above, the foods found to be most likely to cause headaches are beef, yeast, and sugar (corn and cane).

Low blood sugar (hypoglycemia) is another possible reason for migraines. Some people have a defect in the way their bodies utilize glucose, causing dips in their glucose levels even when they eat a healthy diet. Low blood sugar, or fasting, can either prevent or cause a migraine.

If refined sugar, alcohol, potatoes, or other foods that turn into sugar quickly trigger your headache, look to your blood sugar for the cause and solution to your pain. Chromium is a mineral that helps regulate blood sugar levels. Try taking 200–400 micrograms (mcg) of chromium picolinate three times a day. Keep your blood sugar level stable by eating every four to five hours and get some protein at each meal.

SECRET #198 Too little acid can cause migraines.

Alkalosis: Florida dentist Steven N. Green, D.D.S., found that alkalosis (too little acid) can bring on a migraine. His solution is to take two grams of a powdered vitamin C with mineral ascorbates every hour until the migraine subsides. If you're prone to migraines, keep a dozen packets of easily available Emergen-C handy. Dr. Green uses Super Gram III, a comprehensive vitamin C product, which also can be found in natural-food stores, many drugstores, and some supermarkets. It's worth trying.

SECRET #199 A copper imbalance can contribute to migraines.

Copper can trigger a migraine, especially if you have an abnormal copper metabolism or consume high quantities of this mineral. Some alcoholic beverages, such as red wine, beer, and whiskey, are distilled in copper stills. Some water supplies travel through copper pipes. Foods naturally high in copper include shellfish, wheat germ, chocolate, soy, and nuts. Citrus increases your body's absorption of this mineral. Talk with your healthcare practitioner about getting a hair analysis or other assay of your copper levels. Avoid eating too many of the above foods and beverages and make sure your multivitamin and mineral formula is free of copper.

When copper levels are too high, zinc tends to be too low. The result of this imbalance can be anything from fatigue to migraines. For more information on how to identify and correct this imbalance, read *Why Am I Always So Tired?* by Ann Louise Gittleman. When you increase your zinc, copper levels come down.

SECRET #200 This mineral may be all you need for your migraines.

Magnesium: I'm a huge advocate of this mineral. Over the past twenty years, I found that a magnesium deficiency is implicated in an unusually high amount of health problems including migraines. Magnesium helps smooth muscles relax and prevents veins from spasming. It also helps keep blood vessels in the brain open for good blood flow. Since magnesium is depleted when you're under stress, it's no wonder that magnesium levels in the brain were found to be 19 percent lower in people having a migraine headache than in people with no headaches. You also need magnesium to produce serotonin. Insufficient magnesium reduces blood flow to the brain and changes the way serotonin receptors work.

A number of scientific studies found low levels of magnesium in people with migraines. Over two decades ago, my friend Dr. Guy E. Abraham conducted studies on women with PMS and found many women with monthly migraines have low blood levels of magnesium. Magnesium is difficult to measure accurately through regular serum blood tests. Tests that use red blood cells rather than serum to measure magnesium are more accurate, but not all laboratories do them.

Since magnesium is a safe nutrient to take in large amounts, you may want to simply increase your magnesium intake. Take as much as you can without getting uncomfortably loose stools. And remember that the more calcium you take, the more magnesium you need. Try cutting back on calcium while you increase magnesium and see how this change affects your migraines.

SECRET #201 This herb is known for its anti-headache effects, even with migraines.

Feverfew (Tanacetum parthenium) is a member of the daisy family. It is a prolific perennial with small daisy-like flowers and strong-smelling chartreuse leaves. Its leaves contain a chemical called parthenolide that seems to lessen all headaches including migraines. Numerous studies back up feverfew's efficacy. They concluded that feverfew reduces the frequency and severity of migraines and their symptoms, or even stops them completely. It inhibits the release of substances from platelets that cause blood vessels to dilate. Feverfew also reduces the production of inflammatory hormone-like chemicals called prostaglandins and improves blood vessel tone.

Some herbalists suggest you chew a few fresh feverfew leaves, but the bitter leaves have caused mouth ulcers, a sore tongue, and swollen lips. Instead, use a standardized extract or capsules with 0.2% parthenolide. Some commercial products have been found to have little or no parthenolide.

Experts vary in their recommendations for feverfew. Acupuncturist Janet Zand suggests taking either 150 mg of freeze-dried feverfew extract or 200–400 mg of feverfew in capsules two or three times a day to prevent migraines. But naturopath Michael Murray believes that higher amounts—one to two grams a day—might be necessary if you are having an attack. A study reported in the *Lancet* (July 23, 1988) noted that one capsule of feverfew per day was enough to reduce the number and severity of attacks in participants. I suggest you begin with the smaller amounts and increase the dosage until you get the desired result.

You can find feverfew in health-food stores or grow it in your garden. It's easy to grow and quickly spreads from one small, bushy plant into many plants. Dry the leaves, pulverize them, and put them into capsules for a "homegrown" headache solution.

SECRET #202 This "magic trio" often outperforms single headache remedies.

You can be a health detective and see which one or two of the above remedies work best for you. Or you can use a "magic trio" of nutrients developed by a doctor who specializes in migraines. Alexander Mauskop, M.D., director of the New York Headache Center in New York City, and author of a book on migraines, tried each of the three ingredients in his formula both individually and together. He found that his trio outperforms any single nutrient.

Dr. Mauskop used this triple therapy on thousands of headache patients over fifteen years. Like many other combinations, there appears to be a synergistic activity in this formula between the three nutrients that causes them to work better together than alone. He talks about it in great detail in his book *What Your Doctor May Not Tell You about Migraines.* The trio consists of magnesium, riboflavin (vitamin B$_2$), and feverfew.

Riboflavin: I've already told you about magnesium and feverfew, so let me tell you why Dr. Mauskop added riboflavin to his formula. Riboflavin is not a new headache therapy. It's been used to treat migraines for more than fifty years.

A Belgian study published in 1997 found that it took a lot of riboflavin to reduce the frequency of migraines—400 mg! But this amount reduced migraines by a whopping 67 percent. The amount of riboflavin that's needed to reduce headaches is much more than you'll find in any multivitamin, and riboflavin doesn't work overnight. Be sure you take enough of it and give it at least a three-month trial. When it's combined with magnesium and feverfew, it should work more quickly. You can order Dr. Mauskop's formula, MigreLief, with information in the Resources section at the end of this book.

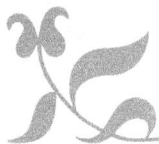

CHAPTER 27

Two Do-It-Yourself Therapies Can Relieve Headaches and Back Pain

What if you could relieve some of your back or headache pain today? Right now? Would you take a few minutes out of your day to give it a try? When it comes to pain, we're willing to do almost anything to get relief. Still, we tend to overlook simple steps within our control in favor of treatments we need to seek out and buy. And when we're in pain, we tend to look for a quick fix. Well, I've found some no-cost therapies that reduce or eliminate pain: specific stretches and foot reflexology. They take more time than swallowing a pill, but once again they can treat the source of your problem. Try them instead of, or to enhance, other therapies. They worked for me, and they could work for you.

Stretch your pain away. I used to wake up most mornings with pain in my lower back. It was from a number of reasons: an auto accident in my twenties, stress, and the positions I get into when I'm sleeping. The stiffness was in my muscles, and heat helped relax them and get rid of the pain. I found that most of my back pain vanished after I began gently stretching the muscles in my lower back.

My mother used to stretch, even when she was in her nineties. She had painful arthritis in her spine and hands, and mornings were particularly difficult for her because of stiffness. She spent the first thirty minutes after waking up doing stretching exercises in bed. Then she could begin to move.

Injuries, various health conditions such as arthritis or fibromyalgia, and stress can all cause muscle pain. Sometimes we forget that stress can contribute to pain, but it does by setting off a set of physical responses leading to muscle tension. Whenever there's constant tension, our muscles lose some of their elasticity and become shorter, causing pain and muscle spasms. Eventually, chronic pain can cause your muscles to deteriorate. Exercise can help discharge this stored tension, but few of us get enough of the right kind of exercise, especially as we get older. Stretching relaxes tight muscles and improves their flexibility, which reduces pain. It increases your range of motion and circulation and it helps prevent you from injuring yourself.

SECRET #203 Stretching can cause back pain.

Some chiropractors I talked to have mixed feelings about stretching. If it's not done properly, or if you overexercise, they point out that you could end up in more pain than before. So here's a word of caution:

Be particularly careful if you have a competitive personality or if you tend to push yourself to your limits. You could injure yourself if you stretch too much or for too long. In fact, there's a name for this phenomenon. It's called "the stretch reflex." When you overstretch, a nerve reflex sends a signal to that muscle to contract so it won't get injured. So overstretching ends up by tightening the muscle you're trying to loosen. This causes more pain.

Stretching shouldn't hurt and it should get easier over time. Begin your stretching exercises at the point where you begin to feel tension. Then hold this position for thirty to sixty seconds. Your muscles should become looser and the stretching easier. If it is not easier, back off.

Too much stretching causes more pain, not less. Your muscles could feel weak, you might have more numbness or tingling, and your hands and feet could feel cold. The very best way to begin a stretching program is after an evaluation by a physical therapist, chiropractor, or medical doctor. Bring the book *Stretching* by Bob Anderson to your physician or chiropractor to ask which exercises are most appropriate for you. It's considered the gold standard of books on stretching.

Because muscles are large tissues with a good blood supply, they respond well to increased circulation and the releasing of tension. Stretching is an effective way to do both. Try it daily for several weeks and see how much better you feel.

SECRET #204 Warm your muscles before stretching them.

This may not be a secret to you, but it's so important I just had to mention it. If you stretch without some kind of warm-up, you can hurt yourself. Cold muscles don't stretch easily. Begin any stretching program very slowly and gradually increase the number of stretches, the time it takes to do them, and the amount of tension in your stretches.

It's best to stretch later in the day when your muscles are warm, but many people find it helps their pain when they stretch first thing in the morning. It doesn't matter as long as you've warmed your muscles. Either do your morning stretches slowly or stretch after taking a hot shower. A gentle stretch that you hold for a few minutes is better in the morning than a strong stretch that causes more pain. It's a good idea to begin your day with a few simple stretches. Then find specific exercises that increase your flexibility after particular activities. Stretch after gardening, walking, or staying in one position for a long time like sitting and watching TV or typing at a computer.

When you're under stress, take five minutes to move around and stretch. Remember to breathe slowly and deeply, visualizing your breath softening the very muscles you're trying to relax. Just stretch enough to feel a gentle tugging. If you stretch past this point, you could cause your muscles to contract and tighten.

The very best way to stretch any muscle is to contract the opposite muscle. This releases the tight muscle. Here's an example from Bob Anderson's book *Stretching*. It's excellent for relieving pain in your shoulder blades.

SECRET #205 This stretch relaxes your shoulders.

With your fingers interlaced behind your head, keep your elbows straight out to the side with your upper body straight. Pull your shoulder blades together and feel the tension through your upper back and shoulder blades. Hold this position for four or five seconds as you breathe into your upper back. Then relax. Do this exercise several times. This is particularly good when your shoulders and upper back are tense or tight. But you don't have to wait until you're in pain.

Sometimes a single exercise will stretch away the pain in an area. Often, like with pain in the lower back or hands, it takes a series of several exercises. Here are a few exercises for hands and wrists from Bob Anderson's book.

SECRET #206 This exercise relieves pain from typing, knitting, and stiffness in your fingers.

First, interlace your fingers in front of you and rotate your hands and wrists clockwise ten times. Repeat counterclockwise ten times. This will improve the flexibility of your hands and wrists and provide a slight warm-up. Use it to prevent painful wrists.

Then separate and straighten your fingers until you feel tension from the stretch. Hold for ten seconds, then relax.

Next, bend your fingers at the knuckles and hold this position for ten seconds. Then relax.

With your arms straight out in front of you, bend your wrists and point your fingers upward. This stretches the back of your forearms. Hold for ten to twelve seconds. Do this twice.

Finally, bend your wrist with your fingers pointing downward to stretch the top of your forearms. Hold for ten to twelve seconds and repeat this exercise one more time.

SECRET #207 Relieve back pain without ever touching or stretching your back.

One evening, many years ago when I was a massage therapist, I was waiting in line for a show with some friends. One of them, a young lawyer, complained, "My upper back is killing me! I can't believe how painful it has been all week. Nothing seems to help."

"I'd be happy to work on you while we wait," I offered.

"Don't touch my back!" he said. "It hurts too much already. If it got any worse, it would be unbearable."

"I don't have to go near your back," I answered. "Take your shoes off and I'll show you."

Intrigued, he took off his shoes and socks. I pressed the spot on the outside edge of his big toe. "Ouch! That really hurts!"

I kept massaging that area until the pain in his toe was gone. Then I worked on the same spot on his other foot. By the time I was finished, and the line we were in began to move, his back pain was nearly gone.

"I don't believe it!" he said. "It's magic! What in the world did you do?"

"It's not magic," I smiled, "just a little foot reflexology."

SECRET #208 Reflexology "talks" to your body and changes its responses.

Your hands, feet, and ears contain tiny invisible maps of your body. Specific points correspond to each organ, gland, and body part. When you stimulate these points, you communicate with that part of your body through the nervous system and increase circulation to the affected area. This changes the way muscles, organs, and glands respond.

When I massaged my friend's foot, I knew that the neck and upper spine corresponds to the outside edge of the big toe. The tenderness was an indication of his pain. As the tenderness went away, his back pain lessened.

SECRET #209 Relax your back with a foot reflexology massage.

You can give yourself a mini-massage that relaxes your neck and back by massaging your feet. The reflexes to your back run along the outside "edge" of both feet. Your big toe corresponds to your neck. If you have neck pain, this area is likely to be tender. Rub it until the tenderness decreases. Don't overdo it, however. More is not necessarily better. Working on any area for no more than three to five minutes a day should be plenty.

The outside edge of your heel corresponds to your tailbone. Think of your spine as running between these two points and massage the entire area. I like working all the points for the back whether I have back pain or not. It's a wonderful way to relax.

Next, massage along the band at the base of your toes on the *top* of your feet. This area corresponds to your shoulders. We all hold so much tension in our shoulders and we can't reach them—except through reflexology! Massage across this band and feel your shoulders relax.

Just about anyone can work with reflexology. Just put your foot in your hands and start rubbing. Whether or not you know the particular areas that correspond to tender spots, massaging them can help your body heal. So if you don't have a hand or foot reflexology chart yet (see the Resources section if you want one), dig in and get started anyway.

If you can't reach your feet comfortably, you have two options. Get someone to work on them for you—which is the more relaxing way to go—or roll your foot around on a golf ball. It's hard enough and small enough to hit those tender spots and work out the kinks. Or use a dog toy—a hard rubber ball with bumps on it. You can find one in a pet store. Use the ball daily to reduce all tenderness and watch your pain melt away.

You may be able to find an experienced reflexologist in your area to work on you. Or you may decide to exchange foot massages with a friend. While most people work on the sole of the foot, the top of your feet have reflex points as well. Make sure that your feet get massaged all over from top to bottom. Hand reflexology also works well, but many people find that massaging the feet gives better results.

You can learn reflexology from a good book. I like *Reflexology: Health at Your Fingertips* by Barbara and Kevin Kunz. It's the most beautiful, clear book on the subject I've ever found. It's filled with dozens of photographs that take you step-by-step through a general reflexology session. Then the Kunzs show you just which points to work on for specific health concerns, such as constipation, headaches, back and neck pain, and heartburn. For more information, see the Resources section.

CHAPTER 28

Beyond Glucosamine Sulfate—More Relief from Your Arthritis Pain

Pain is your body's way of getting your attention. It is often a loud voice shouting that you have an inflammation that needs to be addressed. Inflammation affects your arthritis as well as your heart. But other factors trigger arthritis pain. Let's look at some of them you may have missed along with little-known natural solutions.

SECRET #210 **Glucosamine sulfate may help arthritis pain, but other therapies could be even more effective.**

Arthritis used to be an old person's disease. Now I'm surprised to find that many of my patients in their forties and fifties have it. When any condition ends in "itis" it means that inflammation is present. Chronic inflammation damages tissues and contributes to other diseases. This is why it's vitally important to stop the progression of arthritis today. It could prevent major health problems tomorrow.

If you have arthritis pain and are somewhat knowledgeable about integrative medicine, you may already be taking a nutritional supplement containing glucosamine sulfate. Some people take glucosamine sulfate alone; others take it with chondroitin sulfate. These nutrients do help—especially glucosamine sulfate. Glucosamine is a popular and effective joint-pain remedy. It contains a substance that builds cartilage, and damaged cartilage is a common component of arthritis. It helps stabilize joints in doses of 1,000–1,500 mg a day.

You may think it's all you need to take because it reduces your pain and helps repair cartilage. It's not. As good as it is, it's not the whole solution. Pain medications are not the answer either. They often mask the underlying cause. And they're not necessarily safe. We've learned that some of these pain medications can contribute to other more serious health problems like heart disease and stroke. If you add one or two other natural therapies, you may significantly reduce your pain even further and help your body repair itself at the same time.

I found two remedies that are safer than pharmaceuticals: cetyl myristoleate and hyaluronic acid. Never heard of them? I'm not surprised. They're two nutrients that are currently being researched for arthritis pain. One of them looks more promising than the other. I'll give you the latest information on both to help you make a decision about which to try.

Prolotherapy, which I discussed in Chapter 25, is a therapy that works beautifully with arthritis if the pain is caused by weak ligaments. Often, this is just where arthritis in the knee, for instance, begins. Prolotherapy won't remove calcium deposits that can come from a diet too high in calcium and too low in magnesium. But it certainly has its place in arthritis treatment. When prolotherapy is appropriate, the results are amazing.

Before we look at these therapies, it's important to evaluate your diet, because food sensitivities can trigger arthritis pain. Any food sensitivity can trigger it, but one particular food family causes arthritis pain in a large group of people. Eliminate these foods and you could be pain free!

SECRET #211 Tomatoes and potatoes could be causing your arthritis pain.

Years ago, I had a patient with severe arthritis pain who changed her junk food diet for a healthy one high in fruits and vegetables. No matter what she did, her pain persisted. Then she confessed that she couldn't wait for her glass of tomato juice each morning. She had forgotten to list it on her food diary. As soon as she stopped drinking tomato juice, her pain disappeared.

This patient was sensitive to foods in the nightshade family. Nightshades (*Solanaceae*) include potatoes, tomatoes, peppers, eggplant, some spices, and tobacco—and all foods containing any form of them. Inflammation and pain go hand in hand, and food sensitivities cause inflammation.

Whenever there's inflammation, your body's defense mechanism produces extra white blood cells to clean up debris from damaged tissues. These extra cells make chemicals that produce pain. So the more you eat foods that trigger this white blood cell response, the more your pain will continue.

Any food to which you have a sensitivity or allergy will cause your body to produce more pain chemicals. In many people with arthritis, this is particularly true with foods in the nightshade family. It's difficult to avoid the nightshades because

Don't Be Fooled . . .
Safe foods you might think are unsafe include sweet potatoes, yams, and black pepper.

you may have a physiological addition. You see, foods in the nightshade family actually contain small quantities of powerful druglike substances called alkaloids. These alkaloids can cause an addiction to tomatoes, potatoes, and bell peppers.

SECRET #212 Nightshades are hiding in your processed foods.

Even tiny quantities of nightshades hidden in other foods can contribute to excruciating arthritis pain, and nightshades are everywhere.

For instance, potato starch is disguised in many frozen and processed foods in the form of modified food starch, modified vegetable protein, modified vegetable starch, and hydrolyzed vegetable protein. Look for it in meatballs, mock crab, sausages, and all deep-fried foods that have been cooked in the same vegetable oils as French fried potatoes.

Some prescription and over-the-counter (OTC) medications use potato starch as their filler. Is it in your drugs? You or your pharmacist may need to call the pharmaceutical company to find out. It's a pain, to be sure. But it's not as painful as your arthritis!

Tomatoes are an ingredient in brown meat sauces like Worcestershire and steak sauce, as well as salad dressings, some luncheon meats, gravies, and baked beans, so read labels carefully. Green olives may be stuffed with pimentos, a sweet red pepper, and dried pepper flakes are frequently sprinkled over pasta dishes. Don't forget that many spices contain different varieties of peppers including cayenne, chili, paprika, and curry powder.

Avoid sauces, especially Thai, barbecue, Cajun, Mexican, Southern, and Jamaican dishes as well as Tabasco sauce. Prepared mustards usually contain paprika also. Cayenne pepper is also called capsaicin, an ingredient added to many vitamin and herbal formulas. Yes, it's important for you to eliminate them for now.

Tobacco is a member of the nightshade family. If you smoke, you won't know how much it's contributing to your pain until you stop. If you drink alcohol, avoid vodka. It's made from fermented potatoes, remember?

SECRET #213 You can test yourself for a sensitivity to nightshades.

The connection between arthritis pain and the nightshade family was found accidentally by Norman Childers, Ph.D., a horticulturist at Rutgers University. He noticed that animals that grazed on nightshades became crippled and died. Dr. Childers conducted studies on people and concluded that 74 to 90 percent of people who ache from any cause have a nightshade sensitivity.

You may not react to vegetables in the nightshade family, but if you do, you need to stop eating them. Fortunately, you can test yourself at home. And it will cost you nothing but discipline.

Temporarily avoid all foods with any amount of nightshades. Read labels carefully. Here's how you can make this experiment a little easier. Spend a day or two gradually cutting back, then eliminate all nightshades entirely—100 percent—for two full weeks. Did your pain subside or disappear during this time? If so, nightshades are a problem for you.

At the end of two weeks, eat one food from the nightshade family by itself, like a tomato or bell pepper, and watch for any reactions. You may feel tired, agitated, or your heart may race, or you could have more pain, or other undesirable side effects. If you react, continue to avoid foods from the entire nightshade family for three months or more. If not, bring them back into your diet. Some people with arthritis who have a nightshade sensitivity can eventually add small amounts of them back into their diet—like the amount found in salad dressing. Others can't. But if they trigger your arthritis pain, you'll need to avoid them completely at least for two or three months.

SECRET #214 This fatty acid, found naturally in our joints, prevents arthritis.

Harry Diehl accidentally found a solution to arthritis pain. While employed as a research chemist at the National Institutes of Health (NIH), he happened upon a fatty acid known as cetyl myristoleate (CM), which regulates inflammation and pain from arthritis. Harry had an assignment to research and develop drugs that would be effective against arthritis. He began by injecting laboratory rats with a bacteria-like substance that causes extreme inflammation in their joints. Then he injected this same substance into a strain of mice. Remarkably, the mice remained arthritis free.

After careful examination, the only difference Harry could find between the rats and mice was that the mice naturally had CM in their joints. Could this fatty acid actually have prevented arthritis in the mice? To find out, he gave the rats CM and then injected them with the arthritis-producing bacteria. None of the rats developed arthritis!

For the next few years, Harry experimented with CM on his own and found that it not only prevented arthritis, but relieved its pain and symptoms as well. For some reason, the NIH wasn't interested in Harry's discoveries. Why am I not surprised? After all, you can't patent CM and sell it through pharmaceutical companies. It's simply a fatty acid that lubricates joints and reduces inflammation that's found in fish oils, coconut oil, and other foods.

There are only a few studies on CM, and I prefer recommending therapies that have been subjected to rigorous testing. But one of the brightest doctors in the country, Sherry Rogers, M.D., has had remarkable success using CM with her patients. And the few studies that have been conducted show a significant decrease in arthritis symptoms as well as protection against getting arthritis. In one study, researchers gave sixty-four patients with knee pain either CM or a placebo for two months. Only CM improved their range of motion and overall function. CM works for about half of the people who use it, but when it works it gives dramatic relief.

At present, there are a number of CM products available, but no product standardization. Two products I trust are CM-Plus from Longevity Science, the brand Dr. Rogers uses with her patients, and Myristin, from EHP Products, a company owned by Harry Diehl's family. See the Resource section if you don't find either of these products at your natural-food store. CM is often combined with glucosamine sulfate and other anti-inflammatory products. In addition to CM, there's another "new kid" on the arthritis-supplement block. It's called hyaluronic acid, and while there are loads of testimonials touting its benefits, definitive studies are sadly lacking.

SECRET #215 The pros and cons of hyaluronic acid for arthritis.

As we age, we begin to "dry up." Our joints become creaky and painful, our eyes get dry leading to glaucoma, and our skin gets more wrinkled. Hyaluronic acid (HA) is a protein that helps our tissues retain moisture. It's the normal lubricant in our joints. Inflammation breaks down HA molecules into smaller, less effective, pieces. As our HA declines, an enzyme that breaks it down increases resulting in still less HA than when we were young.

Preliminary evidence suggests that people using hyaluronic acid may experience a slowdown or even reversal of arthritis pain. When HA is present in a joint—even if that joint has very little cartilage—it cushions the joint, which, in turn, reduces pain. This makes sense, because HA is a very long molecule that rolls into a ball like yarn and has a natural electrical charge that causes it to resist compression. It actually suspends the body and allows the joint to glide.

In addition to its unique cushioning ability, HA naturally breaks down into glucosamine. For that reason, if you're taking glucosamine sulfate for your arthritis pain, it should not be necessary to take it along with HA. You're already getting it.

The theory behind using hyaluronic acid (HA) for joint pain makes a lot of sense to me. I've heard a number of testimonials about its benefits from reputable people and have read quite a bit about it. But there aren't many studies on oral hyaluronic acid. HA injections, we know, do work. And they're not the same.

SECRET #216 Hyaluronic acid injections are effective; oral HA may not be.

There are a number of studies on HA injections for arthritis in the knee. All but two of them had positive results. Unfortunately, the same can't be said for oral HA. There are few studies on this form of hyaluronic acid. We can't assume that if one form works that the other one will as well. HA breaks down when it's taken orally. If an HA product can be made that survives through the stomach, it may be an effective alternative to injections. So far, studies do not indicate that this has been accomplished. There are testimonials, but no research published in peer-reviewed journals.

Physician and medical researcher K. Dean Reeves conducted a two-month, double-blind study at his own expense using 2 mg of oral HA a day with people who had arthritis in the knee. I spoke with him after the study was finished, and Dr. Reeves wasn't satisfied with the results. He believes that the amount of HA he used wasn't sufficient.

The participants who took higher doses of HA had a greater improvement than those on a smaller dose, but these improvements were not dramatic. Dr. Reeves believes that we don't have enough information to know the optimum dose for oral HA, and that the issue of purity has not yet been established. These are major concerns that I share.

SECRET #217 Hyaluronic acid products vary greatly.

There's another problem—a discrepancy between various forms of hyaluronic acid. Some companies say their product has a high molecular weight, others say theirs has a low molecular weight. Some are powdered substances containing collagen made from the sternums of young chickens, while others are a liquid made in laboratories from bacteria. Each claims to be superior to the other. The benefits of HA are not necessarily related to its molecular weight or viscosity. There may be something else in it—like cofactors—that are responsible for its efficacy. This assumes that HA does work.

Rather than get into an argument over which product is better, I'm waiting for the researchers and the manufacturers to duke it out in scientific studies. Dr. Reeves won't be conducting any other studies at this time. They're too expensive. Meanwhile, there's a simple and inexpensive oral therapy that works well for arthritis pain. It's called magnesium.

SECRET #218 Too much calcium contributes to arthritis.

For twenty years I've been saying that too much calcium, and not enough magnesium, contributes to arthritis. During this same time, Dr. Sherry Rogers was talking about the importance of increasing magnesium and not overdoing calcium. In fact, for two decades we've been among a handful of health professionals who dared to confront the calcium promoters and make a strong case for boosting magnesium intake. Now, the importance of adequate magnesium is well accepted.

Magnesium helps calcium get into your bones. Unabsorbed calcium doesn't just "go away." It gets stores in joints and becomes arthritis, or in arteries where it contributes to atherosclerosis. If you have arthritis, don't overdo calcium either in supplements or in your diet. Take equal amounts of calcium and magnesium. For most people on a healthy diet, 500 mg of each in your supplements should be enough. You'll get more calcium and magnesium in your diet from whole grains, beans, nuts, seeds, and dark green, leafy vegetables. For more information, see my book *User's Guide to Calcium and Magnesium.*

SECRET #219 Prolotherapy can improve knee pain from arthritis.

I spoke about the benefits of prolotherapy for strengthening weak ligaments in Chapter 25. If you have arthritis, you may not think your ligaments are weak. Yet, that may be precisely what's happening. Take arthritis in the knee, for example. It may begin with weak ligaments. When your ligaments are strong, they hold everything in place and allow the bones in your knee to glide as they move. But if one or more ligaments are loose, the stronger ones have to bear the strain and stabilize your knee. This weakness progresses from one ligament to many. Eventually, you have weak ligaments and unstable joints.

Your body does everything in its power to restore itself to balance. When your ligaments become weak, muscles and tendons contract. This attempt at stabilization fails, and now you're in pain. Then more bone begins to form to further help this stabilization. The additional bone that's formed is called osteoarthritis. And this type of arthritis responds well to prolotherapy.

A randomized, double-blind study was conducted at the Bethany Medical Center in Kansas City, Kansas on a group of people with arthritis in their knees. They were injected in the knee either with a 10 percent solution of dextrose with the painkiller lidocaine in water, or with water alone. At the end of a year (with three bimonthly injections), eight out of thirteen dextrose-treated knees had no ligament weakness. None at all. That's great news. However, there was good news for *all* participants who were given the dextrose treatment. Every one of them had less pain, swelling, buckling episodes, and greater knee flexion.

People who use prolotherapy know it works because they often notice their joints getting stronger after each treatment as more ligament tissue is being formed. They have more endurance because constant pain isn't causing constant fatigue. And they can engage in activities that once caused pain. The reason for using prolotherapy is to stabilize joints. The side effect is having your pain lessen or disappear.

Prolotherapy will reduce arthritis pain when weak ligaments cause or contribute to the pain. Check the Resources section for Chapter 25 for information on where to locate a doctor who uses this technique.

CHAPTER 29

Turn Around Chronic Fatigue and Fibromyalgia

Chronic fatigue syndrome is not a single illness, but a complex cluster of various symptoms including fatigue, muscle pain, impaired sleep, depression, brain "fogginess," headache, anxiety, premenstrual syndrome (PMS), stiffness, and joint pain. Fibromyalgia, or muscle pain, is often a component of chronic fatigue.

Chronic fatigue is known as CFIDS, which stands for chronic fatigue and immune dysfunction syndrome. This means that a suppressed immune system is involved. We suspect that an overgrowth of candida, viruses like Epstein-Barr, herpes, and Lyme disease are all implicated. So are environmental illnesses. There are fewer illnesses more complex than chronic fatigue and fibromyalgia.

Doctors who specialize in CFIDS and fibromyalgia often get poor results with their patients. Why, then, am I discussing them? Because I've found some health secrets that could reduce your symptoms. If you suffer from either condition, you're looking for everything from partial to total relief.

The best advice I can give you is, "don't ever give up." Your condition is not hopeless, it's just complex. A woman I know who has chronic fatigue recently wrote to tell me that her foot pain of thirty years simply disappeared overnight. She has no idea why, but she's been working closely with her doctor to methodically correct large and small imbalances. Chronic fatigue and fibromyalgia can take years to correct. But some relief may be just around the corner in the form of common, inexpensive supplementation.

In 2002, I was asked to speak at a conference on fibromyalgia and chronic fatigue. The conference was for medical doctors and other healthcare practitioners, and I was one of only two speakers who was not an M.D. What an honor. I spoke about a mineral I've been researching and using successfully for over a dozen years for these debilitating conditions. I was asked to speak on this topic because word was getting out that a simple change in supplements can have a profound effect on complex conditions. No matter how complicated your condition may be, there may be a simple solution that gives you some relief.

SECRET #220 Chronic fatigue syndrome is not just long-standing fatigue.

We all get tired at times, but the fatigue that is part of CFIDS hits suddenly and is deep and debilitating. Along with this fatigue come difficulty concentrating, headaches, and pain in muscles and joints. Rest takes care of most types of fatigue, but not if you have CFIDS. It never goes away. The fatigue may let up for a while, but then it returns.

That's not all. Other symptoms accompany this deep fatigue: digestive problems, anxiety, low-grade fevers, and, of course, depression. Who wouldn't be depressed if they felt sick year after year?

The cyclical patterns of chronic fatigue symptoms suggest that their origin lies either in a "bug" like Lyme disease and candida, or in a virus that goes into remission and then becomes reactivated. Explore these possibilities with a doctor of integrative medicine. While you do, keep reading. I may have found a partial solution for you.

SECRET #221 The anti-inflammatory drugs given for fibromyalgia can make it worse.

The American College of Rheumatology defines fibromyalgia as a condition with a history of widespread, chronic, musculoskeletal pain that persists for more than three months in all four extremities, along with pain in eleven out of eighteen tender points. I think of it as "nonspecific muscle pain." If you have extremely sensitive and painful points on various parts of your body, or simply ache constantly, you could have fibromyalgia.

Sometimes fibromyalgia begins after a physical trauma, but a hereditary or biochemical imbalance may also cause it. Or it could be connected to another health condition.

Medical doctors typically prescribe nonsteroidal anti-inflammatory drugs (NSAIDs) like Motrin, Advil, and Naprosyn to suppress the pain of fibromyalgia. Unfortunately, NSAIDs can only treat this symptomatic pain, not the underlying cause. And what's more, they can actually create fibromyalgia by increasing intestinal permeability, also known as "leaky gut syndrome," resulting in additional inflammation. NSAIDs are like a Band-Aid contaminated with bacteria that make your sore worse.

SECRET #222 This single nutrient can reduce your symptoms of CFIDS.

Connie was in her late fifties and exhausted all the time. Her doctor had diagnosed her with chronic fatigue syndrome. Although she had little energy to make any changes in her life, Connie came to see me in the outside chance I knew of a "magic bullet" that could reduce her fatigue. Fortunately for her, I did.

When I first saw her, Connie was unable to get a good night's sleep and was so tired during the day that she couldn't fix a simple meal. She relied on frozen foods and ate out whenever she could. I examined her diet in detail and found that many of the foods she ate were high in calcium (dairy), and low in magnesium (beans, whole grains, and green vegetables).

Magnesium was the single nutrient that changed her life. After increasing Connie's magnesium and eliminating dairy products for two weeks, her symptoms had lessened. She slept through the night and had enough energy to plan and prepare meals. She was less stressed and had a more positive outlook. Connie obviously needed more magnesium. You may, too.

In my opinion—and experience—you just can't find a better single nutrient than magnesium for both energy production and pain control. This is why I think everyone who has fibromyalgia or chronic fatigue syndrome—or even general fatigue—should try increasing their magnesium before turning to more expensive remedies.

Any improvement is important to people with fibromyalgia or CFIDS. While magnesium won't eliminate the condition completely, it often plays a major role in improving energy, reducing pain, and lessening other symptoms.

SECRET #223 You may need magnesium even if tests say you don't.

I've not been alone in getting excellent results by increasing magnesium in my CFIDS/fibromyalgia patients. Sherry A. Rogers, M.D., a specialist in environmental illnesses and complex immune problems, found that 50 percent of her fibromyalgia and chronic fatigue patients had significant relief of their symptoms using magnesium alone. Ten percent of them had reduced chemical sensitivity, as well. Truly, magnesium is a well-kept secret that could significantly improve your uncomfortable symptoms. As you're seeing, it works to correct a number of painful chronic conditions.

Magnesium levels are difficult to measure with serum blood tests. (A test called RBC [red blood cell] magnesium is much more accurate, but it's not performed at many laboratories.) This is one reason why your doctor may say you have enough magnesium when you may not. In a study published in the *Lancet,* several hundred CFIDS patients were evaluated for a magnesium deficiency using three tests: serum magnesium, RBC magnesium, and magnesium retention. Half of the patients were found to be magnesium deficient. You may have a detectible deficiency, or a subclinical one that won't show on even the most sensitive tests. It may be worth trying a program with more magnesium and less calcium to see what effects increased magnesium can have on you.

SECRET #224 Sufficient magnesium is essential for energy production.

Adenosine triphosphate (ATP) is a substance in our cells that is responsible for energy production. If you don't have enough ATP, you don't have enough energy. You need sufficient magnesium to make ATP.

Magnesium plays a role in hundreds of enzyme functions that are involved in producing energy. The problem is, our diets and supplements are too low in magnesium. Also, stress places additional demands on this important mineral. The more stress of any kind that you're under, the more magnesium your body needs. Anyone with chronic fatigue or long-term fatigue needs plenty of the raw materials necessary to keep producing ATP. This begins with stress-depleted magnesium.

Some experts suggest taking 300–400 mg of magnesium for ATP production. I have found that some people need, and can tolerate, more. I recommend taking magnesium to bowel tolerance. This means taking as much as you can without having uncomfortably loose stools. The amount can vary from 100–1,000 mg.

Low levels of magnesium affect energy in another way. It leads to increased insulin resistance. When this happens, blood sugar levels rise and remain high. This can contribute to diabetes. Magnesium's role in insulin resistance translates into low energy. Too much or too little glucose in your blood causes fatigue. If low blood sugar is contributing to your fatigue, be sure to eat a diet low in refined sugars and starches. And get plenty of magnesium.

SECRET #225 A magnesium deficiency relates directly to pain.

Calcium causes muscles to contract while magnesium causes them to relax. This is an important concept for you to understand, since relaxed muscles are less painful than those that contract. A magnesium deficiency causes increased smooth-muscle activity, such as headaches and muscle cramping.

But there's more to magnesium's connection to pain. Sometimes muscles hurt because they don't contain enough potassium. One of magnesium's many important functions is to maintain a balance of sodium and potassium. If your muscles lack potassium, taking more magnesium can raise your level better than taking more potassium. If you need both, try a potassium-magnesium aspartate combination (available from most health-food stores). Aspartic acid carries both potassium and magnesium into the cells quickly and efficiently.

SECRET #226 This substance in apples helps make ATP and reduces muscle pain.

Malic acid is an acid found in apples and other fruits. You need it to make ATP. It also reduces fibromyalgia pain. When you add malic acid to magnesium, you have a powerful supplement that can reduce fatigue in a few weeks, and reduce your pain in a few days.

I first heard about using malic acid more than a dozen years ago from research gynecologist and endocrinologist Guy E. Abraham, M.D. He called to tell me about a randomized double-blind study he had designed that was being conducted at the University of Texas School of Medicine on fibromyalgia patients. This study used a formula he had developed combining magnesium with malic acid to reduce or eliminate muscle pain. Although the study was only halfway completed, he announced, "We know the formula is working." I asked him how he could be so sure. "Half the people are better and half are the same," he replied. It turned out he was right. The combination of malic acid with magnesium does often fight fibromyalgia.

Next, Dr. Abraham gave fifteen fibromyalgia patients 300–600 mg of magnesium along with 1,200–2,400 mg of malic acid a day. Within two days, all of them reported a significant improvement in their pain. After eight weeks, they were given a placebo. All reported that their pain returned within two days. Other studies using these lower amounts of magnesium and malic acid were also ineffective.

Later, Dr. Abraham measured RBC magnesium levels in thirteen fibromyalgia patients and found that twelve out of thirteen had below normal magnesium. Since I first talked with him, I have used his formula with great success on my fibromyalgia patients.

While I don't find that malic acid and magnesium works every time, I have used it successfully with many patients. It's the first supplement I turn to for muscle pain because it's such a simple, inexpensive step to take. I only use Dr. Abraham's Super Malic Plus formula. It contains cofactors to help the active ingredients work even better.

More about Magnesium

To learn more about magnesium, check out my book *User's Guide to Calcium and Magnesium*. It explains in detail why magnesium is an important and often overlooked key to many health conditions, lists numerous studies to back this up, and tells you how to get the balance of calcium and magnesium you need. This is a book every person concerned with osteoporosis, arthritis, CFIDS, and other conditions needs to read.

The Next Steps

If magnesium and malic acid are not enough, it's time to look at other reasons for your chronic fatigue or fibromyalgia. These include taking probiotics to repopulate your intestines (see Chapter 2), candida and parasites (see Chapter 12), intestinal permeability (see Chapter 13), and inflammation (see Chapter 38). Your chronic health problems could also be caused by an underlying condition called Lyme disease.

SECRET #227 Lyme disease may be at the bottom of your chronic fatigue or fibromyalgia.

A number of doctors are now looking at Lyme disease as the reason why some people with chronic fatigue and fibromyalgia fail to get well. Lyme disease is an illness caused by a spiral-shaped microorganism called a spirochete. It is spread not only by ticks as originally thought, but also by mosquitoes, fleas, and mites. While Lyme is more prevalent in country settings where it's passed along from deer to humans, now it appears there may be a Lyme disease epidemic.

Increasingly more doctors of integrative medicine believe it is the underlying cause of many chronic illnesses. The problem with this condition is twofold: Lyme disease is difficult to diagnose and it's even more difficult to treat. The usual treatment is from two to four weeks of strong antibiotics. Unfortunately, this is often not long enough to get results. Patients I know who take the antibiotics complain that they feel much sicker during the treatment. Sometimes it works; other times it doesn't. Even patients taking antibiotics for a full year don't always get better. In fact, many of them get worse from the side effects of the antibiotics.

But antibiotics are not the only treatment for Lyme disease. It's important to eat a sugar-free diet. This prevents feeding any bacteria associated with Lyme. Work with a doctor of integrative medicine who can evaluate you for supportive supplements like probiotics, vitamins, minerals, herbs, and medicinal mushrooms. For more detailed information, read *Chronic Fatigue, Fibromyalgia and Lyme Disease* by Burton Goldberg and Larry Trivieri, Jr.

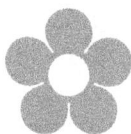

CHAPTER 30

Little-Known Solutions to Shingles

Shingles, also known as herpes zoster, is one of the most painful conditions you will ever experience. Traditional medicine treats shingles with antivirals. This makes sense. If you have a virus, you want to calm it down and inactivate it. There are, however, natural substances that have strong antiviral activity as well. You may want to take them either with, or instead of, antiviral medications.

Doctors generally suggest steroids for the pain. Once more, you should know that you have other options. These options are not only safer, but they're often more effective.

Whatever you decide to do, don't self-medicate without discussing your plans with your doctor. Shingles is nothing to fool around with. If you want to try some of the suggestions in this chapter, ask your doctor to monitor you. I did, and the results astounded both of us.

SECRET #228 **Like its cousin that produces cold sores, the herpes virus is often triggered by stress.**

Several years ago, after a particularly stressful situation that had persisted for months, I noticed a row of painful blisters around my waist. The burning and shooting pain from these tiny spots became so intense I was unable to sleep for five nights.

Exhausted and on the verge of tears, I walked into the office of a doctor friend whose practice was in pain management. He told me the blisters were a sign of shingles and said the pain I was experiencing was the worst pain he knew of. Ordinarily, I don't reach for pharmaceuticals as my first line of defense, but I was exhausted and in excruciating pain. I gladly accepted the painkillers he prescribed, knowing that rest was vital to my recovery. Then I began to explore less toxic options for getting my shingles in remission. In the midst of my intense pain, I vowed I would do everything in my power to prevent them from ever occurring again in me and in my patients.

Like cold sores, shingles is a form of herpes. It occurs when the chickenpox virus, varicella-zoster, reactivates in a different form. If you've ever had chickenpox, or have even been exposed to it, herpes zoster may be lying dormant, waiting for an excuse to erupt. Physical or emotional stress can set it off, especially if your immune system is low. Since stress lowers the immune system, the key to prevention is in managing your stress and supporting your immune system.

SECRET #229 The pain that comes after the blisters disappear can last for years.

Usually, shingles occurs in people over fifty and most commonly breaks out on the trunk or the face. It can begin with flulike symptoms: chills, fever, fatigue, and digestive problems. Then, three or four days later comes the pain, burning, and a red band along the site where the blisters will appear. The burning and painful blisters may be in clusters or in a row and may last for only three to five days, but the intense, unrelenting pain continues. These blisters contain the herpes zoster virus and are infectious for up to a week. Be careful that you don't spread it to those around you during this time. After the blisters dry and disappear, usually in about two weeks, the pain—postherpetic neuralgia—which comes from irritation to the nerves, may continue for weeks, months, and even years.

If you have never had shingles, you cannot comprehend the intensity of this persistent burning pain. The pain is so bad that some people have had surgery to cut the nerves to the affected area. Fortunately, there's a better solution. I found both pharmaceutical and natural ways to reduce the pain and duration of shingles and they should work for you as well.

SECRET #230 Some conventional pain medications work; others don't.

Antivirals, such as acyclovir and valacyclovir, are the traditional treatment for shingles. Talk with your doctor about taking either of them or more natural antivirals. But you need some type of antiviral to stop the virus from replicating.

Oral steroids are often given to reduce the pain of shingles, as well as to prevent postherpetic neuralgia. Take whatever painkillers work for you. Without sufficient rest, you won't get better. Acetaminophen, even with codeine, didn't help me. Neither did topical painkillers such as lidocaine. Take painkillers according to your doctor's instructions, not just when you hurt and can't stand it. It's easier to keep pain under control than to repeatedly get it under control.

If you get a second outbreak of shingles, talk with your doctor about a vaccination with the varicella-zoster virus. It is 80 percent effective.

SECRET #231 To inactivate the herpes virus and keep it dormant, you need to manage your stress better.

Shingles is triggered by stress. So is the less painful but bothersome herpes virus that causes cold sores. Both the blisters of shingles and postherpetic neuralgia can return unless you address your stress. Here's the pattern: Stress lowers your immune system. A lowered immune system allows dormant viruses to become active. The best way to protect yourself from any form of herpes is to have a strong immune system.

Do whatever is necessary to deal with your stress better. If you think you're doing enough, your case of shingles is an indication that you're not. Meditate for a few minutes every day, breathe deeply, drink more water, exercise regularly without pushing yourself too hard, pay attention to your diet and supplements. They either support your immune system or have the opposite effect. Don't underestimate the importance of the right diet. It can hold the key to inactivating the herpes virus.

SECRET #232 Some foods feed the herpes virus; other foods inactivate it.

Shingles and other forms of herpes thrive on sugar. Stop eating sugar for now. If you crave sweets, eat more protein and use stevia, a natural sweetener found in powdered form in health-food stores.

There are two amino acids, components of protein, that affect herpes. One opposes the other. So you need to stop eating some and increase your intake of others. Lysine fights herpes, while arginine feeds it. Eat more foods that are high in lysine, and temporarily eliminate all foods high in arginine.

Lysine-rich foods include fish, chicken, turkey, beef, eggs, brewer's yeast, dairy products and potatoes.

Foods high in arginine include all nuts and seeds, grains, beans, chocolate, and raisins.

Eat a healthy diet with plenty of fresh vegetables to boost your immune system. One warning: Some people get herpes outbreaks when they eat too many acidic foods like tomatoes and oranges. If this is the case for you, eliminate high-acid foods. Avoid alcohol, coffee, and junk foods that can lower your immunity.

SECRET #233 Some supplements inactivate the virus; others support your immune system.

Lysine acts as an antiviral directly on the herpes virus. If you have active herpes, take 1,500 mg of lysine three times a day. My doctor found that lysine was as effective as pharmaceutical antivirals in keeping the herpes virus inactive. After your outbreak is under control, continue to take 1,500 mg three times a day for six months. You need less lysine to prevent an outbreak. Taking 500 mg three times a day is often sufficient.

Medicinal mushrooms are my favorite immune-boosting supplement. For detailed information, see Chapter 3. All medicinal mushrooms strengthen immunity, although some appear to be better than others. You can find mushroom extracts, capsules, and powders at your natural-food store.

Garlic is a strong, inexpensive antiviral. If you like it, add one or two raw cloves to your diet. Or take a few garlic capsules twice a day for a few weeks. Cooked garlic does not have as much antiviral activity, but it's so cheap that it's worth including in your food.

SECRET #234 Homeopathy works on herpes.

Homeopathy is a form of energy medicine that either works or it doesn't. When you find the correct remedy, it seems to work miracles. If you don't take the right one, you just don't have a positive effect.

Homeopathics are not harmful when taken according to directions, so they're certainly worth trying. Individual homeopathics were used historically to treat shingles. One or more of the following remedies may be helpful. If you can't find the dose mentioned, use the one closest to it.

- Mezereum 12X or 6C for severe pain and burning (take one dose four times per day for three days).

- Ranunculus bulbosus 6C for pain, especially on the chest or back.

- Rhus tox. 30X or 15C for a red, swollen rash (take one dose four times per day for three days).

- Staphylococcinium 30C for shortening the length of the outbreak.

- Sulfur 12C for decreasing the risk of future pain (postherpetic neuralgia).

- Arsenicum 30C for intense burning when there is aggravation from cold temperatures.

SECRET #235 Use specific herbs and essential oils topically to reduce pain.

Capsaicin is the active ingredient from cayenne, or chili peppers. It blocks the pain signals from nerves that are right under your skin. I particularly like this herb because it's both effective and easy to find. Many topical preparations found in drugstores to stop pain contain capsaicin. Use any of them containing 0.025% to 0.075% capsaicin topically four or five times a day.

Licorice root extract. Apply it topically at the first sign of any type of herpes, including cold sores and genital herpes.

A number of essential oils with antiviral and antimicrobial properties can be used topically for shingles. They include ravensera, lavender, eucalyptus, oregano, chamomile, tea tree, and sage. But perhaps the most widely used essential oil is lemon balm (*Melissa officinalis*). Always dilute essential oils with olive oil or almond oil to avoid burning or irritation.

Lemon balm contains chemicals with anti-herpes properties. I use ointments with lemon balm at the first sign of a cold sore. Invariably, it stops the blister from forming. Use lemon balm essential oil topically, diluted with a little olive oil. If you can't find the oil, make a strong tea from lemon balm, and apply it gently with cotton balls four times a day. Or get an ointment with lemon balm from the drugstore or natural-food store.

Here are some combination products I've found work well for shingles:

Shingle Aid is a topical essential oil tincture with ravensera made by Simplers Botanicals. I have personally found ravensera to be an amazingly effective treatment for shingles. It relieves pain and is a nerve tonic. You apply it directly to the skin two to three times a day.

Shingle-EEZE by Merix Health Care Products is a topical antiviral spray that is said to stop lesions from spreading, heal blisters in a day and a half, and ease pain in thirty minutes. Both of these products can either be found in natural food stores or through information in the Resources section.

Preventing Shingles

If you don't have shingles now, make avoiding it your primary goal. This is one illness you want to prevent at all costs. If you already have shingles, do everything in your power to keep it from recurring. Since shingles is caused by a virus, you will never completely get rid of it. The idea is to keep it dormant. Here are some suggestions.

Manage your stress: Stressful situations come and go. When they come and stay, you're at risk for any kind of herpes, from cold sores to shingles. Use meditation or prayer, deep breathing, and exercise daily. If you need help, try hypnosis or biofeedback. Eat better during stressful times, even when it's tempting to take the opposite approach. Get extra sleep or rest. Even an extra hour's sleep at night, or a half-hour nap is helpful.

Boost your immune system: Stress, constantly fighting off colds and flu, and chronic health problems all lower your immune system. Supplements, herbs and medicinal mushrooms, and a shift in your attitude can all give your immune system a lift. Review your supplements and look at your lifestyle to see how you can strengthen your natural immunity.

Take an antiviral: If you feel you're at risk for shingles or other viruses, talk with your doctor about taking an antiviral preventively such as lysine 500 mg, three times daily. After having shingles, you may want to take 1,500 mg of lysine, three times daily for six months. Another option is to take an herbal antiviral, such as olive leaf extract or oil of oregano, for two weeks according to the directions on the label. You can find it in most natural-food stores.

Shingles was so painful for me that I found it easy to adhere to a good diet and healthy lifestyle during my recovery. And I remembered to take my supplements, herbs, and essential oils. When I returned to my doctor for a follow-up visit, she was amazed that I had healed so quickly. The proper treatment will give you quick results, and natural products really do work. I've not had a recurrence of shingles or any other form of herpes, nor do I expect to, since my episode three years ago. Pain is a powerful teacher. Learn from mine.

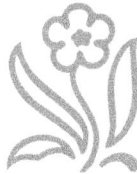

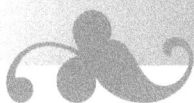

PART 6

HORMONE SECRETS THAT ARE SAFE, SIMPLE, and EFFECTIVE

The biggest area of confusion for menopausal women is whether or not to take hormones. If your decision is yes, the next question is whether or not hormones are safe and effective. If your decision is no, what can you do about your hot flashes and other uncomfortable consequences of hormone deficiency?

There are two reasons to seriously consider taking hormones: If you have menopausal symptoms that can't be eliminated in any other way, and if you feel strongly that hormones will offer you better protection against future conditions than anything else.

Hormones can get rid of hot flashes and night sweats. So can some natural therapies. Hormones can protect your bones. So can certain dietary changes, nutrients, and exercise. But each of us is different in our needs and in what we're willing to do to take care of ourselves. Hormones can be safe and effective when they're used properly. Unfortunately, they're often misused. That's when you run the risk of side effects.

For decades, pharmaceutical companies assured doctors that hormone replacement therapy (HRT) was safe. Then they found that it contributed to breast and uterine cancers. Hormones were said to improve memory. But researchers found that they didn't improve memory.

The UK Royal College of Obstetricians and Gynecologists in England recently issued a handbook on hormones and menopause. They say HRT "should be used only for the short-term relief of menopausal symptoms." They urge women to be assessed by their doctors and informed fully about its benefits and risks.

The World Health Organization (WHO) went one step further when they issued a report that concluded that combined estrogen/progestin therapy, whether it is used in birth control pills or for menopausal symptoms, is carcinogenic. (International Agency for Research on Cancer, press release 167, July 29, 2005.)

Clearly, HRT is not as safe as we once thought. There are so many contradictions that many women throw up their hands. They put up with their night sweats rather than take a chance that hormones will cause worse problems. And they could.

Hormone therapy can be either dangerous or the best gift you can give your body, says Dr. Uzzi Reiss, a Los Angeles-based gynecologist I've known for more twenty years. The trick is getting the right kind of hormones in the right amount. This isn't easy to do. Most traditional doctors are unfamiliar with the safer, natural hormones that are becoming popular with doctors of integrative medicine. Nor are they familiar with the type of tests available that could give them the information they need to prescribe natural hormones.

We think that natural hormones are safer than synthetic hormones, but we don't know for sure. It will take years before we have the results of long-term studies. We do know that just because they're natural doesn't mean that hormones are safe. And we know that it's not smart to self-medicate with hormones—even natural ones. Some people who take natural progesterone have had side effects, and too much DHEA (an estrogen precursor sold in health-food stores) can contribute to breast cancer. In the midst of this confusion, if you're in your fifties or beyond, you need answers today. You can't afford to wait another ten, twenty, or thirty years.

Let me help you unravel the world of hormones, both natural and those made by traditional pharmaceutical companies. The more you understand about hormones, the better able you'll be to make decisions that are right for you. And safe.

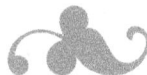

CHAPTER 31

Understanding Hormone Replacement Therapy

You could say, as some doctors do, that estrogen distinguishes women as a gender. Then why would it be harmful to keep taking hormones after menopause? Think about it. Hormones that were protective to us when we are young don't suddenly turn on us as we age.

In fact, they can continue to protect us. It's just that we may need a different amount and balance than before. The key is to find what your body needs now to feel and stay healthy, and then to take just that amount in a safe, effective form.

The subject of hormone therapy is both confusing and frightening, and for good reason. We found that some hormones we thought protected us from diseases are actually contributing to cancer and heart disease. Most medical doctors don't understand the difference between natural and synthetic hormones. They don't realize that some forms are harmful, while others appear to be protective. We all need to understand the value of natural hormones and the dangers of synthetic hormones.

SECRET #236 Reduce your stress and reduce your need for hormones.

Before you decide which type of estrogen and progesterone is best for you to take, consider this: You may not need to take any hormones at all. You may, in fact, need less of a hormone produced when you're under stress. The first step is to stop producing too much cortisol, a hormone made by your adrenal glands. I talked about the connection between high cortisol production and stress in detail in Chapter 19. What you need to know here is that when you lower your cortisol level, you may not need to take other hormones.

Stress upsets your hormone levels. When you're stressed and taking hormone replacement therapy (HRT), your body may not be able to utilize the hormones properly. If you're not taking any hormones, your dwindling reserves will be lower than necessary. So, whether or not you decide to take hormones, you first need to reduce high cortisol levels.

There are two types of stress responses, both triggered by your adrenal glands. One is the more familiar "fight-or-flight" response. It is controlled by epinephrine and norepinephrine, two hormones that give you the extra strength and agility you need to run to safety in an emergency. But too much of these hormones can cause fear and anxiety. This leads to even more stress. Eventually, your adrenal glands become exhausted and unable to function properly.

The other stress response is activated by cortisol, a hormone that results in a big push of energy. But this extra energy comes with a high price tag. It raises your blood sugar to give you the ability to burn more energy (sugar) and it increases your insulin sensitivity. The long-term results can be anything from sudden fatigue to diabetes. Some stressors that increase cortisol levels include heat, cold, pain, radiation, obesity, disease, overexertion, and worrisome events in our lives. In other words, almost everything you experience after menopause. You can't change the stressors in your life, but you can change your response to them.

SECRET #237 Your menopausal symptoms could be caused by too much cortisol, not too little estrogen or progesterone.

Chronically high cortisol levels can affect your memory, because cortisol production is associated with a greater deterioration of the hippocampus, a part of the brain that is related to memory. The single most important step you can take to improve your aging mind is to reduce your cortisol levels by lowering your stress.

Your adrenal glands are designed to produce their hormones as needed—not constantly. When exhausted adrenal glands can't make enough stress-relieving hormones, your body makes them from progesterone. This reduces your storage supply of this important hormone. Before taking even natural progesterone, you need to reduce your response to stress or your progesterone levels will constantly be depleted.

Have you gained weight around your stomach? Are you depressed? Are your muscles weaker than they used to be? Is you skin getting thinner? All of these "menopausal" symptoms may be caused by high cortisol. Surprised? I'll bet you are. It's no wonder that Uzzi Reiss, M.D., gynecologist and author of *Natural Hormone Balance for Women* counsels every one of his patients to lower their stress before they begin any hormone program!

Understanding Estrogens

SECRET #238 Horses have a dozen estrogens. We have three.

When I start talking with my menopausal and postmenopausal patients about estrogen replacement therapy (ERT) their eyes glaze over.

They've heard horror stories about problems with estrogen (breast and endometrial cancers) and horror stories of the consequences of not taking them (osteoporosis and heart disease). So they come to me for a better understanding. I tell them their confusion begins with thinking that there's one hormone called estrogen. There's not. It's estrogens—plural.

It's time to stop thinking about estrogen as being one hormone. The substance we think of as estrogen is really a group of hormones. The number of estrogen compounds that make up what we think of as "estrogen" varies in humans and horses. This is a very important distinction, because many women are taking estrogens made from horse's urine. These formulas (Premarin, Premphase, Prempro) contain a dozen estrogen compounds. Only *one* of them is exactly like one of ours.

Our bodies have three primary estrogen compounds: estrone (E1), estradiol (E2), and estriol (E3). It's plain to see that horse urine estrogens are not in the least identical to ours. They're not even close! For this reason, they can't function like ours. Many of the problems with hormone therapy come from this major difference.

Some estrogens that are now being used in HRT are natural. They're made in laboratories to be identical to those our bodies make. In fact, they're called bio-identical hormones. They may consist of one, two, or all three of the estrogens found in humans.

SECRET #239 There are also estrogens in plants and in the environment.

But there are more kinds of estrogens. Some are made from plants, while others are a result of environmental pollutions. Phytoestrogens are estrogens found in plants, like soy. Some people say they are beneficial; others say they can be harmful, especially if you've had breast cancer.

Xenoestrogens are estrogens found in the environment that can be harmful. So let's unravel the confusion about estrogens and begin by understanding how each of them works.

SECRET #240 Too much or too little estrogen can cause uncomfortable symptoms.

The estrogens I'm talking about here are the three major estrogen compounds found in our bodies: estrone, estradiol, and estriol. They are made primarily in our ovaries starting at puberty, and are made there for the rest of our lives. They play an important role in our menstrual cycle when we're young, and are responsible for our feelings of vitality and sensuality as we age. Estrogens help us feel young, while estrogen deficiency is associated with signs of aging.

In our youth, an excess of estrogens can cause side effects like breast tenderness, swollen breasts, water retention, impatience, nausea, and cramps. Many of these symptoms occur before menstruation each month and are signs of premenstrual syndrome (PMS). After menopause, too much estrogen can increase our risk for some cancers.

After menopause, our estrogen decreases and with it comes estrogen-deficiency symptoms. These symptoms include depression, anxiety, forgetfulness, moodiness, difficulty sleeping, hot flashes or night sweats, fatigue, feeling less sensual, dry skin (and vaginal dryness), weight gain, sagging breasts, heart palpitations, headaches, bloating, and back pain. If you have any of these symptoms, taking the right kind of natural estrogens—in the correct amount for your body—could be helpful.

SECRET #241 Each form of estrogen has different effects.

Estrone (E1): Estrone promotes the formation of bone tissue and is important in preventing osteoporosis. It also reduces hot flashes and other menopausal symptoms. But, estrone is an aggressive estrogen that promotes cancer. To reduce your risk for cancer, never take estrone alone. Be sure to take estriol along with it.

Estradiol (E2): Estradiol is the most prevalent estrogen in your body. It's made in the ovaries from androgens (male hormones). Estradiol is the estrogen that doctors tend to give alone because it's most prevalent and prevents bone loss. After menopause, androgen production drops as much as 50 percent, and so does estradiol. But estradiol is not necessarily safe. Doctors of integrative medicine know that taking estradiol alone is dangerous because it's the most aggressive type of estrogen. Even natural estradiol taken alone can increase your risk for endometriosis and various cancers. Like estrone, estradiol needs to be balanced with estriol.

SECRET #242 Estriol is the safest form of estrogen you can take.

Estriol (E3): Most gynecologists and other medical doctors know little about estriol. This is unfortunate, because estriol is both beneficial and safe. It keeps your skin young, increases vaginal lubrication, reduces hot flashes, and seems to be protective against cancers. Estriol balances the negative effects of other estrogens. It doesn't do everything, however. For instance, estriol doesn't prevent osteoporosis or heart disease (look to magnesium for these conditions). However, my friend and colleague Dr. Reiss has improved mental clarity in many of his postmenopausal patients with estriol when nothing else helped.

If you're afraid of getting breast cancer from taking estrogen replacement therapy, or if you're at a high risk for breast cancer, estriol may be your answer. The few studies that exist suggest estriol prevents breast tumors in rats, and does not cause the formation of a lot of potentially carcinogenic substances (estrone and estradiol do). Estriol may not protect your bones and heart as much as estrone and estradiol, but it offers some protection. You can use a healthier diet and regular exercise to lower your risk for these conditions.

A new patient recently told me her doctor had given her estrogen. Which kind, I asked? Natural estrogen, she replied. The estrogen she was taking was estradiol, the estrogen that increased her risk for cancers. After we spoke about the different natural estrogens available, she talked with her doctor and got a prescription for Tri-Est, a balanced compound of the three estrogens. Some doctors are playing it even safer by using a formula called Bi-Est—estradiol and estriol—via transdermal patches. When estrogens are carried into the body through the skin, they increase other helpful hormone levels, like human growth hormone (HGH).

The World of Natural Estrogens

There are a number of different kinds of natural estrogens. Some are bio-identical hormones made in the laboratories of natural compounding pharmacies. They are available by prescription only. These hormones are chemically identical with those your body makes.

Other estrogens are made by plants. These hormones are called phytoestrogens. Their effect is weak, but it's strong enough to reduce menopausal symptoms in some women. Black cohosh, red clover, and soy are three sources of phytoestrogens used in menopause formulas. Of all of them, only soy is found in our food supply.

You may think that plant estrogens are your best choice. But keep reading. You may change your mind.

SECRET #243 There are pros and cons for taking plant-based estrogens.

Phytoestrogens have a weak estrogenic effect, but they can still activate your estrogen receptors. Estrogen receptors are like parking spaces where all kinds of estrogens can get into your body. Phytoestrogens provide a valuable service by getting into estrogen receptors and preventing more dangerous estrogens (like estradiol and environmental estrogens), from occupying the same space. In this way, they can protect you against the negative effects of some estrogens.

But phytoestrogens in foods and supplements are not the same. There's simply no way to duplicate Mother Nature. Soy naturally contains low amounts of isoflavones, one type of beneficial plant-based estrogen, along with many cofactors. Soy-based supplements often contain high amounts of isoflavones without the same balance of ingredients as the soy in foods. There aren't enough studies yet to satisfy me that isoflavone supplements are both effective and safe. In fact, some studies suggest that they may stimulate the growth of breast and endometrial tissues.

What about the safety of soy foods? There's a big controversy over this subject. I talk about it in more detail in Chapter 44. For now, know that the plant-based estrogens from your foods get into your estrogen receptors and protect you from more harmful estrogens.

I like phytoestrogens. I just prefer getting them from foods than from supplements. If your estrogen levels are already high, phytoestrogens in soy foods won't boost them any higher. But if they're low, like after menopause, they can help increase your total estrogen enough to relieve some of your menopausal symptoms. Until there's more data on soy supplements, my suggestion is to get your phytoestrogens by adding a little soy to your diet. Small amounts of soy have been found to be both safe and beneficial.

A patient of mine who ate half a cup of edamame (green soybeans) a day for two weeks reported to me that her vaginal dryness was greatly reduced. This amount of soybeans contains 70 mg of isoflavones (along with all the cofactors found in soy). This was enough to naturally increase lubrication. You can increase soy in your diet to see if you get similar results.

I wouldn't take high-isoflavone supplements at this point. A recent five-year randomized, double-blind study found that some of the women taking 150 milligrams (mg) of isoflavones a day had a thickening in their endometrial tissues. Could this lead to endometrial cancer? Possibly. We know from animal studies that particular isoflavones stimulate uterine growth. You're always safer using foods over individual substances in supplements. I believe this is especially true with isoflavones.

Supplements made from soy may reduce your hot flashes, but I'm not convinced they will lower your risk for heart disease or improve your brain function. Although they are made from soybeans, Dr. Uzzi Reiss points out they are reconstituted in a way that's similar to horse-urine products. While they're "natural," they are not molecularly identical to the hormones in your body. I asked Dr. Reiss about the difference between Premarin and soy-based estrogen. He replied, "There is no difference. Neither one belongs in your body." The safest, most helpful hormones are those that are exactly like the hormones your body produces. I can't say this often enough. *Only* consider using hormones that exactly mimic your body's hormones.

The Problems with Traditional Estrogens

SECRET #244 Estrogens from horse's urine are not safe.

Until recently, estrogen replacement therapy meant using estrogens from pregnant mare's urine, like Premarin. I think of all of these products as being "foreign" estrogens because they are estrogens that are not identical to those made in our bodies. Doctors have told us for years that they're safe. Then, suddenly, studies found the opposite was true.

Why was anyone surprised? Mare's urine contains a dozen types of estrogens and only one is identical with one of the three in our bodies! The other eleven are foreign estrogens that our bodies don't know how to use. It's true that Premarin and other estrogens made from horse urine have been shown in studies to protect against osteoporosis and heart disease. But this protection comes with a high price. These estrogens have also been associated with endometrial, breast, and other cancers, as well as stroke. They can increase plaque in the arteries of your heart and contribute to heart disease. And they often increase insulin sensitivity, leading to diabetes.

Synthetic hormones are hormones that are unlike those your body makes. The problem with them is that your body lacks important enzymes needed to metabolize certain synthetic hormones. This is true of Premarin, for instance.

Dr. Reiss calls Premarin "the biggest killer of women in this country" because recent data shows it increases breast cancer, closes coronary arteries, and increases insulin sensitivity that can lead to diabetes. Unless the hormones you take are *exactly* like the ones your body makes, in the same ratio, they are foreign to your body and can cause serious health problems.

SECRET #245 Environmental estrogens act like synthetic estrogens.

Some estrogens come from environmental pollutions. They are made outside the body from dioxin, some pesticides, herbicides, insecticides, and residues of plastics and are toxic substances called xenoestrogens that act just like synthetic estrogens—except that they are more aggressive. Exposure to them is one reason why young girls reach sexual maturity earlier than ever before. When you add xenoestrogens to HRT, they increase estrogen levels and contribute to breast and uterine cancers, endometriosis, and uterine fibroids.

You can't escape xenoestrogens, but you can lower your exposure to them. One way is to store safe estrogens—either bio-identical or phytoestrogens from soy foods—in your estrogen receptors. Next, reduce your intake of beef and eat more organic foods. More people are switching from commercial beef to grass-fed beef. Unfortunately, grass is often permeated with dioxin, a xenoestrogen in the air that's a byproduct of waste incineration. Avoid storing or heating foods in plastic containers. Xenoestrogens can get into the food, and the containers leak these substances into the landfill when they're thrown away.

SECRET #246 Natural estrogens can protect you from aging-related symptoms.

Natural, or bio-identical, estrogens provide you with protection against many losses associated with menopause and aging: memory, libido, bone density, and skin moisture, to name just a few. There are certainly other options, but there's no need to exclude using bio-identical hormones. Don't be put off by the frightening information you hear about estrogens made from pregnant mare's urine. Natural estrogens are safer when you're given just exactly what your body needs in the right amounts. They're just not anything to fool around with on your own.

Your particular hormonal needs can be assessed through blood, urine, and saliva tests (saliva tests alone are not accurate). You and your doctor can get specific information on these tests and where to get them from a natural compounding pharmacy or by reading *Natural Hormone Balance for Women* by Uzzi Reiss, M.D.

SECRET #247 Discuss the type and amount of estrogens your body needs with a knowledgeable doctor.

If you don't have a doctor who is familiar with bio-identical hormones, you can find one through any of the natural compounding pharmacies listed in the Resources section. If your doctor is open to learning about them, but isn't familiar with natural hormones yet, these pharmacies will spend a lot of time teaching him or her.

Years ago, I told Dr. Reiss about a pharmacy that made natural hormones. He contacted them and poured through their literature. Whenever he had a question, he would call them for more clarification. Three years later, I happened to be talking with the head of that pharmacy and mentioned Dr. Reiss to him. "Oh yes," he said. "He's become such an expert we call him Dr. Hormone!" Your doctor can become an expert, also. All he or she needs is the interest and the input of knowledgeable pharmacists.

Some doctors believe you should be getting as much estrogen now as your body produced before menopause. I think this is too much. Consider this: Early ancestral women were pregnant or nursing much of their short adult lives. There were relatively few years that their bodies made a lot of estrogens. We're menstruating earlier and stopping later in life than they did. Our lifetime exposure to estrogens is much higher than theirs. The longer you've been exposed to estrogens, the greater your risk is for breast cancer. There's no reason for you to continue taking high amounts of estrogens if smaller amounts are sufficient. This is something for you to discuss with your doctor.

One thing's for sure: The balance and type of estrogens your body needs cannot be found in other mammals. They certainly can't be found in the urine of pregnant horses! The estrogens you need are the exact molecular structure of those your body has been making all your life—in the amounts you used to have—or less.

Jonathan Wright, M.D., did the original research on natural hormones, using three kinds of estrogen along with natural progesterone. The estrogens he used are the ones found in our bodies in the amounts our body naturally produces: 10 to 20 percent estrone, 10 to 20 percent estradiol, and 60 to 80 percent estriol. Of these three, estradiol may be the most procarcinogenic, and estriol may be the most anticarcinogenic. Much of the estrogen used in HRT contains only estradiol!

Dr. Wright has found that 2.5 mg of Tri-Est a day often relieves menopausal symptoms and is the equivalent of 0.625 mg of conjugated estrogens like Premarin. Many doctors have turned to Tri-Est for their menopausal patients. Now, some doctors are opting for Bi-Est, which contains no estrone.

Natural hormones can be beneficial if you really need them. When used properly they can be very safe, as well. Estrogens made from pregnant horse's urine may protect your bones and heart (although we're less sure of its heart-protective abilities right now). But conventional HRT may cause cancers. Don't lump all estrogens into one category and say, "Estrogen is not for me." A combination of natural estrogens may be exactly what you need for a clear mind and healthy body. But keep an open mind and explore the subject more thoroughly.

Progestin vs. Progesterone

There are three kinds of progesterone: synthetic chemical substitutes (called progestins), natural progesterone (identical to those your body makes and made by laboratories at natural compounding pharmacies), and over-the-counter (OTC) progesterone precursors (made from wild yam or soybeans). Each is different from the other. Like estrogens, some are safer than others, as well.

SECRET #248 Progestins are not progesterone.

Progestins, like Provera, are drugs. They are chemicalized progesterone substitutes that have side effects. Progestins are not progesterone. These two hormones act very differently. Progesterone increases immunity. It increases genes that protect against cancer and decrease genes that cause cancer. Progestins contribute to heart disease and breast cancer.

Most progesterone studies have been done on progestins rather than natural progesterone. But progestins are more powerful than the progesterone your body makes, and they have many side effects. They are carcinogenic, cause water retention, nausea, depression, and abnormal menstrual flow. They may affect cholesterol levels, can cause facial hair, and even stimulate estrogen production.

A study funded partly by the National Institutes of Health in 1995 and conducted by researchers at the Johns Hopkins University School of Hygiene and Public Health found that progestins can contribute to breast cancer. This study was not the only one to make such an allegation. Another study in the *New England Journal of Medicine* found that within a group of over 120,000 nurses, those who took progestins alone had more of a risk for breast cancer than women taking estrogen alone.

Lorraine Fitzpatrick, M.D., of the Mayo Clinic, found that Provera closes the coronary arteries and leads to heart disease. Constricted arteries are a major cause of heart disease in women. No wonder heart disease is the number-one killer of postmenopausal women!

SECRET #249 Progesterone creams made from wild yam may not contain any progesterone.

Progesterone creams made from wild yams do not contain any progesterone unless the progesterone hormone, made in a laboratory, is added to them. They contain substances called progesterone precursors that can theoretically turn into progesterone. Unfortunately, these creams, applied topically to your skin, don't convert into progesterone because your skin doesn't have the ability to turn these precursors into progesterone. Without added progesterone, these creams have no hormonal activity.

According to the heads of two natural compounding pharmacies, many of the creams sold in natural-food stores have a little progesterone in them, but the potency is low and the progesterone is poorly absorbed. Dr. Reiss found that his patients who used these creams usually lose any benefits from them over time. He uses a product that contains 10 percent progesterone concentration; the health-food-store brands have around 3 percent progesterone.

While its advocates claim that progesterone creams have no side effects, doctor friends of mine and I have all seen patients with sleeplessness, *increased* hot flashes, increased appetite, and weight gain as a result of using them.

SECRET #250 The most popular progesterone cream may not work.

Progest cream, a heavily promoted OTC cream, was tested by researchers at the

Menopause Clinics at King's College Hospital in London. They found that the absorption of progesterone in Progest is small. It was too small, in fact, to offer endometrial protection from excess estrogen, and too little to help protect against bone loss. These researchers used from two to four times the amount of Progest cream that the manufacturers recommended.

When I read this study, I started searching for a better progesterone cream. The purest, best-quality progesterone I found is Kevala's PureGest Natural Progesterone cream. Most progesterone creams are greasy and don't absorb well. Pure-Gest is not greasy and is absorbed quickly. I have seen better results with women using this cream over the progesterone creams you can buy over the counter. Natural compounding pharmacies make the very best progesterone creams. Why? Because they contain exactly the amount of hormone you need.

SECRET #251 Progesterone creams may contain substances not listed on their labels.

Natural progesterone creams are not regulated and vary considerably. Some have added hormones while others don't. They haven't been studied in sound, scientific double-blind studies, nor is their labeling always accurate.

I heard from a doctor that one of his patients using an OTC progesterone cream was experiencing hirsutism—facial hair. He couldn't understand why, so he sent the cream to a laboratory for analysis at his own expense. The label on the cream did not list any progesterone hormone or other substances. To his surprise, not only did it contain some natural progesterone, it also had some pregnenolone in it as well.

Pregnenolone is a substance that is used by the body to make a variety of hormones: estrogen, testosterone, aldosterone, and progesterone. This means that a progesterone cream with added pregnenolone might cause facial hair or cause some of the problems you're using progesterone to correct. It is very possible that some of the negative side effects women have experienced from natural progesterone creams are coming from these added ingredients. But there's no way to know. Pregnenolone is both safe and effective if you need it and take just the amount you need. But it's not a hormone you want hidden in any other products.

SECRET #252 Without enough estrogen, progesterone can cause problems.

Taking large doses of either progestins or progesterone can lower your immunity, said research gynecologist Guy E. Abraham, M.D. While natural progesterone has been used to reverse vaginal atrophy, if you don't have enough estrogen, progesterone can contribute to this condition.

SECRET #253 **The best progesterone is available from natural compounding pharmacies.**

Natural compounding pharmacies may make progesterone products from soybeans or wild yam, but they're nothing like OTC creams. These progesterone products, which may be in the form of transdermal patches, injections, creams, suppositories, or oral tablets, are identical with your body's progesterone.

To get them, you need a prescription from your doctor. The good news is that these pharmacies work closely with doctors to help them decide which hormone products are best for your particular needs. Belmar Pharmacy (see the Resources section) can send your doctor copies of double-blind studies that have been conducted with their progesterone products. No other natural progesterone has been studied in this manner. These studies may make your doctor more comfortable in learning more about natural hormone products.

SECRET #254 **You need to get tested to see which hormones you need.**

I'm in favor of allowing people to take more responsibility for their health. I like the idea of going to a store and buying the hormones I need without a prescription. But I have heard horror stories from women who did just this. Regulating hormone levels is a complex balancing act. We need help in assessing our individual needs through laboratory tests to find the best form and balance of hormones. And we need to be monitored for the right dosage. Anything else, in my opinion, is playing Russian roulette. It's worth the time and expense to get accurate information.

You may need estrogen, you may need progesterone, or you may need both. Then there are other hormones like testosterone, human growth hormone (HGH), DHEA, melatonin, and pregnenolone. Each is important, but not all women need to take all of them. This is why it's best to work with a medical doctor or other healthcare practitioner to determine what you need and to guide you through the maze of natural hormones.

SECRET #255 **If you're taking hormones, don't test your estrogen levels yet.**

Blood tests designed to measure estrogen levels are not accurate if you're already taking an estrogen replacement made from pregnant horse's urine or from soy. How can it be? These chemicalized hormones are not identical to your body's. It's like comparing apples to oranges. They're both fruit, but that's where the similarity ends.

The results from blood tests taken while you're already using chemicalized hormones often don't match your symptoms. For this reason, the amount of hormones you may be given by your doctor could be based on an inaccurate blood test. To get an accurate measurement, you need to first stop taking these forms of estrogen for two months.

SECRET #256 Saliva tests are not completely accurate. Don't rely on them as your only test.

There's a big disagreement on the use of saliva tests to measure hormone levels. A number of healthcare practitioners are using them because they're easy and inexpensive. But the heads of two natural compounding pharmacies, who have no vested interest in which tests any woman gets, told me that their results often don't correlate with a woman's symptoms.

Saliva tests are most accurate for progesterone alone. If you are using saliva tests, also get your blood levels of hormones tested.

Talk with your doctor, or with one of the many knowledgeable people at a natural compounding pharmacy, for suggestions on which hormones to test and which tests give the best results. You and your doctor can use Dr. Reiss' book as a guideline for determining which hormones you need in which quantities. He has detailed the many tests that can be done to accurately measure the hormones you want to measure. To test estrogen levels, for instance, he suggests the following blood tests: Estradiol (E2), FSH (follicle-stimulating hormone), and SHBG (sex hormone-binding globulin). Let your doctor read Dr Reiss's rationale for various tests and decide together about an evaluation program to determine which hormones you may need.

SECRET #257 Blood and urine tests are more accurate.

Blood tests give a snapshot view of your hormones at any given moment. This means the results may vary from day to day. Since your hormone levels may be higher or lower than the values given by any laboratory, your doctor should combine these results with your symptoms.

Some doctors use a blood test for a baseline, then prescribe hormones and watch what happens. If your hormone levels rise and your symptoms decrease, you're taking the correct amount. This is why you want to work with a doctor skilled in hormone therapy. As limited as a blood test is, the doctors and pharmacists I spoke with agreed that it is the best method we have at this time to measure hormone levels.

Another hormone test that is increasing in popularity is a twenty-four-hour urine test, performed by a few specialized laboratories. The theory behind it is that if you take a full day's amount of urine and have a small amount of it analyzed, it can give a wider view of hormone activity than a blood test. But urine tests don't assess progesterone levels, because progesterone is not excreted in your urine. It may, however, be valuable for measuring other hormones, especially cortisol levels. To locate a laboratory in your area that performs this test, speak with the pharmacists at any of the natural compounding pharmacies listed in the Resources section.

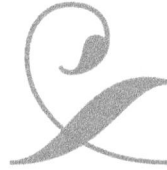

CHAPTER 32

Other Hormones May Be Enough

There's much more to hormone therapy than simply replacing estrogen and progesterone, although many doctors limit their suggestions to these two important hormones. Our bodies contain other sex hormones that are important to our health and feelings of well-being. A comprehensive hormone replacement program consists of evaluating a number of other hormones. This is the only way your doctor can determine whether or not you need to take one or more of them before, after, or instead of using estrogen and/or progesterone. These "other" hormones include DHEA, testosterone, human growth hormone (HGH), melatonin, and pregnenolone. Many doctors of integrative medicine consider them to be the building blocks of their antiaging programs.

Before you jump on the estrogen/progesterone bandwagon, it's important to understand how these other hormones work. Then discuss them with your doctor. He or she can order blood tests and evaluate your symptoms to see which additional hormones could be beneficial to you. Although many conventional doctors are using the same amount of synthetic estrogens and progestins for everyone, as you're seeing, hormone therapy is definitely not a "one-size-fits-all" situation. Your hormonal needs are specific to your body. One or more of these "other" hormones may eliminate the need for taking estrogen or progesterone.

SECRET #258 You need this protein to help regulate your hormones.

Your liver makes a protein that helps regulate hormones. It's called sex-hormone binding globulin, or SHBG for short. SHBG has been called "estrogen's chaperone" because it accompanies sex hormone molecules through the bloodstream. It also regulates a number of hormones. For instance, if your estrogen levels become too high, your liver gets a message to make more SHBG that then binds to, or inactivates, the excess estrogen.

Besides estrogen, SHBG inactivates other hormones like thyroid, human growth hormone, and testosterone. If your SHBG is low, you may need additional amounts of estrogen, thyroid, HGH, and/or testosterone. When you take oral estrogen, your liver produces more SHBG than if it's used as a topical gel or patch. These surges can throw off the balance of your other hormones. This is one reason why I prefer transdermal patches. Before you decide whether or not you need specific hormones, you should ask your doctor to check your SHBG with a blood test. This will help determine just which hormones you might need.

SECRET #259 Low testosterone may be causing your hot flashes.

It's a mistake to think testosterone is just for men. It's not, although it is considered to be a "male" hormone. Just as men's bodies contain a little estrogen, ours contain small amounts of testosterone. After menopause, our male hormones (called androgens) including testosterone decrease by as much as 50 percent. If you've had a hysterectomy that led to menopause, your testosterone level dropped immediately. In either case, the result can be hot flashes and insomnia that remain even after taking estrogen. If this sounds like you, ask your doctor to consider combining a little testosterone with your estrogen.

SECRET #260 A little supplemental testosterone can help your strength and balance.

Small amounts of testosterone can improve your strength, vitality, and emotions. It can even result in better physical balance, reducing your risk for fractures from falls. Testosterone also helps form stronger bones. European studies have shown for years that natural testosterone replacement therapy can lower cholesterol, protect against atherosclerosis, and increase your libido.

But make sure the testosterone you take is natural, not synthetic. The latter is also known as an anabolic steroid, and it can have serious side effects. You may have heard that too much testosterone can cause facial hair, acne, and thinning hair. Not only is this true, some women are very sensitive to normal amounts of natural testosterone, while others get side effects only when their testosterone levels are high. Don't experiment with testosterone. Discuss your possible need for it with your doctor. If you decide to take it, begin with very small amounts to make sure you don't react badly to it.

Tori Hudson, N.D., professor of gynecology at Bastyr University, found that adding 0.5 to 1 mg of natural testosterone to a natural estrogen formula, taken twice daily, is sufficient for the majority of her patients. She has also used a $\frac{1}{2}$ percent, 1 percent, or 2 percent testosterone cream topically every day for two weeks, then just twice a week. This lowers the risk for side effects that could result from taking testosterone every day. Again, discuss these possibilities with your doctor.

SECRET #261 If you don't like taking risks, you may need this hormone.

Do you like to take risks or would you rather play it safe? Your attitude and your energy may be controlled in part by human growth hormone (HGH). High HGH is associated with vitality and an active imagination, while low HGH causes you to not want to change or take risks. Increasing your levels of HGH can give you more mental clarity, reduced irritability, a better immune system, and a more positive attitude. HGH appears to be a significant antiaging hormone.

Declining HGH results in thinner, less elastic skin, falling cheeks, and more wrinkles. Want to age slower? Begin by checking out your levels of HGH with your doctor. Levels for men should be 0–5 ng/mL. Women's levels should be 0–10 ng/mL.

Until recently, HGH supplements were made from the pituitary glands of either animals or human cadavers. Now it's made in laboratories. Unfortunately, HGH is expensive, but you can raise your levels by taking the right amounts of a few amino acids that stimulate its production like arginine, ornithine, and creatine, and by exercising. You can find good information on this method in *Natural Hormone Balance for Women* by Dr. Uzzi Reiss.

SECRET #262 Not all forms of human growth hormone work.

HGH supplements are all the rage. The problem is, many of them are worthless. Take the homeopathic HGH found in health-food stores, for instance. Dr. Reiss tried this form in more than 100 patients and found that it didn't raise their insulinlike growth factor-1 (IGF-1), a measure of HGH, in a single person! It didn't affect their symptoms, either. Based on my conversations with doctors, pharmacists, and nutritionists, his results are not unusual. Save your money. Don't take homeopathic HGH.

If you want to take natural HGH hormone, you first need to find a doctor who is familiar with using it. Contact the American Academy of Anti-Aging Medicine in Chicago for the names of doctors specifically trained in using it. Then, be sure you're getting the real thing, not homeopathic or non-standardized oral over-the-counter HGH.

SECRET #263 This hormone helps you sleep and reduces anxiety.

Melatonin is a hormone made in your brain by your pineal gland. It controls your response to light and dark. It also controls the response of animals to seasons (hibernation and migration). After the age of forty-five, your melatonin levels decrease. The most frequent consequence is insomnia or poor sleeping patterns.

Melatonin is naturally produced around 11 P.M., so taking small amounts of natural melatonin before bedtime may help you sleep better. This hormone is safe enough for you to take it on your own. In fact, it's the only hormone supplement that's safe to self-medicate. Melatonin is more than an anti-insomnia supplement. It also decreases anxiety by stimulating a brain chemical, GABA, that calms you down.

SECRET #264 Melatonin does much more than regulate sleep patterns.

Melatonin is known for its ability to help people sleep better and for its ability to help reduce jet lag. But it also supports your immune system by regenerating your thymus gland—the center of immune function. In one study, breast cancer cells were dosed with the same amount of melatonin you'd find in a young, human body. Growth of these cancer cells was blocked by 75 percent. At the very least, this suggests that melatonin could be an important hormone in protecting against breast cancer.

It also helps your thyroid produce triiodothyronine (T_3), protects your bones, and helps your body use zinc, a mineral needed to lower stress and increase appetite. And it slows down graying hair. Whether or not you want to maintain your looks as long as you can or simply guard against serious health problems like cancer and osteoporosis, melatonin may be one of the best and safest hormones you can take.

SECRET #265 The amount of melatonin you need to take depends on what you want it to do.

From 1 to 5 mg before bed is usually enough to help most people sleep. If you wake up in the middle of the night, you can take another 1 to 5 mg. To eliminate jet lag, try taking from 3 to 5 mg before bedtime for three days before and after flying across time zones. Repeat when you fly home. Melatonin works best when you're sleeping in a dark room. If you take it on a plane, use an eye mask to block out light.

Too much melatonin may give you wild, disturbing dreams or make you sleepy and foggy when you wake up. I take enough melatonin to help me sleep without being foggy in the morning.

Melatonin has also been used in high amounts—from 20 to 40 mg a day—to protect against cancer. These quantities don't usually cause sleepiness.

SECRET #266 You can get a good night's sleep without any hormones at all.

If you don't want to take any hormones, even melatonin, to help you sleep, I have a solution. I'm not talking about barbiturates or other medications. A number of herbs are both safe and effective. Of all herbs, valerian root (*Valeriana officinalis*) has a long-standing reputation for being a strong soporific (a substance that helps you sleep).

It's particularly appropriate for mild insomnia. The American Botanical Council reports that 300–600 mg of valerian root extract is as effective as pharmaceutical sedatives. Take valerian from thirty minutes to several hours before bedtime. Capsules or tinctures are easiest to take but I prefer tinctures. They are absorbed quickly.

You can find a tincture of valerian root at your local health-food store. Or buy some of the dried root and steep it for ten to fifteen minutes in hot water. But I'm warning you now that valerian root smells like dirty socks. You can mix it with other herbs, like mint and chamomile, for a more pleasant, tastier tea. But never mix valerian root with pharmaceutical barbiturates, anesthetics, or central nervous system depressants. It could increase their strength.

Not all products with valerian contain the amount of active ingredients on their labels, says Tod Cooperman, M.D., president of ConsumerLab.com. If the valerian root product you try doesn't work, try another product before reaching for any hormones or sleeping pills.

SECRET #267 Pregnenolone increases other hormone production.

Pregnenolone is made by your adrenal glands from cholesterol and enhances the effects of DHEA. It is a precursor to estrogen, testosterone, and progesterone, as well. By taking pregnenolone, you can support and increase these hormones without actually taking them. This makes pregnenolone an ideal hormone to consider for all women who decide against taking estrogen or progesterone.

Studies show that pregnenolone supports the brain, immunity, and adrenal health. In fact, it's considered to be another antistress hormone. It also seems to contribute to a better memory, alertness, and a feeling of well-being. In fact, some people with depression have low amounts of pregnenolone.

Although there are no specific signs of pregnenolone deficiency, some doctors use it for their patients with memory problems or low stamina. Dr. Reiss suggests taking 50 mg of pregnenolone at breakfast, or using it in a moisturizing cream. But he always gets a blood test to assay its effectiveness and absorption. Normal pregnenolone levels are 70 to 120 mg/dl. If you take too much pregnenolone, you could feel a bit edgy. You could also get undesirable facial hair.

SECRET #268 DHEA may take the place of other hormones.

DHEA is a steroid hormone now being touted as a miracle antiaging nutrient. Structurally, DHEA is similar to other steroid hormones like estrogen, progesterone, and testosterone. In fact, DHEA can be converted into both estrogen and testosterone, boosting estrogen levels. For this reason, DHEA can cause the same side effects as testosterone, like facial hair.

DHEA is a good example of the interconnectedness of all hormones. You may be low in several hormones, but taking this one could boost some of the others. This hormone is made from cholesterol by your adrenal glands, those tiny workhorses that help you handle all the stresses in your life. It is an antistress androgen hormone that supports the immune system and is considered to be anticarcinogenic when it's taken in the correct doses.

DHEA both slows down bone loss and increases bone formation, reducing your risk for osteoporosis. Animal studies indicate it can help prevent diseases such as cancer, lupus, rheumatoid arthritis, Alzheimer's, heart disease, and chronic fatigue. It may even help slow down aging and increase your libido. DHEA is abundant in brain tissue and has been found to increase neurons in laboratory tests with nerve-cell tissue cultures. This means that DHEA may support our brain function as we age.

SECRET #269 Too much DHEA could be dangerous.

A study in the *Journal of the American Medical Association* found a correlation between high DHEA levels and ovarian cancer. Another study showed high DHEA levels in women with breast cancer. Still other studies associate high levels of DHEA with lowered incidence of cancer. There isn't enough research, yet, to know just how DHEA influences cancer. It may affect different people differently. However, it is a good argument for just taking the amount of DHEA your body needs, because too much of this hormone can have either serious or milder side effects. It can produce a testosterone-like effect with symptoms such as facial hair, acne, and irritability.

SECRET #270 DHEA is not the ultimate hormone. It may not work for you.

When you look at the many DHEA studies done you'll find that it sometimes works and it sometimes doesn't. These studies are usually too short and have used high doses. I've found that many women who take DHEA can take only 5–10 mg without experiencing side effects. According to the doctors and pharmacists I've talked with, a lower amount is often enough and is quite effective.

While some women swear that they feel better after taking it, two studies published in the *Journal of Clinical Endocrinology & Metabolism* found that DHEA did not increase any feelings of well-being in women. DHEA may do wonders for you. Or it may do nothing. There's a good explanation for this. Our bodies handle hormones like DHEA differently. In some women, it remains as DHEA; in others, it is converted to testosterone or estrogen. The way your body absorbs and utilizes DHEA will determine whether or not it is a helpful, desirable hormone to take.

SECRET #271 DHEA should be tested and retested.

Only take DHEA if a blood test for DHEA-sulfate, shows that your levels are low. The amount of DHEA your body may need can vary considerably from 5–50 mg a day. However, many doctors are finding that from 5–15 mg is sufficient. Since high amounts of DHEA can have negative effects, begin with a lower amount. Check with your doctor first and discuss dosage with him or her. Discuss a slow method of gradually increasing your levels. Taking too much too soon is more likely to give you undesirable side effects. Then have your blood retested again after taking DHEA for a month or two.

SECRET #272 Not all DHEA products are good quality.

Some DHEA is higher quality than others. The head of a natural pharmacy found that many DHEA products sold in natural-food stores that claimed to be 25–50 mg contained only 5–10 mg of the hormone. "At least people aren't hurting themselves," he told me. Your doctor may know of a supplement company that has high-quality hormones. ProThera (in the Resources section) is one that I particularly like and use. But your doctor may prefer that you get DHEA from a natural compounding pharmacy.

What about precursors to DHEA like the Mexican yam or herbs? They're not a good option. Your body's ability to convert precursors into DHEA diminishes with age. The older you are, the less likely it is that these natural products will have an effect. Any increased feeling of well-being most likely comes from a stimulant effect in these products. The only proven method of raising your DHEA level is by taking DHEA itself.

The benefits of DHEA that many doctors have seen include mental clarity, increased energy and stamina, and better moods. This is definitely a hormone to consider using in any HRT program.

CHAPTER 33

Cool Down
Your Hot Flashes

More women use hormone replacement therapy for their hot flashes and night sweats than for depression, bone loss, or any other reason. That's because heat surges affect the way you feel every day. They can also affect how well you sleep at night. When I was a teenager, I remember my mother telling me that she woke up at night drenched with perspiration. Each night she had to change her nightgown and sheets. During the day—especially in the summer—she would perspire profusely. This went on for many months. At that time, I didn't realize she was going through menopause; I just knew something was wrong.

Now I know that my mother wasn't alone. About 80 percent of menopausal women in this country have hot flashes. Hot flashes are periods of sudden intense heat, while flushes include the obvious flushing or redness. While they usually come and go for a year or two, I've known patients who still have hot flashes ten to fifteen years after menopause. And these hot flashes and flushes can last for a few seconds or up to five minutes.

Fortunately, there are solutions to uncomfortable periods of heat. A change in diet along with particular supplements can often eliminate them completely. Some of these solutions are in your kitchen or at your neighborhood natural-food store. They're inexpensive and may be all you need to do. If you or anyone you know is plagued by surges of heat, read on. Help is on the way.

SECRET #273 Hot flashes may mean that your inner temperature gauge isn't working properly.

One reason hot flashes occur is that the hypothalamus gland, which regulates your body's temperature, isn't able to adjust to changing hormone levels. Even a slight alteration in this thermostat can cause flushing and periods of intense heat. Low estrogen may be one reason for a malfunctioning hypothalamus, or it may be due to an imbalance of naturally occurring brain opiates caused by lowered estrogens and progesterone. This explains why hot flashes appear around menopause.

There may be another reason for them as well. Some researchers believe that hot flashes are caused by too much dopamine, a brain chemical. They are testing the effects of the herb sage to block the neurotransmitter that signals the brain to release more dopamine. Preliminary studies show that sage seems to work well for hot flashes. But there are other things you can do before taking this herb or resorting to hormones.

SECRET #274 Heat-producing foods can trigger hot flashes.

Sometimes the obvious escapes us. It makes sense that your body gets warmer when you eat foods that create heat. When you are warmer, you're more susceptible to hot flashes. The first thing you can do to reduce your hot flashes is to eat fewer foods that create heat. These include fatty foods, sugars, caffeine, and spicy foods. If you like spicy foods, tone them down from "very hot" to "warm."

Drink decaffeinated coffee or tea for now. Or try Teeccino, a caffeine-free herbal beverage you can find in natural-food stores. Teeccino is high in potassium, which means it may give you an energy boost and reduce any heart palpitations you may have. It's brewed just like coffee and can be drunk hot, iced, or as a latte.

SECRET #275 Cooling foods and plant estrogens help reduce hot flashes.

Fruits, vegetables, and dairy products all cool the body. Lemon water is particularly effective—which is why lemonade is such a popular drink in hot weather. Sweeten yours with stevia instead of sugar (for more information on this sweetner, see Chapter 16). It doesn't produce heat or affect your blood sugar. Eat more salads and fewer cooked foods. And don't forget to drink plenty of water throughout the day. Water puts out all kinds of fires.

Eat more soy. In Japan, where soy is a common part of most people's diet, there is no word for "hot flashes." The phenomenon simply doesn't exist. The reason for this is that isoflavones, plant-based estrogens found in soy, have a very weak but positive estrogenic effect. This amount is frequently enough to prevent hot flashes.

Numerous studies found similar results. One concluded that the amount of soy needed to reduce hot flashes was equal to two daily servings of tofu or soymilk. These foods, by the way, are rather low in isoflavones. Edamame (green soybeans) and roasted soynuts, found in natural-food stores, are higher in isoflavones.

Next, Consider Taking Supplements

When dietary changes are not enough, it's time to look at supplements. Most hot flash formulas contain black cohosh or isoflavones, but I've discovered others that may work even better.

SECRET #276 A substance found in vitamin C can help regulate your temperature.

Hesperidin is one of a number of bioflavonoids (parts of the vitamin C complex) found in the skin of lemons and oranges. I stumbled upon it more than a dozen years ago. It works like a miracle for many women, eliminating hot flashes and night sweats. Hands down, hesperidin is my favorite nutrient for excessive menopausal heat.

Hesperidin seems to act directly on the hypothalamus, helping it to regulate temperatures more easily. Studies show that it also decreases the permeability of tiny blood vessels. This makes it a valuable nutrient for all vascular conditions from hot flashes to hemorrhoids. Simply put, hesperidin supports the integrity of the vascular system that is often weakened by hormonal fluctuations.

A placebo-controlled study on hot flashes using hesperidin with extra vitamin C found that hot flashes were eliminated in 53 percent of women participants and were reduced in 34 percent of them. My patients take 500 mg morning and night. You most likely will need that much to reduce your hot flashes.

Although hesperidin is a bioflavonoid, you can't get enough of it in bioflavonoid supplements. Instead, look for a hot flash formula with high amounts of hespiridin (see the Resources section).

SECRET #277 Lydia Pinkham included this herb in her menopause formula in 1875.

Black cohosh (*Cimicifuga racemosa*) is best known today as being the main ingredient in Remifemin, an OTC herbal supplement. Remifemin was originally made and distributed by a supplement company. Now a major pharmaceutical company, GlaxoSmithKline, is making it. But black cohosh was one of the original herbs in Lydia Pinkham's Vegetable Compound, a formula developed in 1875 for "female complaints." It's been used for more than a hundred years.

This herb appears to reduce hot flashes by suppressing the secretion of luteinizing hormone (LH), which is released by the pituitary gland. Black cohosh alone works well for many women, but if it doesn't, there are other single nutrients you can try, or a combination formula to see what works best for you. The herbal supplements listed in the Resources section contain both hesperidin and black cohosh.

SECRET #278 The solution to your hot flashes could be in your garden.

Sage (*Salvia officinalis*) is a common herb that's been overshadowed by more highly processed anti-hot-flash ingredients. Sage has been used since ancient times to stop hot flashes. And it works! In fact, many herbalists know sage as the "hot flush herb" for its ability to reduce all kinds of excessive perspiration.

It's long been licensed in Germany as a tea to treat night sweats and is used extensively in England for this purpose. Almost all of the health practitioners surveyed in England found that sage tea or sage tincture helped hot flashes and night sweats. One Scottish survey showed that women taking sage had 85 percent fewer hot flashes after three months.

This is good news. It means that the answer to your uncomfortable heat and night sweats could be growing in your garden. If not, you may want to plant some.

SECRET #279 Sage has been sold as a nonprescription drug in Europe for the past ten years.

In the early 1990s, a group of German scientists and herbalists evaluated more than 300 herbs and herbal combinations for safety and effectiveness. These monographs were published by the Commission E in 1995 and they permitted the herb to be sold throughout Europe as a nonprescription drug. They are called the *Commission E Monographs*. Subsequently, a group of expert herbalists, headed by Mark Blumenthal, executive director of the American Botanical Council, updated and expanded these monographs. These expanded monographs reissued in 2000 as the *Expanded Commission E Monographs* now contain the most objective, science-based information on herbal medicine currently available.

Both monographs found sage to be safe and effective for hot flashes. Sage is licensed in Germany as a medicinal herb tea for intestinal inflammation and night sweats, as well as for coughs and to improve memory. Its astringency may be why it works so well for excessive perspiration. There's more information on using sage to reduce hot flashes than any other herb. In my opinion, it should be in every formula for hot flashes and night sweats.

SECRET #280 From one to three cups of sage tea can reduce your hot flashes.

You can drink a few cups of the tea a day or take the herb as a supplement. Sage tea is the safest and least expensive solution. Steep a tea bag of sage, or a teaspoon of the dried herb, for five to ten minutes. Allow the tea to cool down for best results. Then drink from one to three cups a day in between meals. You can increase this amount, if you like, to four or five cups a day. You may need much less. In fact, just one serving of sage tea can cool down some women within two hours and last for a day or more.

Tinctures or capsules containing sage are good options if you don't want to drink the tea. An Italian study gave thirty women with hot flashes, insomnia, night sweats, headaches, and palpitations an extract of sage and alfalfa. Hot flashes and night sweats disappeared in twenty of them, and the other ten had a reduction of their symptoms. This study used 120 mg of sage a day, the same amount found in the formulas listed in the Resources section.

Sage is an attractive plant that's easy to grow, even in poor soil with very little water. It could make a valuable addition to your garden. Whether you'd rather drink sage tea every day for awhile or try a product with sage, this herb may be the solution to your uncomfortable heat.

SECRET #281 A combination formula may work best.

If you want a broader supplement containing several anti-hot flash ingredients, you may want to give a formula containing hesperidin, black cohosh, and sage a two-month trial. You can find several listed in the Resources section. Look in natural-food stores for other combination formulas using some of these ingredients. They could be a quick, simple end to uncomfortable hot flashes with the right dietary changes and supplements. In fact, modifying your diet may be all you need to do!

SECRET #282 The right kind of oils can reduce hot flashes.

Vitamin E and evening primrose oil may reduce hot flashes, but you could need to take as much as 1,200 international units (IU) of vitamin E each day. This is a lot, especially since vitamin E thins the blood. It's definitely not a good choice for anyone taking coumadin or other blood-thinner medications. Evening primrose oil, on the other hand, is quite safe in any quantity and is high in gamma-linolenic acid (GLA), an essential fatty acid. You may want to try one capsule of evening primrose oil twice a day and gradually increase it up to six or eight capsules a day until you get relief.

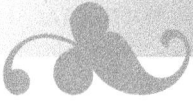

PART 7

SURPRISING BREAKTHROUGHS THAT CAN SAVE YOU from OSTEOPOROSIS

I think of osteoporosis as being the greatest misunderstood women's health problem of modern times. No matter what you've heard—and I'm sure you've heard this often enough to believe it—taking a lot of calcium is not the answer. If it were, fewer women today would have broken bones.

Think about it. Doctors have been pushing calcium supplements on women for decades, and osteoporosis continues to plague us.

While taking calcium may help preserve bone density, it also makes your bones more brittle, and brittle bones break easily. Taking too much calcium also has other consequences. It contributes to heart disease and arthritis, diseases that are becoming more common in women ever since calcium has been emphasized. Not only is calcium not the answer, in many cases it's the problem.

The right diet can help by carrying calcium into your bones where it belongs, and by having enough of another mineral to keep your bones more flexible. What you don't eat may be just as important as what you do eat. Some foods actually pull calcium out of your bones and should be eaten only in small quantities if at all.

Exercise is vital to the formation of strong bones, but not all exercises give the same results. You want exercises that help you keep your balance, and others that strengthen your bones, not just your muscles. I discovered an easy-to-do set of exercises with an inexpensive and portable piece of equipment that has been shown to reverse osteoporosis—not just slow down its progression.

We think of osteoporosis as being a disease that only affects our arms, legs, and spine. But there's more. Gum disease (periodontitis) can cause you to lose the bones that keep your teeth in place. Dental problems affect the foods you're able to eat, like crunchy fruits and vegetables. I'll give you some simple tips your dentist may not have mentioned that could keep your teeth where they belong—rooted firmly in your mouth.

When all else fails, you may want to consider taking prescription drugs. But not before you have more information. If you are tempted to take any of these medications, you'll want to read a little more about them so you can make a more informed choice.

Stress reduction, diet, and the right kind of bone-stressing exercises all help build strong, flexible bones. So does the right balance of minerals. Let me explain some of the myths surrounding osteoporosis and suggest some real solutions that can keep your bones from breaking, even if you take a tumble.

FOUR WAYS TO PREVENT YOUR BONES FROM BREAKING

1. Keep them supple. Take 500–1,000 mg of magnesium a day and 500–800 mg of calcium to build strong, flexible bones.

2. Strengthen them with bone-stressing exercise.

3. Learn to balance. People break bones when they fall.

4. Reduce your stress. Stress hormones, such as cortisol, pull calcium out of your bones.

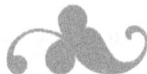

CHAPTER 34

Major Myths about Osteoporosis

I've learned that if you live long enough, just about everything changes, even definitions of diseases. Sometimes these definitions help by telling us more specifically what's going on and what we need to do to correct a situation. Other times they just add to our confusion. I know of no disease—or condition—that fits this latter category as well as osteoporosis. The definition of osteoporosis has changed, and with this change has come more confusion.

SECRET #283 Brittle bones, not a loss of bone density, are a sign of osteoporosis.

Gillian Sanson, author of *The Myth of Osteoporosis,* says, "Calling low, bone-mineral density osteoporosis is like calling elevated cholesterol heart disease, or calling high blood pressure a stroke." There's a connection between the two, but bone density alone does not define osteoporosis.

Doctors still define osteoporosis as a condition where bones have lost some of their density—which is a normal part of aging. This suggests that aging is a disease, not a process. At one time, osteoporosis was considered to be a disease characterized by broken bones. If you broke your hip, you had osteoporosis; if you had no fractures, you didn't have this disease. This original definition makes the most sense to me.

If osteoporosis simply indicated a loss of bone density, it would mean that everyone over the age of fifty has this disease and needs to take something to increase it—whether or not their bones are fragile and break easily. Not true at all! We all lose some bone density as we age, but the majority of people never have fractures as a result of this loss.

It's time to go back to the original definition and understand *why* our bones break.

Bone brittleness is a key factor in whether or not your bones will break when you fall, but it's a subject that's rarely discussed. One reason is that there's no way

241

to measure brittleness and the medical community is reluctant to talk about any subject for which it has no answers. But to ignore a primary cause for fractures, like bone fragility, is dangerous and unconscionable.

Increasing bone density is big business. Pharmaceutical companies are getting rich selling hormones to frightened women. Supplement companies are making a fortune pushing calcium pills even when supplemental calcium is unnecessary and can contribute to heart disease and arthritis. Unfortunately, neither hormones nor calcium are the answer to fragile bones that are an integral part of osteoporosis. Excessive calcium makes bones more brittle and more likely to break.

SECRET #284 Bone-density tests only give limited information.

Measuring your bone density is not an accurate way of predicting future fractures. It doesn't take into account the structure of your bones. Flexible bones are less likely to break than fragile bones, regardless of their thickness and size.

Bone density is commonly measured with dual energy x-ray absorptiometry (DXA). The problem is, this test doesn't measure your bone density at all. The DXA test measures the amount of calcium you have in your bones.

Now, listen carefully to this next part. If the calcium in your bones is a little low, but you have plenty of magnesium, the bone you build will be strong and flexible. However, a DXA test can measure only the low calcium content. It will most likely indicate that your bones are at risk for breaking when the opposite may be true. Sufficient magnesium (up to bowel tolerance, with a maximum of 1,000 milligrams (mg) a day, even with a lower calcium intake (500–800 mg a day), helps form more flexible bones that don't break easily.

Another problem with bone-density tests is that they measure only the density in one particular bone. Bone is living tissue, and the mineral content in one bone is rarely identical with the minerals in another. If you happen to have any calcium deposits in the area that's being tested, your results will inaccurately reflect dense bones.

Bottom-line: The problem is not bone mass, but bone strength. DXA only measures the amount of calcium in your bones.

SECRET #285 Progesterone, not estrogen, helps build bones.

It's true that estrogen can prevent the loss of bone tissue. But to reduce your risk for osteoporosis, you need to begin taking it right at menopause. Estrogen doesn't have any effect on the formation of new bone tissue, just its loss. What's more, if you begin taking estrogen and then stop using it, your bone loss can accelerate.

All of us go through menopause, but not all of us break bones—even women who are not on hormone replacement therapy (HRT) who have serious falls. Why is this? It may not be a lack of estrogen at all, but rather low levels of progesterone. Estrogen helps prevent bone loss, but progesterone appears to promote bone formation. We don't yet know if there are any long-term side effects from taking natural progesterone. I suggest using it only as a last resort and after your hormone levels have been checked. Then take it under the direction of a qualified health practitioner who can monitor you for any side effects.

SECRET #286 Magnesium, not calcium, helps prevent osteoporosis.

Repeat after me: "High calcium intake causes bones to form that are brittle. Magnesium causes bones to form that are strong and flexible. I need plenty of magnesium and enough, but not too much, calcium."

Here's why. The calcium crystals in bone tissue help determine how brittle or supple your bones will be. Abnormally large, smooth calcium crystals can't grab onto one another and form strong bones. That's why the bone they make is brittle. Magnesium helps form crystals that are smaller and irregular in shape. These crystals bind to one another and create stronger, more flexible bones.

Let's use chalk and ivory to illustrate this bone-building phenomenon. Chalk is pure calcium carbonate, one of the forms of calcium added to many osteoporosis supplements. Ivory, on the other hand, contains calcium with magnesium. If you took a three-inch long, thin piece of chalk and dropped it, it would break. The same size piece of ivory would bounce. Do you want your bones to be more like chalk or ivory?

SECRET #287 The calcium/magnesium ratio in your supplements may be causing more problems than it solves.

Most multivitamin/mineral formulas are based on old information saying that women need twice as much calcium as magnesium. This isn't enough magnesium to help carry calcium into your bones and form strong bone tissues. But that's not all. In addition to forming brittle bones, this ratio creates other health problems. You see, unabsorbed calcium doesn't just "go away." Instead, it can collect in your joints where it becomes arthritis or in your arteries where it contributes to atherosclerosis. No wonder so many women suffer from heart attacks and painful arthritis as they age!

Meanwhile, vested interest groups continue to give out old information. The dairy industry and supplement companies that profit from selling millions of dollars' worth of calcium pills are two of them. A review of nearly sixty studies on the effects of dairy consumption on bones published in the *American Journal of Clinical Nutrition* concluded that there was not enough evidence to support recommending dairy products for osteoporosis prevention.

So how much calcium and magnesium do you need in your daily supplement? Around 500 mg of each, added to a healthy diet, should be plenty. Many foods in a healthy diet contain both of these minerals, so the amount you get each day is much higher than this. If you're eating dairy every day, you may want to add more magnesium to your diet and supplements. For more information on calcium and magnesium, along with numerous references, read my *User's Guide to Calcium and Magnesium.*

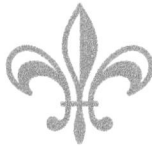

CHAPTER 35

The Two Missing Links: Diet and Exercise

SECRET #288 **These foods pull calcium out of your bones.**

Bone is mostly made from calcium. You want calcium to get into them, not to be pulled out of them. Some foods and beverages actually leech calcium from your bones. They include alcohol, refined sugar, and caffeine. Limited quantities should cause no problems. Two cups of coffee (or four cups of green tea) a day and one glass of wine, with an occasional cookie or dessert, is not going to affect your bones. But four or five cups of coffee and a lot of sugar may. Don't take the risk. Keep your intake low.

Phosphorus is a mineral essential to healthy bones. You can find it in nuts, corn, eggs, whole grains, and dairy products. But you don't want too much phosphorus or it will keep calcium from being absorbed. Some colas are particularly high in phosphorus. It doesn't matter which ones. They either contain a lot of sugar, caffeine, or sugar substitutes, none of which are beneficial. Avoid soft drinks, please. If necessary, put an inch or two of fruit juice in a glass of mineral water and make your own soda.

SECRET #289 **Eat a diet containing a balance of calcium and magnesium.**

Remember, too much calcium and not enough magnesium forms brittle bones and increases your risk for arthritis and heart disease. Most of us get too much calcium and not enough magnesium in our diets. Milk, cheese, yogurt, and other dairy products are the culprits. They're high in calcium with no magnesium. To balance the calcium in dairy, you need to eat huge amounts of whole grains, nuts, seeds, and dark green leafy vegetables. Limit your dairy consumption to one small portion a day and be sure to eat magnesium-rich foods regularly. Otherwise, you may need to take supplemental magnesium.

A study on cyclists, runners, and non-athletes found absolutely no association between calcium intake and bone density. I've said it before: To get calcium into your bones you need enough magnesium and not too much calcium. Most diets and supplements are too high in calcium and too low in magnesium. The majority of supplements contain twice as much calcium as magnesium. You need equal amounts—or more magnesium than calcium—along with specific exercises that build strong bones. You don't need more calcium.

By the way, foods high in magnesium are also high in boron, a mineral found to protect against osteoporosis. The amount found to be helpful is 2 or 3 mg of boron a day, the amount found in a healthy vegetarian diet. Make sure that your daily multivitamin and mineral formula contains enough of this mineral. Getting just 1 mg won't give you the protection you want unless your diet regularly contains high-boron foods.

SECRET #290 You need enough, but not too much, protein.

Too much protein increases your risk for fractures; too little protein causes low collagen and brittle bones. So how much is enough? What's too much? You need as much as 15 to 20 grams of protein at each meal, at least for a while. This is not easy for a vegetarian like me! But it's possible.

In a three-year study with 500 women participants in their sixties and seventies, those who ate the most protein had significantly better bone density than those who ate the least. This study is good news for all of us. It says that we can improve our bone health even if we start later in life. Bone is living tissue. It's always breaking down and being rebuilt.

Pay attention to your sources of protein and don't overdo protein from animal sources. They usually contain harmful hormones and pesticides. The more animal protein you eat, the more likely you are to get serious chronic illnesses like cancer. In addition, animal fats increase inflammation and can contribute to heart disease. Eat some animal and some vegetable protein each day. Don't fool yourself by thinking you can get away with eating protein only occasionally. You'll survive, but your bones won't be strong. Eating protein once a day is not enough. Many of the women I counsel eat small amounts of protein once or twice a day. This won't support muscle strength and tone. Here are some hints to help you increase your vegetable protein:

- Add a scoop of soy or rice protein powder to your morning cereal or juice.

- Choose the soy products highest in protein. (One Boca brand meatless Italian sausage has 13 grams of protein, while a larger veggie burger may contain only 10 grams.)

- Add beans, nuts, or slices of pressed tofu to salads. Even the small amount of protein found in beans is better than no protein at all.

SECRET #291 Protein and exercise build muscle, and muscle mass affects bone strength.

You're taking your calcium—but not too much of it. And you're getting plenty of magnesium, boron, and vitamin D to drive that calcium into your bones.

You've eliminated large amounts of refined sugar and stopped drinking colas. You even walk four or five times a week. So your bones should be strong, right? Well, maybe! If you're getting enough protein and using it to build muscles through the right kind of exercise.

Muscle mass is directly related to muscle and bone strength. Building muscles through resistance exercises protects you from osteoporosis. It also helps with weight control. Here's why: The more total muscle mass you have, the more calories you burn—even when you're just sitting around or sleeping. When you increase your muscles, you increase your metabolism.

> Weaker, smaller muscles are associated with osteoporosis, falls, fluctuating blood sugar levels, and an increasing sensitivity to heat and cold.
>
> —AMERICAN JOURNAL OF CLINICAL NUTRITION, JUNE 2003

As we age, exercise becomes more than important—it becomes essential to good health. Aging causes our bodies to produce fewer hormones like DHEA and testosterone that help maintain muscles. This means that the older we get, the more we lose muscle mass, quality, and strength. We also lose our balance, making it easier to fall and break bones.

Hormone therapy, like DHEA, can help. But it certainly isn't the first step for you to take. Begin with the proper diet and the right kinds of exercises first. They're inexpensive solutions. They'll work for you if you're willing to make the necessary changes.

SECRET #292 Only full-body, weight-bearing exercises help build bones.

Not all exercises are equally effective in protecting you against osteoporosis. Some build bones, while others don't. Swimming is excellent for your flexibility but not for building bones. Dancing and calisthenics are excellent aerobic exercises for your heart health, but they're not the most effective ones to protect against osteoporosis. Neither are running and biking which primarily stress the legs. Daily cardiovascular exercises such as walking or running, or using a stationary bike or treadmill, strengthen your heart and lungs. Resistance exercises strengthen your muscles and bones.

An eighteen-month study on runners, bicyclists, and women who didn't exercise found that the non-exercisers had more bone loss in their necks than the runners and bicyclists. But neither running nor biking completely prevented bone loss in the upper spine, indicating that their "neck bones" weren't being stressed enough.

If you're not doing full-body, weight-bearing exercises, you're losing bone density no matter how much calcium you take and how much exercising you do. To increase your bone density, you need exercises that stress all your muscles where they attach to your bones. I was surprised and delighted to find that the best exercise you can do for your bones is *gardening.*

SECRET #293 For gardening to build bones, you need to do more than plant and weed.

Several years ago, I heard about a study claiming that gardening can build bone density. I immediately contacted the head researcher, Lori W. Turner, associate professor of health science at the University of Arkansas. Her team had begun studying how various exercises affect bone density. "We're not ready to release our statistics," she said. "But it looks like yard work is one of the best exercises a woman can do to protect and build her bones."

Later, Dr. Turner sent me her completed study. Sure enough, yard work topped the list of bone-building exercises! Now, kneeling and weeding may not be enough to stress all your muscles and help create strong bones, but if you push a lawnmower or rototiller, dig holes, spread mulch, and carry compost or soil around, you've got a winning combination.

I've loved gardening all my life, ever since my parents grew a victory garden in the 1940s. As an adult, I've usually had my own vegetable garden. Now there's not much sun on my property, so I've coordinated a community garden with my neighbors. We till and amend the soil and make huge piles of compost. We move huge planter boxes for raised beds. And soon we'll put up a tool shed. As we garden, we're getting plenty of weight-bearing exercise to build strong bones. And by working outdoors, we get the vitamin D we need as well that also contributes to strong bones. If you don't have a place to garden, find a friend or group of friends and garden with them.

SECRET #294 Walking has its place in preserving bone density . . . if you add arm weights.

Walking is a form of weight-bearing exercise for your legs. Dr. Turner and her team found it to be moderately protective for bone density. But it wasn't as good as weight training. Still, if you like to walk instead of garden, you can buy a set of one- or two-pound weights with Velcro fasteners and attach them to your wrists and ankles before your walk. You can also find inexpensive handheld weights with foam padding at sporting goods stores. Either will work, especially if you move your arms back and forth, and up and down as you walk. You can even do exercises at home holding cans of beans!

I like the idea of weight training, but I prefer a safer, more precise method than free weights. Several years ago, I discovered an excellent exercise program using a partially inflated vinyl ball with handles called the OsteoBall. Robert Swezey, M.D., the rheumatologist who developed the ball and exercises, studied their effect on bone density for more than fifteen years and published his findings in the *Journal of Rheumatology* a few years ago. He heads the Sweezy Institute, an osteoporosis prevention and treatment center in Santa Monica, California, which I visited. I'm impressed with his findings and am convinced that his program is a safe and inexpensive way of building bone and muscle strength. The OsteoBall uses resistance training rather than heavy weights. I tell you more about it next.

SECRET #295 Resistance training is your key to bone-saving exercises.

Resistance training means pushing against gravity. This increases muscle strength and endurance. It also strengthens your muscles at each end where they attach to bones. When you strengthen muscles at these attachment points, it makes your bones stronger. This is why resistance training is essential in your exercise program.

Holding two- or five-pound weights and raising, then lowering your arms is one type of resistance exercise. But it's not enough. You need to work other muscle groups as well. You can buy large, inexpensive latex resistance bands ($8–$30) from sporting goods stores. Most of them include instruction booklets containing a number of exercises. Use these bands to strengthen your arms and legs. Or, if you would use it and can afford the cost and space, you can buy a multipurpose exercise machine like the Bowflex (around $800) that works both arms and legs, and all other muscle groups in the body. Or you can join a gym and use their machines.

My favorite home equipment for resistance exercises is small, light, and affordable. It's Dr. Swezey's OsteoBall—an inflatable ball with handles. The OsteoBall comes with a videotape and instruction booklet of simple resistance exercises that target all muscle groups, including the neck. More importantly, it comes with a dozen years of sound research. Ten minutes of exercise a day with the OsteoBall builds muscle and protects your bones.

Dr. Swezey found that when you stress your muscles at the place where they attach to the bone, your body builds denser bones as well as strengthens your muscles. Let me give you an example. If you want to build strong biceps, you can do a "biceps curl" and strengthen your upper arm. What you're doing is stressing your biceps in the middle of your upper arm. But Dr. Swezey found that if you stress the biceps at its attachments—to your elbow and shoulder—then you encourage your bone to grow at those sites. So, which would you prefer? Do you want a big bulging muscle in the middle of your upper arm, or would you rather have nice muscle tone and stronger bones?

Dr. Swezey looked over the entire body and came up with exercises that build bone not only in the legs and arms, but the hips and spine as well. He found that the easiest way to do these exercises was with a partially inflated ball. The ball could be used with very specific exercises to increase a person's range of motion as well as strengthen muscles. And the end result was denser bones.

When I work out with free weights or machines at the gym, I just have to prove to myself how strong I am. So sometimes I use heavier weights than I should. That's when I get hurt. The OsteoBall won't let me do this because all I'm doing is using my body's pressure to resist against movement in a particular direction. These resistance exercises don't lend themselves to injury, even when done by smarty-pants overachievers like me.

The OsteoBall uses resistance training to stimulate formation of stronger bone, help prevent "dowager's hump," improve your posture, and strengthen muscles. It does this through a series of ten exercises that work on your body from your neck to your ankles. You do a set of five alternating exercises each day for just two repetitions each.

What I like most about Dr. Swezey's specific resistance exercises is that they can reverse not only osteoporosis, but also frailty. You see, you're not "stuck" with poor balance. When you improve your balance, you reduce your risk for falling. And you can strengthen your muscles throughout your body even if you have physical limitations that prevent you from walking, running, or using heavy exercise equipment.

The quality of your muscles indicates whether or not you're doing the right kind of exercise often enough. If you think you are but you're not progressing, look at your protein intake. You see, there's no way you can have strong, toned muscles without eating enough protein. If you're doing the right kind of exercise and not eating much protein, you're fooling yourself. You may be healthy in other ways, but you're not protecting your bones.

SECRET #296 You can prevent and reverse frailty.

Frailty is a huge factor of aging. By age seventy, most people have at least 20 percent less muscle than they did at age thirty. *About 70 percent of elderly women are too frail to lift just ten pounds, and 60 percent cannot perform such household work as vacuuming.* About 35 percent of men are equally frail.

The good news, though, is that you're not destined to become frail. And if you're already so frail you can't do the things you really enjoy, there's even more good news—frailty doesn't have to be part of your life. In fact, studies have found that even ninety-year-olds can rebuild lost muscle and bone structure with some careful exercise.

I realized this for myself when I was flying across the country. I had my usual rollaway suitcase that fits in the plane's overhead bin, and when I tried to lift it up I found I couldn't. I asked another passenger for help in getting the bag into the bin and down. But I wasn't happy about this new finding. Shortly after that trip, I joined a gym. I've been exercising there four to five times a week ever since. Half of the time I'm at the gym I do cardiovascular exercises on a treadmill or an exercise bike. The other half of my program consists of weight-bearing, muscle- and core-strengthening exercises.

Six months after that plane trip, I was once more heading back east with the same suitcase. This time it was heavier. I had no problem lifting it up or down. None at all. In six short months, I had reversed this sign of frailty.

SECRET #297 You need to stress your muscles to keep your balance.

The three main factors related to frailty are muscle and bone deterioration and balance. (Other factors such as ligament and cartilage damage also contribute, but not to the same degree.) While most people are aware that muscles are strengthened by exercise, few people realize that bones are also strengthened by exercise. Now you're aware of this and can take steps to preserve your bones.

Just like with your bones, in order for your muscles to grow in strength and help you keep your balance, you have to subject them to a certain degree of stress. The difference is in the type of stress each responds to. While your muscles respond to contractile stress, your bones must undergo bending, compression, and twisting to experience stress.

If your bones and muscles don't undergo at least a minimal amount of stress on a regular basis (three times a week), they begin to atrophy. The adage "use it or lose it" definitely applies here.

The degree of stress your bones and muscles must experience in order to grow is called the minimal essential strain. This is the point that if surpassed often enough will cause the bone or muscle to call in help to deal with the stress. This help comes in the form of osteoblasts, which migrate to the area being stressed and help build more muscle and bone tissue.

As we age, our muscles and joints tighten, arthritis often sets in, and years of neglecting our body begins to take its toll. The exercise we know we need gets harder and harder to do, so a sedentary lifestyle sets in (or continues). Let's face it. Very few of us enjoy getting out of our comfort zones, especially when it hurts.

But that inactivity is a prime cause of frailty.

SECRET #298 Balance is the key to avoiding broken bones.

Most people break bones when they fall. The better your balance, the less likely you are to take a tumble. Any exercise that tones your muscles will help you keep your balance. Yoga is particularly good. If you can't find a beginner's yoga class near you, you can find books and videotapes that can show you simple poses.

My favorite method of improving balance is an exercise concept known as Pilates. It focuses on strengthening you at your core—in your mid-section—and in improving your balance. I began using Pilates exercises using a large inflated rubber ball at my gym. At first, I couldn't balance myself at all! Within a few months the changes were dramatic.

You can get books and videos that will show you Pilates exercises to strengthen your abdominal area and support your balance. The DVDs I particularly like and use are the *Pilates Powerhouse DVD Collection,* available from Gaiam (see the Resources section for more information).

TIPS TO REDUCE YOUR RISK FOR FALLS AND FRACTURES

- Increase your level of physical activity. Exercise at least three times a week.
- Spend at least four hours a day on your feet.
- Engage in exercise that may improve your coordination like yoga and Pilates.
- Decrease your caffeine intake. More than two cups of coffee a day can affect your bones.
- Avoid long-acting sedative or hypnotic drugs that affect your balance.
- Quit smoking.
- Get regular eye exams and treat visual problems.
- Secure loose rugs, electrical wires, and other falling hazards.
- Use light-colored carpet, paint, or other finish on stairs to increase depth perception visibility.
- At night, use a small, plug-in nightlight to light up path from bed to bathroom.
- If necessary, install grab bars, stair rails, and other structures that can help prevent falls.

CHAPTER 36

The "Other" Bone Loss

We're so focused on not breaking our hips, arms, and legs that we ignore dental bone loss. Yet, without strong jawbones, we can lose our teeth. Bone loss from periodontal (gum) disease can be just as devastating as osteoporosis.

SECRET #299 You can lose your teeth from this bone-destroying disease.

If you lose density from the bones that hold your teeth in place, that bone becomes more vulnerable to periodontal disease and accelerates the rate at which this disease destroys bone. When this happens, you're more likely to lose your teeth and your ability to chew well.

As you've seen, every cell in your body needs good nutrition, including those in your bones. Your mouth is the doorway to your health and all the nutrients provided by your diet must pass through this sensitive doorway. But the only way you can get vitamins and minerals from your food is if you can efficiently chew the nutritious foods you eat, releasing their nutrients.

The older you are, the more likely it is that you already have some form of gum disease. Fortunately, not all gum disease leads to bone loss. If you act on its warning signs, early stages of gum disease can be reversed. Do this and you can save your teeth and bones, and improve your general health.

SECRET #300 The damage from this early indication of periodontal disease is irreversible.

Gingivitis (inflammation of the gums) is an early warning sign and the most common type of periodontal disease. By the time you progress to periodontitis, bone loss has already begun. And while this infection can be stopped, its damage can't be reversed.

Gingivitis often occurs in the most neglected areas in the mouth, like in the gums around and in between your back teeth. Early stages are marked by tender red or inflamed gums, and possibly bleeding with any pressure. Advanced gingivitis, or trench mouth, consists of painful swollen gums with more bleeding and requires immediate professional attention. You can slow down and often reverse gingivitis by having a thorough periodontal examination by your dentist or hygienist, having your teeth cleaned regularly, eating a nutritious diet, and with an effective daily oral hygiene program. If you don't, you may be heading towards periodontitis—and bone loss.

SECRET #301 Plaque contains the food and bacteria that feed periodontal disease and its bone loss.

When bacteria mix with food, saliva, and other oral debris, they form a sticky substance called plaque. Left alone for even a few hours, the acids produced by these bacteria begin to etch microscopic holes in your enamel—the first stage of tooth decay. As plaque grows and hardens, it can eventually make its way into the space between your teeth and gums (called a periodontal pocket), infecting the gum tissue. Once there, they have an almost unlimited amount of food—your teeth, gum tissue, and jawbone.

SIGNS OF PERIODONTITIS

- Teeth and gums sensitive to heat, cold, sugar, or acid foods
- Sudden throbbing pain made worse by tapping tooth
- Constant or frequent gum bleeding
- Deep, dull pain
- Toothache
- Loose teeth
- Bad breath

Source: From *Tooth Fitness* by Thomas McGuire, D.D.S. (St. Michael's Press, 1994)

If untreated, they will eat away at your teeth and their supporting bones. Periodontal disease needs three things: teeth, bacteria, and food—especially refined foods, such as sugar and white flour products. Remove or reduce any of these three and you can stop or reduce the progression of periodontal disease and bone loss. The obvious place to begin is to reduce your oral colonies of destructive bacteria and the food they love so much—sucrose. It's also time to reevaluate your personal and professional dental program.

SECRET #302 These tips to control bacteria in your mouth can save your jaw bones and teeth.

You may have been told by your parents, as I was, that all you need to do is brush your teeth twice a day. But brushing isn't enough to prevent gum disease and possible bone loss. It's just the beginning.

The next step is to floss or use a proxy brush to get in between your teeth. You should also use a rubber tip or toothpick to stimulate your gums, and a good mouthwash to prevent food or bacteria from sticking around. If you have advanced periodontal disease with deep periodontal pockets, you'll need to use a water irrigator in addition to everything else.

Toothbrushes trap bacteria, reintroducing them into your mouth. Rinse your toothbrush in very hot water after each use and let it dry thoroughly in an upright position before reusing it. Change your toothbrush often, especially if you have gum disease.

All of the dentists I spoke with agreed that the electric toothbrushes are best. The problem with them is that you can't always change their heads as often as less expensive ordinary toothbrushes. And toothbrushes get dirty over time. Very dirty. They hold on to bacteria from your mouth, and they can pick up some of the nasty bacteria that are in the air in bathrooms.

Fortunately, there's a way to keep your toothbrush super clean. It's a device I discovered called the Germ Terminator. This handy plug-in sterilizer destroys any bacteria on your toothbrush after every use with steam, and keeps it clean until the next time you use it. Each Germ Terminator can sanitize either one or two toothbrushes at a time. It works with ultrasonic toothbrush heads and handheld toothbrushes. Please check the Resources section for contact information.

How good is it, really? Tests showed that the Germ Terminator kills the cold and flu viruses, salmonella, listeria, *E. coli*, candida, staph infections, herpes virus, and even hepatitis and HIV. This is one powerful little sterilizer!

SECRET #303 nvesting in professional cleaning once or twice a year can save your teeth.

It's easy for debris to collect in your gums next to your teeth, especially in areas that are difficult to brush. Your best protection against bone loss is to have a regular deep cleaning by a skilled dental hygienist. Some people need their teeth cleaned once or twice a year. Some, like me, need more. But even though prices for cleanings keep rising, they're much less expensive than losing a tooth! Discuss your cleaning treatment program with your dentist after a thorough exam, and follow through with better oral care. You may find that you become inspired to work even harder to save your teeth.

I did.

Last year I saw a new dentist who told me the same things that every other dentist had told me: brush, floss, use an antibacterial mouthwash, and use a rubber tip. All I had done in the past was to brush twice a day and occasionally floss or use a rubber tip. But my pockets were getting deeper, and while I'm lazy at times, I'm not stupid. I realized it was within my control to improve my condition. So I did a little experiment. I followed his instructions for three months. The improvement was huge and I was hooked. An extra five minutes a day meant I could save my teeth. What a good investment of my time! Now I have my teeth cleaned three times a year instead of four, and my mouth is getting healthier, not deteriorating.

SECRET #304 Your diet can feed bone-destroying bacteria.

Any diet can contribute to the formation of plaque, which as I mentioned, is a sticky substance that contains dead cells, live bacteria, and saliva. When plaque hangs around, it keeps harmful bacteria on your teeth and in your gums. Sugar, refined grains like white rice and white flour, and sticky foods encourage bacterial growth and tooth decay. After eating any of these, finish your meal with something raw and fibrous like a carrot or apple, and rinse or brush your teeth.

Of all substances in your diet, the biggest threat to your gum health is sucrose. It increases the bacteria in your mouth. The reason sucrose is so damaging is that it consists of small enough particles for harmful bacteria to eat. The major source of sucrose is refined sugar. Unrefined complex carbohydrates, like whole grain bread and brown rice, contain particles that are too large for these germs to digest.

The waste product these bacteria produce is often acidic enough to dissolve your tooth's enamel, the hardest substance in your body. The more they eat, the more they multiply and the more acid they produce. If you can't completely avoid eating sucrose, rinse your mouth or brush your teeth right after eating any sugar.

Any source of sucrose contributes to feeding bacteria including white, brown, and turbinado sugars, molasses, cane sugar, and "pure cane sugar juice" present in so-called "health foods." Many foods, including some fruits, naturally contain small amounts of sucrose. Grapes are especially high.

Fructose, lactose, glucose, maltose, corn syrup, and other sugars may be low in sucrose but can also contribute to tooth decay and inflamed gums, although the progress is slower.

SECRET #305 Some supplements can help improve your gums.

Vitamins C and A help your mouth heal if you already have gum infections, while a deficiency of B vitamins can worsen gingivitis. You can get these and other supportive nutrients in a good multivitamin/mineral formula. But there's more you can do.

I had a history of inflamed gums until I began taking resveratrol, a powerful antioxidant made from grape skins, to protect myself from colds and the flu. I kept taking it for several months. When I had my next tooth cleaning session, my dental hygienist was astonished. My gums were normal. The only change I had made was to take a resveratrol formula twice a day.

It's important to remember that there's a direct connection between periodontal disease and osteoporosis. Both affect your bones. Periodontal disease proceeds more rapidly and is more destructive in people who have decreased bone density, and people with a decrease in bone density are more vulnerable to periodontal infection. Because periodontal disease is a serious infection that affects bone and soft tissue, it often contributes to other health problems like heart disease. Gum disease is potentially serious.

To reevaluate your personal hygiene program, I suggest you read Dr. Tom McGuire's book *Tooth Fitness*. It's filled with easy-to-understand information and tooth-saving tips.

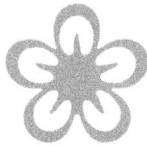

CHAPTER 37

What Osteoporosis Drugs Can and Can't Do

You may be able to avoid taking medications designed to stop osteoporosis through diet, weight-bearing exercise, and bone-building supplements. But if you feel you need to do more, it may help to understand the pros and cons of a few of the more recent drugs. Each new drug claims to work miracles and each has its limitations. Some have uncomfortable side effects.

The most important thing you can do is to not be pressured into taking any-thing—either natural solutions or pharmaceuticals—without sufficient informa-tion. Take your time to understand the risks and benefits from any therapy. Then make the best choice you can for your particular condition.

Before you can make this choice, you first need to understand how bone is made. Bone is living tissue that is constantly being broken down and rebuilt. The idea is to build it up as quickly as it's torn down. Plus, you want your bones to be flexible, not brittle, so they won't break when you fall. This is where the balance of calcium to magnesium becomes critical. As I explained earlier, calcium causes bones to become more brittle and magnesium makes them more flexible. Take at least as much magnesium as calcium (about 500–800 mg of each a day).

Osteoporosis occurs when more bone is broken down than is rebuilt. Estrogen protects against osteoporosis because it blocks this breakdown. The less estrogen we make, the less protection we have against this phase of bone loss and remodel-ing. Other substances slow down bone loss as well, but they don't directly stimu-late bone growth.

SECRET #306 This class of drugs can destroy cells that break down bone, but they also slow down the ability to build bone.

Bisphosphonates are a class of drugs that kill cells in bone tissue called osteoclasts.

Osteoclasts remove bone, but they do much more. They also work in a delicate balance with osteoblasts to increase bone density. Balance is the key here. If you stop bone loss by killing osteoclasts, you also limit their bone-building benefits.

Alendronate (Fosamex) is a bisphosphonate that can significantly reduce hip and vertebral fractures. The problem is that no one knows how much you need to take. One two-year study showed a 7.21 percent increase bone-mineral density in the spine and a 5.27 percent increase in the hip with women who took 10 mg a day.

If your doctor prescribes more or less alendronate than this, there's a good reason. According to a study published in *Obstetrics and Gynecology* (April 2003), women who took 35 mg of alendronate once a week for a year had the same benefits as those who took 5 mg a day.

Alendronate may be best for women who already have osteoporosis in the neck. There was an increase in bone density—but, interestingly, no reduction of fractures—in a group of people who had no prior fractures in their spine who took alendronate for four years. This suggests to me that while some drugs may help maintain bone density, the quality of the bone that is formed is too brittle to prevent fractures.

Risedronate (Actonel) is another bisphosphonate that looks good on paper. It decreased fractures in older women with previous spinal fractures. But again, it had little effect on women with no prior spinal fractures, even when their bone-mineral density was low. In addition, risedronate has been associated with a significant increase in lung cancer, a finding currently being disputed by regulating authorities. The bottom-line is: We don't know enough about this drug's connection with lung cancer for me to consider it safe.

Ibandronate (Boniva) is a new bisphosphonate that has shown a significant reduction in fractures when taken in a large dose followed by a two-month or more dose-free interval. However, once again, there's no agreement as to the best amount to take. Studies show that 20 mg taken once a week gives the same benefits as 2.5 mg every day. It's confusing because we're just beginning to understand just what these new bisphosphonates can do and their limitations. It may take decades to identify all their side effects. However, if you need an answer now and have nowhere else to turn, bisphosphonates may offer some solutions.

Bisphosphonate side effects include blurred vision, swelling, and pain in the eyes. Alendronate has also been associated with ulcerative esophagitis and esophageal erosion. In other words, it's a pretty strong irritant to that tube that carries food into your stomach. You may be able to take a bisphosphonate safely, but be aware of possible side effects and speak with your doctor immediately if you experience any of them.

SECRET #307 Various forms of strontium may prevent osteoporosis.

Strontium ranelate is a non-radioactive trace element found in the atmosphere. Studies dating back to 1910 suggest it may have wide implications in preventing osteoporosis. Based on laboratory studies, it appears to slow down the breakdown of bone while stimulating new bone-tissue formation. Animal studies suggest it may be able to prevent the type of bone loss caused by estrogen deficiency.

One promising finding came from a three-year study where participants were given two grams of Strontium ranelate a day. It reduced the risk of a first vertebral fracture by 41 percent. Other human studies showed a 2.5 to 3.2 percent increase in bone-mineral density, but these benefits come with a price—gastrointestinal side effects in a full 15 percent of the participants.

Currently, some supplement companies are selling formulas with strontium as nutrients to prevent osteoporosis. They don't contain the same form, however. Still, other forms of strontium look promising, and it may be that they work just as well. Time . . . and additional studies . . . will tell. If your doctor recommends strontium ranelate, ask him or her if another form of strontium, like strontium lactate, would be a possibility for you. It may give the same results without digestive side effects.

SECRET #308 This hormone could build bone or have the opposite effect depending on the dose.

Parathyroid hormone (PTH) is released when calcium levels are decreased. It helps restore mineral balance in our bones. PTH can either help build bone or break it down, depending on the dosage. When it's used intermittently in low doses, it helps build bones. When it's used continuously in higher doses, it has the opposite effect. Clearly, since we are not all alike, it is important to use the proper dose of PTH.

When PTH is used along with estrogen therapy, bones become denser. After PTH is stopped and estrogen continued, the density is maintained. But we don't know what will happen if you stop both PTH and estrogen. A dose of 20 micrograms (mcg) of PTH increased bone density by 2 to 4 percent, which admittedly isn't much. Increasing the dose to 40 mcg worked better, but resulted in more nausea and headaches. PTH looks promising, but there's still a lot we don't know about it. Please, only use PTH under the supervision of a doctor experienced in hormone therapy.

SECRET #309 The problem with osteoporosis medications is conflicting studies.

Several studies point out the confusion with using these medications. One study found that alendronate increased bone density by decreasing the rate at which bone breaks down without increasing bone mass. It's still too early to know which pharmaceuticals will keep your bones from breaking without putting you at risk for other side effects. That's the bottom-line.

Bone density is measurable. Bone fragility or flexibility is not. If your bones are dense and brittle, they'll break. If they're less dense and not brittle, they won't. All of us—patients, doctors, and researchers—need to look at all aspects of osteoporosis. We need to evaluate our bones' probable strength and flexibility based on our diet, stress reduction, and exercise, not just their density. Until we do, I think we're looking at only half of the issue.

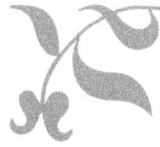

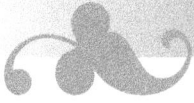

PART 8

BEAT HEART DISEASE
and STROKE

Both stroke and heart disease are striking postmenopausal women without warning. In fact, heart disease has become the number one killer of women in their fifties and beyond. Doctors tell us to watch our cholesterol and blood pressure, get plenty of exercise, and eat a healthy diet. Obviously, this is not enough. We continue to have heart attacks and brain attacks (stroke).

In some cases, simple blood tests can identify risk factors and we can be treated before a disease takes place. In other cases, little-known nutrients offer protection.

I've expanded this section beyond the length of the others because heart disease and stroke are so prevalent today among women. Unnecessarily so in many cases, I might add. I feel compelled to explain to you some of the steps you can take to protect yourself from future heart problems. I'd be surprised if your doctor has done this. He, or she, may not even be aware of all of them.

Is Cholesterol the Culprit?

You've undoubtedly heard about the connection between high cholesterol levels and heart disease. First we were told that a high cholesterol level was predictive of heart disease. Then cholesterol was broken down for us into HDL (high-density lipoprotein) and LDL (low-density lipoprotein). One is healthy (HDL), one is not (LDL).

The ratio of the healthy, slick cholesterol to the unhealthy, sticky stuff was, we were told, a better predictor of heart disease. But that's not the last word about cholesterol. It's oxidized cholesterol that's the culprit, not just LDL. In time, perhaps we'll find yet another component of cholesterol that can lead to heart disease.

Next came the role of hormone replacement therapy (HRT), which kept calcium deposits on arterial walls at bay. Nutritional studies later showed, however, that this calcium buildup was due to unabsorbed calcium, and that magnesium, the mineral that helps with calcium absorption was an effective blocker of these deposits and also helped keep the heart muscle relaxed.

Magnesium and other nutrients, along with specific dietary changes, can protect your heart and normalize your blood pressure. Some herbs, like hawthorn, are proven heart tonics that can strengthen the heart. Other substances, like coenzyme Q_{10}, can alleviate heart arrhythmias (rapid heartbeat).

We're finding that excessive amounts of two substances, homocysteine and fibrinogen, put us at increased risk for heart disease and stroke. Homocysteine is a substance made from some of the foods we eat, especially when some of our vitamin intake is low. Yet, a few supplements and simple dietary changes can lower our homocysteine to safe levels.

Add fibrinogen to the mix. Too much fibrinogen, a substance that clogs our arteries, can cause both heart disease and stroke. But several nutrients you probably haven't heard about, Padma (a Tibetan herbal formula) and nattokinase (an enzyme in a Japanese food), can dissolve blood clots and clogged arteries. You don't necessarily need any medications to do this.

But before I begin to unravel all of these, we should take a closer look at inflammation. I'd like to explain to you why an inflammation anywhere in your body could contribute to heart disease. By now, you know that any illness ending in "itis," like arthritis, tendonitis, and gingivitis, is an inflammatory disease. So where does heart disease come in? It, too, can be caused by chronic inflammation, and there are blood tests that will give you and your doctor information about whether or not you're at risk.

If you are at risk for heart disease, a change in diet could help, especially if you've been eating a diet that emphasizes animal protein. A high-protein diet could actually be contributing to heart disease and stroke. You don't have to give up this type of diet, just make a minor dietary adjustment that could make the difference between reducing inflammation and increasing it. Since soy has been shown to lower the risk of heart disease, and there are many vocal critics of soy products, we'll take a look at just how safe it is to eat.

Your diet should support a healthy heart, but few of us are on an ideal eating program. This is where supplements can come in—anything from magnesium and hawthorn to green tea and fish oils—can make a difference in your health. I'll help you decide which ones might be most beneficial to you.

Is your blood pressure climbing? If so, you can take medications to lower it or make some dietary and lifestyle changes. Even if you take drugs, lifestyle modifications are wise. They may allow you to take a lower dose of medications. Sometimes hypertension is caused by a buildup of a heavy metal that you can eliminate safely without expensive therapies. Learn which heavy metal affects you and how to remove it safely and inexpensively.

Stroke and heart disease are often silent killers. Chances are you haven't been given all of the information you need to protect yourself against them. This section may be the most important one you can read. It could save your life. It has already helped me save mine.

THEY'RE ALL CONNECTED

"Itis" means inflammation, so arthritis, gastritis, dermatitis, pancreatitis, bronchitis, colitis, dermatitis, gingivitis, and hepatitis, have a common denominator: chronic inflammation. So do other conditions like some forms of cancer, asthma, diabetes, inflammatory bowel disease, psoriasis, and coronary heart disease. When you reduce chronic inflammation, all of these conditions can improve.

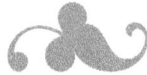

CHAPTER 38

Inflammation—
The Silent Killer

Janet was fifty-two when she came to me worried and confused. Her doctor had diagnosed her with high cholesterol and coronary artery disease, a narrowing of the arteries in her heart. He wanted to put her on cholesterol-lowering statins—drugs that would address both of her symptoms, but not the underlying cause.

Janet wanted to reverse her condition and knew that medications were not the solution, but she wasn't sure what to do next. After taking a lengthy health history, it was clear to me that her problem was due, in part, to chronic inflammation—something her doctor had missed.

Janet was overweight, didn't exercise, and had a lot of allergies, tendonitis, and a gum infection. She thought these problems were minor and separate from one another. They weren't. They were interrelated. After Janet went on a diet and supplement program designed to lower chronic inflammation, she began to feel better—and her plummeting cholesterol numbers proved it wasn't just emotional.

Recent studies are pointing to chronic inflammation as being a major risk factor for heart disease. Because inflammation can be painless and frequently goes undetected, its relationship to disease has been overlooked. If you have several diseases caused by inflammation, you may have a low-level chronic inflammatory process that could eventually lead to heart disease. This is preventable.

SECRET #310 Inflammation can either be protective or harmful.

All inflammation isn't bad. It can be a useful process that protects us by helping our bodies get rid of foreign matter like bacteria and toxins. This keeps these harmful substances from spreading into other tissues and organs. Inflammation's protective responses—redness, heat, pain, and swelling—help the body get rid of foreign substances and prepare injured tissues for repair. Occasional acute inflammation is a necessary part of the normal healing process.

But like just about everything, excessive inflammation has its downside. Chronic inflammation is destructive. When tissues that have been inflamed repeatedly become damaged and break down, they contribute to diseases. Health problems caused by chronic inflammation don't just suddenly "happen." They can lie hidden for years until one day the fire that has been smoldering suddenly becomes too hot and bursts into flame. Since many illnesses, including heart disease, begin with chronic inflammation, we would all be wise to address it as early as possible. But first you need to find the cause for any inflammation.

SECRET #311 Here are three often-overlooked causes for heart disease.

The blood vessel walls in your heart can become inflamed from three sources: a low-level infection anywhere in your body, high levels of homocysteine (an amino acid made from methionine), or oxysterols (rancid cholesterol).

Like Janet, many of us have mild chronic infections that we ignore. They don't bother us and we learn to live with them. Unfortunately, a slight infection in your mouth or a touch of tendonitis in your elbow can cause blood vessels in your heart to become inflamed. Now you're heading toward possible heart disease.

The subject of homocysteine is more complex. I'll talk about it in more detail in Chapter 41. For now, just understand that normally, methionine—an amino acid found in abundance in some foods—is converted into homocysteine. Homocysteine, in turn, is normally converted into an obscure and harmless amino acid called cystathionine. In this way, homocysteine levels are kept from being too high.

But some people don't have the enzyme that's necessary for this process to occur, and the result is high homocysteine. Red meat and dairy products are high-methionine foods. In small quantities, they usually pose no problems. But when you eat large amounts of them, your body can make too much homocysteine. This is the beginning of a vicious cycle, because excessive homocysteine produces free radicals that, in turn, make oxysterols.

SECRET #312 Food allergies contribute to inflammation.

Food sensitivities and food allergies reduce immunity, contribute to digestive problems, and produce inflammation. Even eating healthy foods like oranges, barley, and seafood could conceivably cause an inflammatory response that can eventually affect your heart and brain if you're sensitive to them. Environmental allergies have the same effect. So can sensitivities to aspartame, MSG, nitrites, sulfites, food coloring, and a host of other chemicals found in prepared foods and the environment. Begin by cleaning up your diet and eat more whole foods. Then, if you need more information on food and other allergies, read *Stopping Inflammation* by Nancy Appleton, Ph.D. It contains solid information on identifying and dealing with allergies.

PRO-INFLAMMATORY FOODS INCLUDE . . .

- Omega-6 fats (vegetable oils like corn, safflower, peanut)
- Trans fats (hydrogenated or partially hydrogenated vegetable oils, margarine)
- Refined sugar, grains, and high-glycemic foods

ANTI-INFLAMMATORY FOODS INCLUDE . . .

- Omega-3 fats (fish oil, flaxseed, green leafy vegetables)
- Omega-9 fats (olive oil, avocados, macadamia nuts)

Source: Jack Challem, *The Inflammation Syndrome* (John Wiley & Sons, 2003)

SECRET #313 **Learn which foods promote or reduce inflammation.**

Some foods reduce inflammation while others promote it. The foods you choose to eat are your foundation for a healthy heart program. The type of fats in your diet will either increase or decrease inflammation. So will your choice of sugars.

To reduce inflammation, replace refined sugars with whole grains and fruit, and watch the balance of fats in your diet. The amount of individual dietary fats has a direct influence on chronic inflammation.

Prostaglandins are hormonelike substances made from fats that either promote or reduce inflammation. A high animal-protein diet contains arachidonic acid (AA) that, in turn, makes a pro-inflammatory prostaglandin, PGE2. A diet high in fish and green leafy vegetables makes an anti-inflammatory prostaglandin, PGE1. Popular high-protein diets can either promote inflammation or contain too much mercury from fish. Be sure the fish you eat is wild Alaskan salmon or small fish from cold waters—not farmed fish.

Earlier, I mentioned that oxidized cholesterol is the culprit, not just total cholesterol levels. Oxysterols are the harmful, oxidized form of cholesterol that can cause plaque to form on artery walls. Oxysterols are not only created from homocysteine, they are found in some processed foods like powdered eggs and milk, reheated lard (donuts anyone?), and gelatin products. Some nutrients, like beta-carotene, folic acid, and vitamins B_6, B_{12}, C, and E, can neutralize both homocysteine and oxysterols. Be sure you're taking a good quality multivitamin/mineral formula, especially if you eat a diet high in animal protein. You may need stronger anti-inflammatory nutrients as well.

SECRET #314 Your toothbrush can cause inflammation.

Think about it. Your toothbrush is a breeding ground for microscopic bacteria that live off food particles. In addition, it sits in most bathrooms, head in the air, gathering bacteria from the air after each time you flush your toilet. Finally, it makes tiny cuts into your gums as you brush your teeth, allowing these bacteria into your bloodstream. This can contribute to inflammation and a lowered immune system.

Rinsing your toothbrush after each use doesn't get rid of these bacteria. Few people want to rinse their toothbrushes after each use with hydrogen peroxide. Fortunately, there's another answer that I mentioned in Chapter 36: a toothbrush-sanitizing device called the Germ Terminator.

Put Out That Fire
An inflammation is like a fire. If you don't put it out, it spreads. It may lie smoldering so you don't even know it's there. But if you don't put it out, it continues to burn slowly.

James Song has written an excellent book about inflammation, *Why Your Toothbrush May be Killing You.* Unlike all the other books on the subject, James speaks at length about the role your toothbrush plays in this inflammatory cascade from gum infections (periodontal disease) to chronic infections, heart disease, and arthritis. He offers a number of suggestions that will keep nasty bacteria from getting into your bloodstream via your mouth. This is a very important little book.

Bottom-line: Keep your toothbrush sanitized and use soft toothbrushes. They are less likely to cut your gums than stiff-bristled brushes.

SECRET #315 This simple blood test can detect inflammation.

The problem with inflammation is that often it can't be seen or felt. This is why you may want to have a blood test that measures the levels of a particular protein called C-reactive protein (CRP). Inflammation is a major source of increased CRP. A CRP test is often used to detect inflammation associated with arthritis. But it identifies inflammation associated with other conditions as well.

Two comprehensive studies, the Physician's Health Study and the Women's Health Study, found that people with the highest CRP levels were three times more at risk for having a heart attack and two times more likely to have a stroke than those with normal CRP levels.

If you suspect you have chronic inflammation anywhere in your body, or if you just want to make sure you don't, talk with your doctor about being tested for CRP. This blood test costs between $20–$50 and is now widely available. If your CRP level is over 0.20 mg/dL, it's time to take action and reduce it.

My friend Jack Challem wrote an important book on inflammation called *The Inflammation Syndrome.* In it, he "connects the dots," as he calls it, and makes the association between chronic inflammation and dozens of illnesses. If you have one or two of these conditions, chances are you'll end up with more of them if you don't make some important changes now. Jack's book is a good guide for cooling down the inflammatory process. If you need more information or support (including recipes), pick it up.

SECRET #316 Free radicals can contribute to inflammation.

High levels of homocysteine's damaging oxygen molecules make free radicals. So do contaminants in our air and food. Some free radicals are even made in our bodies from substances in the foods we eat like fried, barbecued, and charbroiled foods. And free radicals are increased when we drink coffee and alcohol. They're found in our environment in pesticides, solvents used in cleaning supplies, and radiation from sunlight. What's more, some are internally generated. It's obvious that you can't escape free radicals, but you can limit your exposure to them.

Free radicals damage, or oxidize, other molecules in our bodies just like iron causes rust in the presence of oxygen. An overabundance of free radicals can lead to inflammation. They do this by activating substances called "adhesion molecules." These molecules attach themselves to infectious microbes and damaged cells to tag them as cells that need to be eliminated. But in the presence of chronic inflammation, these molecules also stick to healthy cells, often resulting in blockages in arteries.

You may not be able to control the contaminants in the air, but you can limit contaminants in your food by eating more organic fruits and vegetables. They are high in antioxidants, nutrients that counteract the formation of harmful oxidants. In addition to dietary changes, consider taking supplemental antioxidants like essential fatty acids, vitamins C and E, and flavonoids (compounds found in vitamin C).

SECRET #317 Anti-inflammatory drugs called NSAIDs have been found to be unsafe.

If you still think that NSAIDs (nonsteroidal anti-inflammatory drugs) like Celebrex and Vioxx are safe, you've been on an information vacation for a long time. From Food and Drug Administration (FDA) findings that some NSAIDs have caused heart attack and stroke, to warnings against using these anti-inflammatory drugs for inflammatory bowel disease, NSAIDs are emerging as an unsafe class of drugs for many people with inflammation. Without a doubt they have more side effects than natural anti-inflammatory products.

NSAIDs (including aspirin and ibuprofen) commonly cause headaches, dizziness, fatigue, diarrhea, nausea, swollen legs and feet, and urinary tract infections. Less frequent but more serious side effects include sudden stomach and intestinal bleeding, serious allergic reactions, and liver or kidney problems. Even aspirin can cause heartburn, nausea, irritation, and bleeding in your stomach.

Recently, acetaminophen, an ingredient in many over-the-counter (OTC) pain medications, was found to cause injury to the small intestines in more than 70 percent of the people who used them. Why take something that damages your stomach and intestines when other effective solutions cause no irritation?

Instead, try some of the more natural supplements that block inflammation before rushing to your doctor or the pharmacy. Always discuss your decision with your doctor and ask him or her to monitor your progress. If natural anti-inflammatory products, along with dietary changes, are not sufficient, you can always reach for a pharmaceutical.

Control Inflammation Naturally

SECRET #318 Begin taking two common anti-inflammatory nutrients—vitamin C and fish oils.

Vitamin C: If you have inflammation, without a doubt you need more vitamin C. The reason for this is that inflammation leads to a vitamin C deficiency by causing the vitamin to break down in our bodies and be excreted at greater than normal rates. This is unfortunate, because vitamin C and the flavonoids it contains are important anti-inflammatory agents. They destroy damaging free radicals as well as reduce inflammation. Be sure you get at least 500 milligrams (mg) of vitamin C with bioflavonoids each day. You can take as much as 1,000 mg every hour for a week unless this amount causes loose stools or irritates your stomach. Buffered, or Ester C, is less likely to cause these side effects.

Fish oils: Earlier, I talked about the harmful effects of a diet high in animal protein. This is because meat and dairy products contain a pro-inflammatory fat called arachidonic acid. When arachidonic acid is released, it interacts with enzymes called cyclooxygenase—commonly known as COX-1 and COX-2. COX-2 produces inflammation. You have heard of drugs that are called "COX inhibitors." They include Vioxx, Celebrex, and aspirin. Well, there are natural COX inhibitors, too, like fish oils.

Fish oils are high in omega-3 fatty acids, essential fats that block COX-2 enzymes. Omega-3 oils function in a manner similar to aspirin but without side effects. If you have chronic inflammation, you'll want to increase your fish-oil supplements to around 3 grams a day. But be careful: Some fish oils may contain mercury or pesticide residues.

Only buy fish-oil supplements guaranteed to be free from contaminants.

Since animal fats are pro-inflammatory, and fish oils are anti-inflammatory, any high-protein diet should consist of more fish and less animal fats.

Anti-Inflammatory Herbs

Numerous herbs have anti-inflammatory properties, but instead of choosing one or two of them at random, I suggest you use an anti-inflammatory formula. Often, a formula is more potent than any single herb because of its synergistic effects. This has been proven with traditional Chinese and Tibetan medicine, where single herbs are rarely used. I found two very different types of anti-inflammatory formulas, each with good studies supporting their effectiveness. One is a formula based on Western herbs, and the other is based on Tibetan medicine.

SECRET #319 These two herbal formulas of varying strength contain effective anti-inflammatory herbs.

Zyflamend and InflaThera are two Western herbal formulas that block inflammation by preventing the excessive stimulation of COX-2 enzymes. Each formula contains such well-researched anti-inflammatory herbs as turmeric, holy basil, oregano, rosemary, green tea, ginger, Chinese goldenthread, and skullcap.

Of all of these, turmeric may be the most important. It contains curcumin, an ingredient that stops inflammation by blocking COX-2 and by stopping the production of inflammatory hormonelike substances called prostaglandins.

InflaThera is stronger than Zyflamend. One capsule contains 375 mg of turmeric with 95% curcuminoids while Zyflamend has just 50 mg of turmeric with 7% curcumin. When I compared the other ingredients in these products, I noticed that InflaThera has twice as much of other ingredients. However, each is worth trying since the balance of herbs differs slightly and one might work better for you than the other.

SECRET #320 This herbal formula is used throughout Europe to reduce inflammation.

Padma Basic is an herbal formula of twenty plant-based ingredients derived from traditional Tibetan medicine and made under strict quality conditions in Switzerland. It is known throughout Europe as Padma 28 and has been highly researched for decades. Padma has many impressive applications, including extremely strong anti-inflammatory properties. It's a powerful antioxidant that also strengthens the immune system, allowing the body to heal more quickly.

We don't yet know how or why the antioxidants in particular plants work the way they do. Pharmaceutical companies are reluctant to fund studies that investigate the effects of substances they can't patent, and good studies are too expensive for many supplement companies to fund. So the pharmacology of each herb used in Padma is not completely understood at this time. We do know, however, that many of the herbs in this formula have known anti-inflammatory properties.

When you cool down an inflammation in one area in your body, you put out fires in other areas, as well. This explains why your dermatitis may clear up when your inflammatory bowel disease is treated with anti-inflammatory drugs. Similarly, the cooling properties in the antioxidants in Padma work on all inflammatory processes simultaneously. As one inflammation subsides, so do others.

SECRET #321 Some herbs warm the body; Padma cools it.

Padma is a cooling formula that is particularly effective in supporting circulation and reducing inflammation. It consists of twenty different plants along with calcium sulfate. These ingredients are rich in antioxidants, containing plant compounds including polyphenols such as bioflavonoids and tannins, as well as other plant chemicals. The antioxidants promote good circulation and a healthy heart, while the combination of ingredients reduces inflammation and supports the immune system.

Padma Basic has been tested on patients with chronic hepatitis B. In a one-year study of thirty-four hepatitis patients, more than 75 percent improved or had normal T-cell counts. Padma Basic has been tested on more than 300 children with chronic bronchitis (remember, "itis" means inflammation), and more than 70 percent had a noticeable improvement. This formula is good! It's also more expensive than the others. But if you have a tough case of chronic inflammation, start with a strong formula that has a lot of science behind it. In this case, I would personally use Padma Basic. In milder cases, you can either use another formula or less Padma Basic.

A full daily dose of Padma is typically two tablets taken three times a day, but two tablets twice a day will be sufficient for some people depending on their weight and the severity of their health problems. Begin by taking one tablet twice a day for a few days, then increase to two tablets two or three times daily.

CHAPTER 39

Lower Your
Dangerous Cholesterol

High cholesterol itself is not necessarily dangerous. At best, it's only a secondary risk for heart disease. What's important is the breakdown of cholesterol into HDL and LDL. If your LDL cholesterol is high, even if your total cholesterol is normal, you're at risk for heart disease. And if your LDL contains oxidized cholesterol, it's time to make some changes. Oxidized LDL is the most dangerous form of cholesterol.

It's unconscionable that women are being frightened into taking medications without even looking at their HDL and LDL levels and asking them to make sensible lifestyle changes. Especially since many medications given for high cholesterol have undesirable side effects.

SECRET #322 High cholesterol is not necessarily dangerous.

Judith, a patient in her mid-seventies, called me in a panic. "My cholesterol is over 240 for the first time," she said. "In the past, it was always under 200. Now my doctor wants me to take medication to bring it down. What should I do?"

I asked Judith about her HDL and LDL levels, but she didn't know what they were. "I just see cholesterol and triglycerides on the lab report," she answered. "There's nothing here that says HDL or LDL and I don't remember what you told me they meant."

Cholesterol is a necessary fat contained in all cell membranes that's needed to make sex hormones such as estrogen, progesterone, and testosterone, as well as bile, which is needed to digest fats and utilize fat-soluble vitamins. HDL and LDL are parts of cholesterol.

I think of HDL (high-density lipoprotein) as "healthy" and LDL (low-density lipoprotein) as "lousy." HDL is slick, while LDL is sticky. To keep the sticky fat from sticking to your artery walls and causing a buildup of plaque, you want plenty of HDLs (above 45) and low LDLs (under 100). The dietary and lifestyle changes that raise healthy HDLs also lower LDLs. HDLs gather up LDLs and recycle them and collect cholesterol from arterial plaque.

Estrogen raises HDL levels. This is why postmenopausal women not on hormone therapy are more susceptible to heart disease than women on HRT. However, low dietary fat, aerobic exercise, and keeping your weight down also raises your HDL. Smoking, obesity, a diet high in animal fats, and a lack of exercise lower it.

SECRET #323 Oxysterols (oxidized cholesterol) from your diet and the environment are the danger.

LDL cholesterol is harmful when it has combined with oxygen and become oxidized. This form of cholesterol is called oxysterols. Oxysterols can form plaque in arteries and lead to heart attacks and stroke. Think about it. What are some of the most important nutrients for a healthy heart? Antioxidants. Antioxidants fight and destroy oxidants. You want more anti-oxidants and fewer pro-oxidants.

You get oxysterols from your diet and from environmental exposure. Dietary sources include powdered milk and powdered eggs. You never eat them, you say? You do if you eat a lot of processed foods and salad dressing. It's time to start reading labels and avoiding products that contain eggs and milk. Reheated oils are filled with oxysterols. They're used to make French fries, potato chips, donuts, and other deep-fried foods. When hamburgers and eggs are cooked at high temperatures, they produce oxysterols. Cook your foods with a lower flame to avoid producing these pro-oxidants.

Pesticides and chemicals like chlorine and fluoride also generate oxysterols. These are pretty much impossible to avoid, but you can reduce your exposure to them. Eat more organic foods, and remove chlorine from your tap water and shower water with filters. Make sure you get filters that really work. You can find some through the Resources section under Chapter 1.

High cholesterol is a warning sign. But that's all. If your cholesterol is high, look at its components, HDL and LDL. After that, look at your diet and your exposure to substances that cause oxidation to see whether or not you should make a few lifestyle changes. Don't just reach for a prescription.

SECRET #324 Statins have side effect you want to avoid.

Statin drugs, the usual treatment for heart disease, don't always work and may do more harm than good. Several clinical trials found that while they lowered cholesterol, they didn't reduce cardiac events significantly. In spite of these findings, most doctors take the easy way out and prescribe statins like Lipitor, Zocor, Mevacor, and Pravachol instead of reviewing their patients' diet and exercise program.

Statins do block your body's production of cholesterol, raise HDL, and lower LDL. But they also can have nasty side effects. They can cause liver toxicity, dizziness, nausea, headaches, constipation, diarrhea, fatigue, blurred vision, heartburn, abdominal pain, and insomnia. Some statins actually raise harmful LDL levels in people whose LDL is already high!

One answer is to take the lowest possible dosage of a statin. Large doses may be both harmful and unnecessary. Two-thirds of the cholesterol-lowering effects from statins occur at their starting dose. So if your doctor suggests you take a higher amount, ask if this is necessary.

When high doses of statins are combined with other medications, they can lead to life-threatening complications. Talk with your pharmacist about all of your medications to make sure there are no negative interactions. Most importantly, if you are at a low-to-moderate risk for heart disease and are willing to make lifestyle changes, talk with your doctor about a more natural, safer approach than taking drugs.

SECRET #325 Statins reduce your body's stores of an important heart-protective nutrient.

Coenzyme Q_{10} (CoQ_{10}) is a vitaminlike substance found in all cells. The largest concentration of this nutrient is in your heart. Needless to say, CoQ_{10} is essential for good heart health. In fact, studies have shown that heart function deterioration is associated with low amounts of CoQ_{10} in heart tissues. The more severe a person's heart disease is, the higher their deficiency of CoQ_{10}.

We've known that low levels of CoQ_{10} frequently lead to congestive heart failure. One study revealed that 75 percent of people with heart disease not only had low levels of CoQ_{10}, but also their condition improved after they took it in supplement form. Supplemental CoQ_{10} has also reduced irregular heartbeats (arrhythmia) in many people. In fact, they dramatically reduced mine. Bottom-line: Your heart wants more CoQ_{10}, not less.

Unfortunately, statins lower your stores of this important nutrient. So while these cholesterol-lowering drugs reduce your cholesterol, they also reduce a primary nutrient that supports your heart. If you take any statin, or if you just want to protect your heart, you may want to take at least 100 to 200 mg of CoQ_{10} daily! Some doctors suggest their heart patients take much more. But before you take massive doses of this nutrient, talk with your doctor.

SECRET #326 Diet and exercise can lower your LDL.

Exercise: Inactivity is not an option. If you expect or hope to live a long life, you simply must make regular exercise a priority. It will make a huge difference in your health. It doesn't matter whether or not you like it. If you don't exercise at all, you're at twice the risk for developing heart disease. If you exercise five times a week, you dramatically reduce your chance of dying from heart disease. Find something to do that is active enough to protect you from heart disease.

Exercise strengthens your heart, reduces high blood pressure, raises HDL, and lowers LDL. Any form of exercise including walking, yoga, and tai chi will help your heart. Don't put it off. Begin today with a five-minute walk. Do this every day for a week. Then increase your exercise to ten minutes, five times a week. Gradually build up the length of time you exercise, maintaining a five-day per week schedule. Your goal is thirty to forty-five minutes of cardiovascular exercise. This means any exercise that increases your heart rate

Diet: Soluble fiber (beans, brown rice, oat bran, fruit pectin, and psyllium seed) binds to cholesterol and carries it out of your body. This lowers your cholesterol and your LDL. But fiber interferes with the absorption of some statins like lovastatin. That's right. A healthy cholesterol-lowering diet interferes with some cholesterol-lowering drugs! Try eating a diet high in soluble fiber for three months before resorting to medications if your doctor agrees that this is an option.

Sugars can increase your cholesterol. A liver enzyme stimulated by insulin controls the production of cholesterol in your liver. Sugars, including alcohol, fruit, and fruit juices, can trigger an insulin response. If you eat a lot of sugars and trigger an insulin response, your cholesterol can rise. This is why some people on a healthy diet who drink a lot of juices or eat large quantities of fruit have high cholesterol.

Reduce all fats. When your liver is overworked by handling a high-fat diet, it's unable to lower your cholesterol and LDLs. The best fats for your heart are from wild (not farmed) fish high in omega-3 fats, walnuts, and flaxseed. Olive oil keeps healthy HDL levels high.

SECRET #327 Any of these four nutrients can lower your LDL.

Grape seed extract (GSE) has reversed atherosclerosis in animals. It lowers cholesterol and LDLs while raising HDLs. Use grape seed oil daily in your salad dressings, or take a GSE supplement. The active ingredient in grape seed is called resveratrol. You can find resveratrol supplements, GSE supplements, and grape-seed oil in health-food stores.

Green tea and green tea extract support the heart and help stabilize blood sugar. Chemicals naturally found in green tea stimulate bile salt secretion and help your body eliminate excessive cholesterol. Drink one or two cups of the tea a day, or take it in supplement form.

Guggulipid is a waxy substance used extensively in India for the heart. It lowers

LDL and raises HDL. One study showed that when people took guggulipid (500 mg, twice a day) for three months they lowered their total cholesterol by more than 23 percent. Guggulipid can be found in many cholesterol-lowering supplement formulas.

Pectin from citrus and apples reduces the stickiness of LDLs, keeping them from sticking to artery walls. PectaSol Modified Citrus Pectin is more effective than ordinary apple and citrus pectins because it has smaller particles that are better absorbed into your bloodstream. Most pectin contains large molecules that remain in your intestines. Studies showed that PectaSol lowered total and LDL cholesterol between 7.6 percent and 10.8 percent in three and a half months.

SECRET #328 This supplement outperformed statins.

Policosanol is a mixture of fatty alcohol molecules (not fatty acids) that has been studied extensively. In one three-month double-blind study using policosanol (10 mg a day) versus statins, policosanol reduced LDLs by 24 percent. Even 5 mg a day lowered LDLs nearly 17 percent. Policosanol outperformed both Mevacor and Zocor. It also raised HDL levels when the statins didn't.

A double-blind study with more than fifty participants compared policosanol with Mevacor; other studies compared it with Pravachol and Zocor. Ten mg/day of policosanol improved HDL, LDL, and total cholesterol levels better than any of these drugs and was found to be safer and better tolerated. In a two-to-four year study of over 25,000 people who used policosanol for at least one month, the most severe adverse effect was weight loss in less than 1 percent of the participants. You can see why I like policosanol so much! Policosanol is effective in amounts of 5–20 mg a day. I have found a number of patients who responded to 5 mg twice a day, while others needed double that amount.

SECRET #329 The one "natural" supplement I wouldn't take to lower cholesterol.

Red yeast rice is a popular new product I don't trust. Although it's been used in China for centuries, it is effective because it contains a natural statin chemically identical to Mevacor and other lovastatins. It's a food product that acts exactly like a drug. The FDA has been vacillating between calling red yeast rice a drug or a supplement since 1998. Since statins lower CoQ_{10} levels, this product has the same negative side effects as pharmaceutical statins. In addition, red yeast rice powders are not standardized. Their active ingredients can differ from company to company, and from batch to batch. Until I have more information on its safety, I wouldn't use red yeast rice.

CHAPTER 40

Eat Fat and Protect Your Heart

Fats have gotten a bad rap, and the misinformation surrounding them is costing women their health and their lives. Fats can contribute to heart disease or they can protect your heart. It all depends on the type and quantity of fats you eat. Fats are not your enemy as long as you get the right type in the correct amount and balance. Do this and you can lose weight and protect yourself from heart disease at the same time. Sound too good to be true? I can assure you, it's not.

SECRET #330 A low-fat or no-fat diet can harm your heart.

The problem is that many people are either eating too much of the wrong fats or are opting for a fat-free or low-fat diet. Either choice results in a deficiency of important essential fatty acids (EFAs)—fats your body needs but can't make.

No-fat diets won't give you enough of these EFAs. Low-fat diets may not, as well. Just eating more fats is not the answer. You need two types of EFAs for a healthy heart: omega-3 and omega-6 fats. And you need the proper ratio of the two. This is another one of many delicate balancing acts that can either lead to increased health or disease.

SECRET #331 Omega-3 and omega-6 fats are EFAs found in healthy foods, but keep omega-6 fats low.

The balance of omega-3 and omega-6 fatty acids is critical to your health. Our ancestors ate equal amounts of omega-3 and omega-6 fats, but over the last 100 years, our diets have shifted. People used to eat twice as much omega-6 to omega-3 fats (a 2:1 ratio), but we're now eating 20:1! This is far too much omega-6.

Omega-6 fats are essential fats, but too much of them causes the blood to get thicker, stickier, and more likely to clot. Omega-3 fats have the opposite effect. To prevent heart disease, you need essential fats with more omega-3 and less omega-6.

Omega-3 fats are found in fish oil, flaxseed, walnuts, pumpkins, and green leafy vegetables. Soy contains both omega-3 and omega-6 fatty acids, so it belongs in both categories. Populations that eat a diet high in omega-3 fats historically have a low risk for heart disease. If you eat a lot of green vegetables and fish, you may be getting enough of these beneficial fats. If not, consider adding freshly ground flaxseed to your morning cereal or breakfast drink, sprinkling raw walnuts on salads and cereals, or taking a supplement containing higher levels of omega-3 fats. Buy eggs that say they are high in omega-3 fats. Add flax oil to salad dressings and use it instead of butter on steamed vegetables or potatoes.

Omega-6 fats are found in vegetable oils like corn, safflower, sunflower, cottonseed, peanut, sesame, grape seed, borage, black currant, primrose, and soy. Omega-6 fats have protective effects only when they're combined with sufficient omega-3 fats. Otherwise, they contribute to the stickiness in blood. Keep their amount reasonably low.

This means watching the amount of oils you eat. If you cook with any of the above oils, switch to olive oil. It doesn't contain any EFAs, but its monounsaturated fats have a positive effect on HDL and LDL cholesterol.

Omega-9 fats are the monounsaturated fats like olive oil. They're beneficial, but not called "essential" because your body can make them from other fats. Include them in your diet as safe fats, but don't use them to achieve a balance of EFAs.

SECRET #332 Monounsaturated and polyunsaturated fats are both unsaturated fats that contain EFAs.

Let's look at it another way. Unsaturated fats, the ones you want to emphasize in your diet and supplements, are liquid at room temperature. There are two kinds of unsaturated fats: monounsaturated and polyunsaturated. Both contain EFAs, but polyunsaturated fats, which remain liquid at any temperature, have more of them.

Monounsaturated fats: These are liquid at room temperature but become more solid when they're refrigerated. They include olive, canola, and peanut oils. Monounsaturated fats are beneficial to your heart because they're the only fats that lower LDL (harmful) cholesterol and raise HDL (protective) levels. Keep them in your diet. Since they're more stable in heat than other oils, use them for stir-frying, baking, and other situations where oil is heated.

Polyunsaturated fats remain liquid at any temperature. They include corn, flaxseed, safflower, sesame, soy, and sunflower oils. They're also found in fatty fish, walnuts, pumpkin seeds, and some oils used in supplements (borage, black currant, and evening primrose). Polyunsaturated fats contain both omega-6 and omega-3 EFAs in varying ratios. The ratio of omega-6 to omega-3 fats in your diet determines how beneficial they are, so some polyunsaturated fats are better than others for your heart and weight control. EFAs are needed to make hormone-like substances, known as prostaglandins, that regulate metabolism.

SECRET #333 Butter and coconut oil do not cause heart disease.

This may come as a big surprise, but it's true. Both butter and coconut oil are saturated fats, but not all saturated fats are alike.

Remember, the more solid any fat is, the less protective and more harmful it tends to be. Saturated fats, which include butter, cheese, beef, pork, lamb, chicken, and both coconut and palm kernel oils, are either solid or semisolid at room temperature.

All fats are made from chains of atoms. The longer the fat chain, the longer it takes to burn. The longer any fat takes to burn, the stickier it is. The stickier it is, the more likely it is to clog arteries. Now, here's where butter and coconut oil come in. They are *short-chain* and *medium-chain* saturated fats. This means that they burn quicker and don't contribute to weight gain or heart disease. Which is the short chain fat? If you thought it was coconut oil, you're wrong. It's butter!

SECRET #334 Trans fats make more harmful cholesterol and reduce helpful cholesterol.

Trans-fatty acids, known as trans fats, are fats that began as oils and had hydrogen added to them. You know them as margarine and shortening. This procedure causes the oil to become either solid or semisolid. Trans fats are primarily found in artificially solidified (hydrogenated) oils.

The reason that trans fats became so popular is that they're more stable than other oils. This means that cookies and crackers made with trans-fatty acids won't spoil as quickly as those made with butter. But when oil becomes more solid, it contains fewer EFAs. Besides, they're not good for you.

While trans fats lower total cholesterol, they also raise harmful cholesterol (LDL) and lower helpful cholesterol (HDL). What's more, they raise blood-sugar levels and cause more weight gain than the same amount of other fats. "Partially hydrogenated" or "hydrogenated" on a food label means the food contains trans-fatty acids. Watch out for them, especially in cakes, cookies, crackers, artificial cheese, and margarine.

SECRET #335 These simple dietary tips will help you get the right balance of fats in your diet.

Let's keep it simple. EFAs speed up your metabolism, support your immune system, and guard against the buildup of sticky arterial plaque. Other fats have the opposite effect. Keep your intake of foods with EFAs high, and your saturated fats low.

Tip 1: If you eat meat daily, avoid eating any foods with trans-fatty acids, or foods containing hydrogenated or partially hydrogenated oils. And it means limiting your intake of meat to one serving per day.

Tip 2: Eat a Mediterranean diet. This type of diet is high in fruits and vegetables, and includes copious amounts of olive oil, which raises the good cholesterol and lowers the bad. It's rich in omega-3 fatty acid food such as fatty fish, walnuts, pumpkin seeds, flax seeds, and some green leafy vegetables. Other nuts have some omega-3 fats, but not as much as walnuts. Of all vegetables, purslane, a low growing, fleshy "weed" is highest in EFAs. It's excellent raw in salads or cooked as a side dish and may be lurking in your garden. I found huge patches of purslane in mine last year.

A Mediterranean diet is also high in vegetable protein (beans, soy, peas, and lentils) and low in animal protein. The soluble fiber in these beans and legumes lowers cholesterol. Choose low-fat animal protein such as lean meats, low-fat or fat-free dairy products, and white-meat poultry.

Reduce or avoid vegetable oils high in omega-6 fats (corn, soy, sunflower, and safflower) and trans fats (cookies, crackers, cakes, chips, and many convenience foods). And of course, avoid deep-fried foods.

Tip 3: Eat more fish. The American Heart Association suggests eating two 3-ounce servings or more of fatty fish each week—the more the better. Some fatty fish include catfish, halibut, herring, lake trout, mackerel, pompano, salmon, striped sea bass, albacore tuna, and whitefish.

Studies show that people who consume more canned tuna have significantly less arrhythmias than those who don't, therefore fresh fish isn't required to protect your heart. When these people switched to a diet higher in animal fats, their arrhythmias worsened.

Researchers studying Eskimos in Greenland found their high-fish diet kept their blood from getting sticky and clotting, and lowered their triglycerides as well. And when postmenopausal women (some on hormone therapy, some not) were given fish-oil supplements, the risk for heart disease in both groups was reduced by 27 percent. Eating fish or other foods high in EFAs, or taking supplements protects your heart.

Theoretically, fish is an excellent food. It's high in protein and contains essential fatty acids that support your immune system, nervous system, brain function, and vision. But more and more news is showing how fish and fish oils can actually poison you.

This means you should avoid fish, right? Wrong. It just means you have to be extra careful! As you know, our waters are polluted. Increasing numbers of fish have been found to contain pesticides and mercury. These toxins get stored in your fat cells where they're difficult to eliminate. Eventually, they can lead to serious health problems. The toxins in fish are even more dangerous for women than for men, since as we age, we tend to gain weight. It's no longer easy to find fish that are free from contaminants. But you can find fish with fewer toxins.

SECRET #336 Here's how to find better quality fish.

The amount of pesticides in fish depends on how contaminated the waters are that they come from. The larger the fish, the more mercury it is likely to contain.

Eat small fish: Avoid shark, swordfish, king mackerel, marlin, and tilefish. These large fish are high in mercury. The Environmental Protection Agency (EPA) recently added tuna steaks and canned albacore tuna to this list. Canned light-meat tuna has less mercury and is safer. Other cleaner fish include cod, haddock, and pollock.

Eat wild, cold-water fish, such as trout and salmon. The frigid waters where they live tend to be lower in contaminants. But be aware that rivers may contain industrial wastes or mercury residues from gold mining. Don't eat these fish exclusively.

Avoid farmed fish: They are often crowded and fed a diet lower in healthful fats than fish found in the wild. Farmed salmon has less omega-3 fats than wild salmon, because they are fed soybean oil in their diet, rather than the high omega-3 oils found naturally in algae. Most restaurants serve farmed salmon, and farmed salmon has the highest antibiotic residue of any animal-based protein, according to fats and oil expert, Mary G. Enig, Ph.D. Whenever possible, choose salmon that has been frozen at sea (FAS).

In addition, farmed salmon was found to have higher concentrations of thirteen pollutants than wild salmon. Some of these pollutants are associated with a higher risk for cancers. Skinning the fish before grilling it greatly reduced the toxins, but it didn't remove them. Hint: Atlantic salmon is farmed. Avoid it!

Eat only cooked fish: Raw and undercooked fish can contain parasites, worms, and flukes. Doctors have seen a huge rise in patients with parasites since sushi became popular. Parasites are expensive to identify and difficult to eliminate. Raw Pacific salmon and red snapper (Pacific rockfish) have been specifically linked to anisakiasis, a parasite infection from anisakid worms. But no raw fish is completely safe. If you love sushi, stick to cooked eel and vegetarian sushi.

Limit your fish intake: Eat one or two small servings a week. The EPA also suggests you eat a variety of fish rather than one kind to reduce your exposure to contaminants.

SECRET #337 Add fatty acid supplements to your daily regimen.

Fatty acid supplements are a good investment because these fats are needed to reduce inflammation and support your heart, immune system, and reproductive system. Instead of eating more fish, some people prefer taking supplements to be sure they're getting enough. Make sure that yours are the best quality available. An evaluation of nineteen different brands of fish-oil capsules by ConsumerLab.com concluded that one-third of the products tested did not have the amount of active ingredients they claimed to have.

The following brands contained the amount of DHA and EPA (the primary EFAs in fish oil) claimed on the label: Health From the Sun, Jarrow, Member's Mark, Pure Encapsulations, Puritan's Pride, Shaklee, Solgar Omega-3, Spectrum, Trader Darwin's, The Vitamin Shoppe, Vitamin World, and ZonePerfect. Nature's Way Neuromins, which is an algae product containing only DHA, also passed this evaluation. None of the tested products contained mercury. To my knowledge, they were not tested for pesticide residue. Several supplements guaranteed to be free of both mercury and pesticides are listed in the Resources section.

How much do you need?

The type of EFAs found in fish oils differs from those in vegetable sources, and both are important. The EFAs in fish oils are particularly protective, so I suggest you either eat fish two times a week or take daily fish-oil supplements. If you're a vegetarian who objects to any amount of fish, increase your vegetable sources of EFAs. Personally, I find the research on the benefits of fish oils so compelling that I do take fish-oil supplements daily, although I consider myself a vegetarian and don't eat any fish.

To protect yourself against heart disease, I suggest that you get about 1 gram of fish or flax oil a day. If you have high blood pressure, high triglycerides, or other signs of heart disease, 3–5 grams may be more helpful. One tablespoon of flax oil equals 1 gram. Talk with your doctor or pharmacist if you're taking medications to make sure there are no negative interactions. Fish oils thin the blood just like aspirin, ginkgo biloba, and garlic. You don't want to thin your blood so much that it causes bleeding.

For more information on fats and oils, most people turn to *Fats & Oils* by Udo Erasmus. I prefer *Know Your Fats* by Mary G. Enig, Ph.D. Dr. Enig is a nutritionist and biochemist known for her expertise in this area. While I disagree with her position on soy (she says it's harmful, I and my respected colleagues say it's beneficial and safe), I think she knows more about the subject of fats than any other writer or researcher.

SECRET #338 Eating fats can help you lose weight.

Obesity contributes to heart disease, so you may be asking how you can eat these fats without gaining weight. Actually, foods high in EFAs speed up your metabolism whether you're obese or just a little overweight. They do this by causing brown fat to burn calories more quickly. Adding more fish, walnuts, pumpkin seeds, and flaxseed oil to your diet can actually help you lose weight. Also, because dietary fats burn slowly, a meal with fats feels more satisfying. Slow-burning fuel gives you energy over a long period of time—up to five or six hours.

Your body contains two kinds of fats: white and brown. White fat insulates you from cold and is what you think of as "fat" when you look in the mirror. It is stored fat, used by your body for emergencies. Brown fat surrounds various organs and protects your spine, burning calories instead of storing them. Foods high in EFAs speed up your metabolism and help you burn calories faster.

Remember to keep foods containing vegetable oils (omega-6 fats) low in your diet. This is extremely important. Israelis eat more omega-6 fats than any other population and they have a high proportion of obesity. Studies show that people with a low intake of omega-3 and high omega-6 fats are likely to be both insulin-resistant (diabetic) and obese. Unheated, unprocessed vegetable oils high in omega-3 fats (like the Spectrum brand found in health-food stores) are safer.

Bottom-line

- Fat-free or very low-fat diets are not the answer.
- Reduce animal fats.
- Eat more fish, walnuts, green vegetables, and flax seed.
- Add omega-3 supplements to your diet (fish oil, flax seed oil, black currant seed oil).

CHAPTER 41

How You Can Avoid
Strokes and Heart Attacks

Three weeks before her fifty-fifth birthday, my friend Lindy had a stroke. As a result, I wanted to know what causes some young women to have strokes and what risk factors exist for women of any age. Through my investigation, I became more aware of how vulnerable we all are to risks that can frequently be reduced.

There are known lifestyle choices that can increase your risk for having a stroke. Some may surprise you; some you may know or suspect and could be ignoring. But even one risk factor is enough to land you in the hospital. When you combine two or more, you're pushing the odds. I know a lot of people beat the odds, but many people don't. Even with Lindy's youth, strength, and determination, the road to wellness after a stroke is a challenge.

SECRET #339 **To prevent a stroke, you need to understand what causes one.**

Stroke is the third leading cause of death in most Western countries. In many cases, it's avoidable. A stroke is really a "brain attack" that occurs when blood flow to the brain is interrupted by a blood clot or burst blood vessel. This results in a lack of oxygen to the brain, which, in turn, causes some brain cells to die.

Fortunately, healthy brain cells often take over the job of those that have died, and recovery can be quite good—or a stroke can leave the person with permanent damage. Depending on which part of the brain is affected, disabilities may include speech problems, paralysis, and even dementia.

There are several kinds of stroke. One is a hemorrhagic stroke that results in bleeding in the brain. When this happens, the blood that accumulates in the brain may cause pressure on some of the tissues, interfering with brain activity. When the blood supply to the brain is reduced, some brain cells lose their food supply and die. Damage from this type of stroke is permanent. Once brain cells die, they can't be revived.

An embolism causes another type of stroke. This is the most common type, accounting for 70 to 80 percent of all strokes. It typically occurs at night or early morning when blood pressure is lowest and is frequently preceded by a mini-stroke (a transient ischemic attack, or TIA). Embolisms occur when a blood clot or another particle that can form in a blood vessel in the heart—like a piece of arterial plaque—moves through the bloodstream and gets stuck in an artery to the brain, blocking the blood flow. Strokes can also occur if small blood clots form during rapid heartbeat (atrial fibrillation).

SECRET #340 These six risk factors can lead to a stroke. Avoid all of them.

Genetics: Naturopath Tori Hudson says if your father had a stroke before age fifty or your mother before age sixty-five, you may have a genetic predisposition to stroke. While you can't change your genetics, a genetic factor means you need to work even harder to reduce other risks.

High cholesterol: Elevated cholesterol is a risk, especially with low HDL (high-density lipoproteins—the healthy fat). HDL helps pick up pieces of cholesterol in the blood and recycles them in the liver. So if your HDL is low, it means your body is not able to collect as much cholesterol from the plaque in your arteries. To raise your HDL, keep your animal fat intake low and your fats from fish oil, raw walnuts, and flax higher. A normal weight program and regular aerobic exercise (like walking or biking) for at least half an hour, five days a week, raises HDL.

Smoking: Cigarette smoking pretty much doubles your risk and, when combined with any other risk factor, it increases your chance for stroke more than the two combined. Breathing secondhand smoke also increases stroke risk. If anyone in your family smokes, ask them to smoke outdoors.

The Framingham Heart Study discovered that people who smoked two packs of cigarettes a day had twice the risk for stroke as those who smoked half a pack daily. The more a person smoked the greater their risk. When they stopped smoking, their risk started to decrease within two years. Five years after stopping, ex-smokers had the same low risk as a non-smoker. As difficult as it may be, I implore you to stop smoking.

Alcohol: Alcohol consumption can either increase or decrease your risk for stroke, depending on how much you drink. Studies have shown that one or two drinks a day may be protective in a similar way as taking aspirin, since both reduce the clotting ability of platelets. The less clotting, the fewer blood clots there are to get stuck in arteries. But heavy drinking has the opposite effect. One reason is that it tends to increase blood pressure. Heavy drinking can also reduce platelets and thin the blood too much. Perhaps the most important reason to keep alcohol consumption low is heavy drinking or binge drinking can cause a rebound effect after you stop. At this point, blood gets thicker and platelets increase dramatically, sky-rocketing your risk for stroke.

Migraines: Young women with migraines have a three times greater risk for stroke than those who never have them, according to a study reported in *Therapy Weekly.* Forty percent of strokes in young women were associated with migraines. However, when their blood pressure was under control and they stopped smoking (or didn't smoke), their risk was reduced to no more than that of anyone else. This study also found that oral contraceptives added to stroke risk for women with migraines.

Cocaine: This drug causes blood vessels to constrict and reduces blood flow to the brain by up to 30 percent. It prevents blood vessels from relaxing, which can lead to narrower arteries. We think these blood-vessel changes increase blood pressure and block or reduce flow to the brain. All you need for a cocaine-related stroke is for one blood clot to form when blood vessels constrict and then pop free to clog up an artery. If you've used cocaine with no serious side effects, consider yourself lucky. If you use it, it's time to stop, especially if you have been a smoker. Why? Smoking increases vascular fragility and, with cocaine use, increases the risk for stroke.

SECRET #341 These dietary changes can lower your risk for stroke.

Eat whole grains: These whole foods lower your risk for stroke, says the Nurses' Health Study, a twelve-year study of 75,000 women. This study found that even when women ate saturated fats (animal fats) and trans-fatty acids (margarines), those who ate more whole grains had fewer strokes than those who ate refined flours and white rice.

Eat more protective fats: Sources of good fats such as fish, raw walnuts, and flax oil are all high in essential fatty acids (EFAs) that support your immune system.

Increase your vitamin C. The amount of vitamin C in your blood may be a predictor of a low stroke risk, according to a study published in the journal, *Stroke.* The amount of vitamin C was evaluated in the diets of over 1,000 women. Women who ate vegetables six to seven days a week had a 58 percent less risk for stroke than women who ate them twice a week.

Most fresh fruits and vegetables are high in vitamin C, but it's a fragile vitamin, losing its potency when exposed to light, air, and heat. Cutting, processing, and bruising also reduce its levels in foods. If you drink a lot of water, you could also be depleting your body of vitamin C. Stress, smoking, and even smelling petroleum fumes can reduce absorption of this important vitamin.

Add to this the fact that your body doesn't store vitamin C, but needs some every day, and you'll see why it is so important to include fruits, vegetables, and possibly an additional supplement to reduce your risk for stroke. It may be the vitamin C itself, that is protective, or other nutrients found in fruits and vegetables could have a protective effect. So eat your veggies daily, and consider taking an extra 500 to 1,000 mg of vitamin C as well.

Too much iron: Large stores of iron can increase the production of free radicals in your brain cells and the tiny blood vessels in your brain. If your iron levels are too high, your brain cells can release a brain neurotransmitter called glutamate that can trigger chemical reactions causing brain-cell death.

To see if your glutamate levels are high, have a simple blood test to check your ferritin (iron) level. Ferritin, a protein in the blood that contains iron, indicates how much iron is stored in bone marrow. Sixty percent of people with high ferritin levels have been found to have high glutamate levels. If your ferritin level is higher than 275 ng/mL, you should lower your iron intake in food and supplements.

Stored iron normally increases as we age, but in a few people, it is very high. The next time you have a blood test, ask that your ferritin level be tested. It's a simple and inexpensive aspect of stroke protection.

SECRET #342 You need these three tests to evaluate your risk for heart disease and stroke.

With knowledge comes power. If you know you're heading towards a stroke or heart disease, you can take action and lower your risk. Three simple blood tests can help determine your present and future heart health. Although they're inexpensive, doctors still rely on cholesterol levels. I'm telling you that you need more. You should have your homocysteine, C-reactive protein, and fibrinogen checked every year.

Homocysteine is an amino acid that occurs naturally in our bodies. In small quantities, it's safe. In large amounts, it can produce free radicals that can lead to a buildup of plaque in the arteries and heart disease. It is also an independent predictor of heart problems. The right amounts of certain vitamins can turn off homocysteine's damaging effects. But some of these vitamins, like vitamin C and vitamin B_6 are depleted when you're under stress. This is one way stress contributes to heart disease.

A simple, inexpensive homocysteine blood test indicates inflammation. Make sure you get this test the next time you see your doctor. A change in diet, stress reduction, or vitamin therapy can all reverse it.

C-reactive protein (CRP) is a protein made in the liver that promotes inflammation and helps predict your risk for atherosclerosis and heart attacks. One study found that the higher your CRP, the more your heart disease is likely to progress. Once again, a blood test can measure your CRP.

Fibrinogen levels, however, are not tested as routinely as homocysteine or CRP. They should be. Fibrinogen is a protein that is part of our blood's clotting system and viscosity (its stickiness and thickness). You want just the right amount and not too much more.

Fibrinogen stimulates the growth and movement of some of our muscle cells into the walls of the arteries, causing these arteries to become clogged. During blood-clotting, fibrinogen turns into fibrin. The more fibrin or fibrinogen you have, the thicker and stickier the insides of your arteries are likely to become. And the higher your risk for heart disease and stroke.

Studies have found that people with high fibrinogen levels had the most damage from stroke. And too much fibrinogen can also be an indication that someone who had one stroke is likely to have another. This is why so many doctors put their patients on Coumadin, a blood thinner.

There are other options to Coumadin. Some you have heard of and some will be new to you. All have their place in reducing clot-forming proteins.

Homocysteine

High amounts of homocysteine, an amino acid, damage cell membranes, make collagen unstable, and lead to the formation of atherosclerotic plaques. It is also an indicator of inflammation and predicts your risk for heart disease.

SECRET #343 Lower your homocysteine with diet and supplements and help prevent heart disease.

Homocysteine is made with the help of other nutrients and from the breakdown of methionine. These nutrients, like betaine, vitamins B_6 and B_{12}, and folic acid, convert homocysteine into other chemicals and then either turn them back into methionine or excrete them. When you have enough of these nutrients, you can keep your homocysteine level low.

Aging is a factor in high homocysteine levels. One reason for this is that as we age, our diets contain less of the vitamins B_6, B_{12}, and folic acid needed to "deactivate" harmful homocysteine. Studies found that elderly people in the Framingham Heart Study had lowered consumption and blood levels of these particular nutrients. I'm not surprised. Try going to New England and find lots of vegetables in restaurants. They're not there. Green leafy vegetables are the primary source of folic acid (the name comes from "folate," or leaves). What would a study of vegetarians who eat plenty of fresh produce show? Low homocysteine.

Folic acid may be the most important nutrient to keep your homocysteine levels low. It is most abundant in legumes (beans) and green leafy vegetables. Few people eat enough of them every day. A salad plus a serving of broccoli, spinach, or chard is an easy way to get plenty of greens. The way you cook vegetables can also either reduce or retain folic acid. When you stir fry, you seal in a number of nutrients and retain more folic acid than if you steam or boil them. Aim for a total folic acid intake of 400–800 micrograms (mcg) a day.

Some medications and other substances block the absorption of folic acid. They include oral contraceptives, alcohol, nicotine, anticonvulsants, antibacterials, and some chemotherapy drugs. If you are on medication, check with your doctor or pharmacist to see if the medication you are taking or have taken blocks folic acid metabolism.

In a European study, normally healthy people with elevated homocysteine who took 1,000 mcg a day of folic acid responded with lowered homocysteine during the first five days of treatment.

Vitamin B_{12} often becomes lower as we age because it needs a substance called "intrinsic factor" before it can be absorbed. Intrinsic factor is made in the large intestines. Intestinal bacteria also affect the amount of intrinsic factor. If you have digestive problems or not enough friendly bacteria like *L. acidophilus* and *Bifidobacterium*, you may not be producing enough intrinsic factor to have sufficient vitamin B_{12}. This means you need to pay attention to your digestion as part of a homocysteine-lowering program. To correct digestive problems, begin by chewing your food well. Next, consider taking enzymes and/or hydrochloric acid. Check with your health care practitioner about these supplements before taking them.

Vitamin B_{12} is lacking in a vegan diet. However, many vegetarians who eat eggs and dairy products get sufficient B_{12} from their diet and a healthy digestive system. The amount of B_{12} found in most multivitamins is sufficient to meet your daily needs of 5–8 mcg a day.

Vitamin B_6 also helps lower homocysteine, according to the Framingham Heart Study. This is the lengthiest evaluation of heart problems and nutrients ever conducted. In this study, low folic acid and vitamin B_6 correlated with high homocysteine in people who had heart attacks. Vitamin B_6 is found in meats and whole grains, but the amount in food may not be enough to lower your homocysteine. Consider taking a multivitamin with 25–50 mg of B_6.

Alcohol can be a problem if you drink too much, but not if you have one or two drinks a day. Alcoholics tend to have twice as much homocysteine as non-drinkers. All alcoholics have low folate levels, which could be the reason their homocysteine is high. Malnutrition is rampant among alcoholics. And chronic alcohol abuse contributes to inflammation. It's a vicious cycle. If you drink one or two alcoholic drinks a day, keep your vegetable intake high and supplement your diet with a multivitamin.

SECRET #344 You can even lower genetically high homocysteine.

Men usually have higher levels of homocysteine than women. But as we women age, our homocysteine levels rise. This is why postmenopausal women usually have higher homocysteine levels than premenopausal women.

Genetic factors can cause a high homocysteine level in people of any age. This just means you have to work harder to bring it down. A healthy diet and a few supplements are usually sufficient. Remember, folate is an important nutrient in lowering homocysteine, and folate comes from leaves. Eat at least one serving of dark green leafy vegetables a day.

Tea also contains a lot of folate. Drink a couple of cups of green tea daily. If your homocysteine is high, tea is a much better choice than coffee. Authors of a Norwegian study found that all caffeinated coffee contributed to elevated homocysteine, while caffeinated tea did not.

In addition, friendly bacteria in your intestines lower homocysteine. Take probiotics and add dietary sources of friendly bacteria like plain yogurt, sauerkraut, and miso soup.

SECRET #345 Get a blood test to check your homocysteine.

Every time you have your cholesterol tested, tell your doctor to check your homocysteine. Many laboratories are now routinely performing these blood tests. Just like for a cholesterol test, you need to fast for about twelve hours (nothing but water from 9:00 p.m. until you have your blood drawn in the morning).

This test is accurate if you have a clear-cut high homocysteine level. If you don't, and many people do not, you may want to have a more reliable test. It's called a methionine-loading test. This test consists of taking 100 mg per kilogram of body weight of methionine and then having your blood drawn six hours later to test your homocysteine levels. Speak with your doctor about either of these tests. Why would you get the methionine-loading test? If your diet has been low in vegetables, you take no supplements, and have been under a lot of stress.

David Perlmutter, M.D., who heads the Perlmutter Health Center in Naples, Florida, says that homocysteine levels should be from 8–14 µmol/L, and ideally less than 10 µmol/L. In his book *BrainRecovery.com,* he cites a study that found 10 mg of vitamin B_6, 400 mcg of vitamin B_{12}, and 650 mcg of folic acid are enough to reduce homocysteine by 50 percent.

One of the earliest researchers in the link between high homocysteine levels and heart disease is Kilmer S. McCully, M.D., author of *The Heart Revolution.* His book offers an extensive explanation of this formerly obscure amino acid and its effects on heart disease, aging, and hormone levels in both men and women. If you're looking for a more thorough explanation, you'll want to read this book.

SECRET #346 Homocysteine affects much more than your heart.

More than 1,000 articles on homocysteine have been published in scientific journals over the past five years. We've seen that when homocysteine is high, cell damage occurs and plaque builds up in the arteries of the heart, leading to atherosclerosis. But there are more reasons for wanting low homocysteine levels, especially since you're a woman. High levels have been implicated in neural tube defects, osteoporosis, diabetes, and rheumatoid arthritis—conditions which, when added together, affect just about all women.

Homocysteine and pregnancy: Folic acid supplementation is now being touted as the nutrient that will prevent both neural tube defects and miscarriages. Research currently in progress in the Netherlands suggests that a defect in the metabolism of methionine and homocysteine may be both the cause of these problems and the reason folic acid corrects them.

Homocysteine and bone loss: The connection between high homocysteine and osteoporosis is less well defined. A number of authors of scientific studies have suggested that because children with genetically high homocysteine commonly have osteoporosis, the same pathway that causes this condition in children may well contribute to bone loss in adults. At present it is only a theory, but one based on sound scientific principles. Until there are further studies, we won't know for certain. But this connection may explain the reason for more osteoporosis in women whose homocysteine levels rise after menopause. Until we have more information, the wise approach would be to keep your homocysteine levels low, especially after menopause.

Homocysteine and diabetes: Homocysteine metabolism seems to be impaired in people with type 2 (non-insulin-dependent diabetes mellitus)—as opposed to those with type 1 diabetes. This can lead to diabetic retinopathy. Elevated homocysteine is also a risk factor for this eye condition. Remember, high homocysteine causes cell damage, and injured cells within small vessels like the eyes appear to lead to retinopathy, as well as heart disease.

Homocysteine and arthritis: Rheumatoid arthritis patients also tend to have high homocysteine levels. This isn't surprising, since high homocysteine levels point to inflammation. When a number of these patients were given an arthritis medication that assists the conversion of homocysteine to methionine, their homocysteine levels dropped and their pain was reduced. Again, it's too early to do more than postulate, but for those of us who don't have the time to wait for research on these diseases, it is clear that there are numerous benefits in lowering homocysteine levels, especially as we grow older.

C-reactive Protein (CRP)

CRP is a protein made in your liver that both indicates systemic inflammation and appears to promote inflammation. But your liver is not the only generator of CRP. Large amounts of this protein are made by abdominal fat cells. If you're overweight, and carrying this weight around your middle, you need to get a CRP blood test.

SECRET #347 If your CRP is high, you're 4½ times more likely to have a heart attack than if it was normal.

I predict you'll hear much more about CRP in the future. Not necessarily because doctors are taking a closer look at its connection to heart disease, but because pharmaceutical companies have found a way to lower it—statins. There's big money in lowering CRP.

CRP is an indication of general inflammation throughout your body. It seems to be a risk factor for atherosclerosis and heart disease. In fact, high levels of CRP place you at a 4½ times greater risk for a heart attack than someone with normal levels! In the Women's Health Study, CRP was a stronger predictor of heart problems than any other test.

Fortunately, fewer women are choosing hormone replacement therapy (HRT) after menopause. Here's another reason to avoid it. In a trial of women taking estrogen and progestin (synthetic hormones), HRT significantly increased CRP in women who already had heart disease. What did it do to the other women? We don't know.

Normal CRP levels are less than 0.11 mg/dL. If your CRP is moderate, the levels will be somewhere between 0.12 and 0.19 mg/dL. This is a warning sign to take steps to lower your CRP. When your CRP is between 0.20 and 1.50 mg/dL, begin to lower it immediately. However, you do have options other than statins, drugs that have many side effects.

SECRET #348 Statins are not the only way to lower CRP.

Doctors give drugs called statins to women with high CRP. They work, but as I've explained before, they also have side effects. What if I told you that a common, inexpensive vitamin could lower your CRP and allow you to bypass these expensive and potentially dangerous medications? Well, several studies found that vitamin E does just this. In one, a group of fifty-seven people with diabetes were given one of three antioxidants—800 international units (IU) of natural vitamin E, 500 mg of vitamin C, or tomato juice—for one month. The vitamin E cut CRP levels in half. The other antioxidants didn't.

Another study was less dramatic but still gave good results. That group included some people with diabetes, some with heart disease, and some who were healthy. They took 1,200 IU of natural vitamin E for three months. Although CRP levels "only" dropped 30 percent, they did so in each and every group.

Fibrinogen

Fibrinogen, a protein made in your liver, is one of the greatest predictors of heart disease and stroke. Too much of it makes your blood thicker, stickier, and more difficult to move through your veins. High levels of fibrinogen often contribute to dangerous blood clots that lead to heart attacks and stroke, as well as varicose veins and deep vein thrombosis (DVT).

SECRET #349 Fibrinogen can be measured by a blood test, but most doctors don't bother.

One reason why doctors don't measure fibrinogen levels routinely is that there are no treatments for elevated levels. That's right. If they don't have a pill to give you for a problem, why identify the problem? Instead, they may measure homocysteine or CRP, because they know how to treat them. Well, there are natural ways to lower your fibrinogen, but few doctors are aware of them. Since high fibrinogen can contribute to heart disease, stroke, and major illnesses for postmenopausal women, I think it's essential for all of us to be tested.

Ask your doctor to order a blood test that measures your fibrinogen levels. Normal levels are from 200 to 400 mg/dL. More than these can indicate a tendency toward too much clotting.

SECRET #350 High fibrinogen causes excessive clotting.

Fibrinogen is an important protein, as long as you don't have too much of it. It helps prevent excessive bleeding by helping blood to clot, and it does this by making the blood sticky. Fibrinogen makes fibrin, and fibrin makes blood clots. Too much fibrinogen and fibrin results in excessive blood clotting.

Obviously, we all need enough fibrinogen. When we have a cut, we want the bleeding to stop within a reasonable amount of time. If we have surgery, we want our blood to clot appropriately. But too much of this protein can cause more blood clotting than you need. Fibrinogen can cause clots that cause heart attacks and stroke if they break loose.

As with just about everything, our body has checks and balances. But aging slows down numerous body functions, and as we get older our bodies may not make enough of the substance that keeps fibrinogen levels in check.

SECRET #351 Any of these six factors can increase your fibrinogen.

- Estrogen
- High blood sugar
- Mental or psychological stress
- Obesity
- Smoking
- Very high LDL cholesterol

SECRET #352 Begin lowering your fibrinogen with these simple lifestyle changes.

Exercise is the most important thing you can do to reduce your fibrinogen. This means more than an occasional walk. Take some time to plan a weekly exercise schedule and stick to it. Join a gym, buy an exercise bike, or find a friend to walk with every day.

Some people find their fibrinogen is reduced slightly when they drink a glass of wine at night. Don't depend on this. It's an extra benefit.

Fish-oil supplements, and eating fatty fish, might lower your fibrinogen. Again, don't depend on it, but include it in your supplement regime.

Garlic lowers fibrinogen, but you have to eat a lot of it. Or you could take garlic capsules.

Olive oil works. Use it for cooking and salad dressings.

A vegetarian diet is extreme for some people. For others, it's an easy and natural way to eat. This diet lowers fibrinogen.

Vitamin E reduces fibrinogen, and a common herb I'll talk about shortly increases vitamin E's action.

SECRET #353 You may have genetically high fibrinogen.

When I told my doctor about a decades-long arrhythmia that had improved with increased supplementation, she didn't just make a note in my chart like I thought she would. She scheduled a barrage of tests for me. She wanted to rule out any other problems. My doctor, Terri Turner, is one of the smartest docs out there. Am

I fortunate to have found her! One of the tests she ordered was fibrinogen. Not only was it high, it was part of a pattern that emerged indicating genetically high factors that can lead to heart disease and stroke.

I was shocked, and at the same time grateful. Without this knowledge, I could have had a heart attack or stroke for no apparent reason. I immediately took steps to lower all of my risk indicators that were too high. And then I shared my information with friends who do a lot of traveling. You see, a number of people who take long plane flights get deep vein thrombosis (DVT), where blood clots can form, break loose, and travel to the lungs. Long-distance traveling is one risk factor because it's so easy to remain immobile and to cross our legs, cutting off our blood supply.

High fibrinogen levels would raise their risk of DVT while traveling. This is a surefire way to have a terrible vacation!

I suggested they get tested for fibrinogen since their mothers, like mine, all had some form of heart disease. We could have a genetic factor that caused elevated fibrinogen. Also, the three of us are in our sixties and seventies, so our bodies might not be making enough antifibrinogen substances. We had two good reasons to get our fibrinogen checked.

Their blood tests indicated that they, too, had high fibrinogen. In itself, this didn't mean they would get blood clots from long plane rides. But it did increase their risk. The three of us are now on supplementation to lower our fibrinogen. If you're planning a vacation that includes a long plane ride, be sure to either have your fibrinogen levels checked, or take an antithrombotic supplement to prevent a blood clot from forming in your leg. I'll talk about one in the next chapter.

SECRET #354 Some nutrients can help break down fibrin and fibrinogen.

Cayenne (capsicum), garlic, onions, ginger, and the enzyme bromelain (500 mg between meals twice a day) all help break down fibrin. Add them to your diet on a regular basis. Fish oils decrease the stickiness of your blood. This makes it more difficult to stick to the walls of your arteries.

And there's more.

A common household herb may hold the key to lowering both fibrin and fibrinogen. It's called curcumin, and it's the active ingredient in turmeric. Turmeric is the herb found in curry powder that turns rice yellow.

Curcumin is a powerful anti-inflammatory substance that's packed with antioxidants. Some of these antioxidants reduce damaging free radicals and can normalize fibrin and fibrinogen. Curcumin "turns on" natural vitamin E and helps it clean out arteries. You can't get enough curcumin by eating a lot of curry. Try taking 500 mg of either turmeric or curcumin. You can find both in health-food stores.

SECRET #355 Yes, you can take too many blood thinners.

The idea is to dissolve fibrin and fibrinogen, not just to thin your blood. Don't overdo it. After all, your blood can not only be too thick, it can also be too thin.

Helen is in her eighties and has been taking prednisone for years for her arthritis. It takes away some of the pain, but leaves her with very thin skin. Recently, she bumped her leg, and it began to bleed. Her blood was so thin it wouldn't clot. Hours later, when the cut wouldn't stop bleeding, she had to go to the hospital emergency room to have it dressed. One of Helen's problems was her thin skin, but her excessive bleeding compounded the situation.

Helen wasn't taking Coumadin or any other blood-thinning medications, but she did take a baby aspirin every morning. In addition, she had increased her vitamin E to protect her heart, and was taking ginkgo for better memory.

While all of these have their benefits, they are all blood thinners. The total amount of blood thinners you're taking needs to be considered to make sure your blood isn't too thin.

Helen had watered down her blood too much. It cost her a trip to the hospital, where she ended up getting an infection in her leg. This was unfortunate, but not surprising, since hospitals are notorious breeding grounds for bacteria. When her infection refused to heal, even with oral antibiotics, she was admitted to the hospital and given intravenous antibiotics. Taking too many blood thinners almost cost Helen her life. It was months before she was back to normal.

SECRET #356 Your pharmacist is the best person to evaluate your nutrients and medications for their blood-thinning properties.

Doctors aren't always savvy about drug, food, and nutrient interactions. Pharmacists frequently have access to an up-to-the-minute database that tells them which substances combine well together and which can cause problems. You need to know whether or not the nutrients you're taking thin your blood too much, especially if you're scheduled for surgery.

The American Association of Nurse Anesthetists (AANA) are very concerned. They published a study in the *AANA Journal* evaluating the interactions of various nutrients with anesthetics. They caution that people who take blood-thinning nutrients can dramatically increase the time it takes for their blood to clot. This means you could bleed uncontrollably during surgery if your blood won't clot!

The nutrients they mentioned that may prolong coagulation time include alfalfa, chamomile, fish oils, garlic, ginkgo biloba, kava kava, licorice root, and vitamin E. But there are more. An article in a German journal, *Perfusion,* talks about a host of herbs that increase the effect of medicinal anticoagulants. For instance, in large doses (300 mg), the natural hormone DHEA was found to increase clotting time. We don't know how little you can take without getting this effect. Individually, these nutrients may not thin your blood too much. But in combination, you, like Helen, may experience problems.

What if Helen had been in surgery? Her uncontrollable bleeding could have ended her life. I think it's vital to talk with several people in your healthcare team: your pharmacist, physician, and any practitioners of complementary medicine, to look carefully at the actions and interactions of everything you're taking. Ask them to make sure you're not thinning your blood too much. You or they can also consult the new *Physicians' Desk Reference (PDR) for Nutritional Supplements,* an excellent up-to-date reference on the actions and adverse reactions of hundreds of nutrients.

SECRET #357 These four common nutrients thin your blood.

Fish oil supplements are good for your heart partially because they decrease blood clotting. Fish oils contain several fatty acids, but it appears to be the EPA (eicosapentaenoic acid) that has this antithrombotic effect. EPA also reduces blood pressure. If you're taking supplements high in EPA, you may want to stop taking them two weeks before surgery. Check with your anesthetist to determine whether or not a fish dinner is advisable the night before any surgery.

Vitamin E reduces platelet adhesion and aggregation. Simply put, it thins your blood and keeps it from sticking to artery walls. It's an excellent protective vitamin, but if you're taking as much as 400 IU of vitamin E a day, you may want to stop taking it before any surgery. If your multivitamin contains 400 IU, ask the anesthetist or your doctor if this amount is safe for you to continue right up until surgery.

The *PDR for Nutritional Supplements* suggests that people who are already on blood-thinning medications should not take much more than 100 IU of vitamin E a day. This indicates that more than 100 IU of vitamin E a day has measurable blood-thinning capabilities. If you're taking blood-thinning medications, be monitored by your doctor to make sure the amount of vitamin E you're taking is consistent. This ensures that your medications thin your blood to the same degree each day.

Garlic is used by people with atherosclerosis to help prevent their platelets from sticking. This can both increase bleeding and accelerate bleeding time in people on medications. There have been reports of garlic extracts that increased the effect of blood-thinning medications like Coumadin. The World Health Organization (WHO) has stated that, "Patients on warfarin (Coumadin) therapy should be warned that garlic supplements may increase bleeding times. Blood-clotting times have been reported to double in patients taking warfarin and garlic supplements." Eating a clove of garlic a day, or adding it to your food, should not be a problem.

Ginkgo biloba is used to increase memory and circulation. It does this, in part, by increasing blood flow to the brain and by increasing the tone of blood vessels. Blood flow is increased when the blood is thinner. Individual cases of excessive bleeding have been seen with people who combined ginkgo with aspirin. One patient who took just 40 mg a day of a standardized 50:1 ginkgo extract along with aspirin experienced bleeding from her iris. I think ginkgo is a valuable herb, but for now I have enough reasons to be cautious about who uses it, in which amounts, and with what other nutrients and medications. I don't think it's as safe, across the board, as people think.

SECRET #358 Goldenseal and echinacea are blood thinners.

Other nutrients that could affect clotting include alfalfa, chamomile, feverfew, echinacea, dong quai, willow bark (natural aspirin), goldenseal, and horse chestnut. This doesn't mean you shouldn't use them. It means you should talk with your doctor and pharmacist about your supplements so that any doctors associated with a scheduled or unscheduled surgery are aware of your blood's clotting abilities. Perhaps you'll decide to use some herbs with anticoagulant properties on an as-needed basis, instead of daily—such as echinacea and goldenseal. Or you may find that you don't need aspirin if you're taking a number of nutrients with a similar activity.

SECRET #359 Your diet affects your blood viscosity.

Vitamin K causes blood to clot. It's found in abundance in dark green vegetables and vegetable oils. This does not mean that if you have high fibrinogen you shouldn't eat spinach or salads. Nor does it mean that if you're taking a blood thinner you cannot enjoy some of these foods. Remember, there are checks and balances. Garlic balances greens. If you're taking nutrients with anticoagulant properties, eat plenty of veggies to increase your vitamin K and reduce your risk for bleeding.

If you're taking Coumadin or any other blood thinner, you may have been told to reduce your dietary intake of vitamin K. Actually, if you're willing and able to eat the same amount of vitamin K-rich foods daily, ask your doctor if he or she can adjust your medication to allow for this. Olive oil is another food high in vitamin K. Take the time to design a healthy diet with your doctor—one that allows reasonable amounts of foods high in vitamin K along with blood-thinning herbs or medications.

SECRET #360 What you should avoid for two weeks before any surgery.

Two weeks before any surgery, including dental surgery, stop taking all blood thinners except for those given by your physician. Talk with your doctor to see if it would be wise and safe to stop any prescribed blood thinners prior to surgery. Never make this decision on your own. For more information both for you and your doctor, contact the American Association of Nurse Anesthetists (AANA) at 847-692-7050 or www.aana.com.

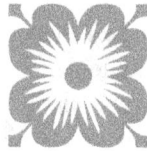

CHAPTER 42

This Japanese Nutrient Protects Your Heart and Brain

When I first wrote about this nutrient, I had no idea that I was at risk for a sudden heart attack or stroke. My doctor found a hidden genetic pattern that could have struck me down at some time in the future without any notice. Thank goodness, I had found an alternative to medications with unpleasant side effects. It's a substance made from soy and bacteria that protects the heart and brain.

Blood clots can be deadly. They can block blood flow to muscle tissues, causing them to die. They can trigger a heart attack or chest pain. They can get in your brain and cause a stroke or senility.

Some people take natural blood thinners like ginkgo biloba and vitamin E to prevent blood clots, but there's more you can do, especially if you're at risk for getting blood clots or have had them in the past.

SECRET #361 This nutrient can break up blood clots and keep them from forming.

There's a superfood from Japan that can keep blood clots from forming. If you have any existing blood clots, whether you know about them or not, it can dissolve them. And it does so even more effectively than blood-thinning drugs. How? Well, blood thinners stop working shortly after you stop taking them. The active ingredient in this food is an enzyme that works for hours after you stop taking it.

Natto is a fermented glutinous cheeselike food with stringy fibers that's made from soybeans. The Japanese love it, although other cultures find it tastes too much like smelly cheese. They eat natto for breakfast on top of rice, so they get plenty of this clot-busting food regularly. You may be one of a select few people who enjoys eating natto. If you want to try some, you can probably find it in an Asian market. Let me know what you think of it!

If you don't like natto, can't find it, or don't want to try it, there's another solution—a supplement containing its active enzyme, nattokinase. This is what most people are doing based on dozens and dozens of studies on the enzyme alone.

SECRET #362 Your body makes an enzyme to thin your blood. Nattokinase is an enzyme in a Japanese food that does the same thing.

Your blood needs to be just right—not too thick, not too thin—and your body with its infinite wisdom knows this. It makes a number of enzymes that cause blood to clot so you don't keep bleeding after surgery or when you cut yourself. But it makes only one primary enzyme to thin your blood. This enzyme is called plasmin. If your blood is too thick, or if blood clots have formed, you need more plasmin. Or something that has the same effect.

Natto, and the enzyme it contains called nattokinase, works a lot like plasmin. Actually, it's even better. It doesn't cause excessive bleeding like some blood thinners and it doesn't have any side effects. All the research has shown it is exceptionally safe. Nattokinase is only found in natto.

SECRET #363 Nattokinase can dissolve blood clots in less than a day.

Blood clots form when red blood cells and platelets are bound together with a protein in the blood called fibrin. If you have a cut, this clotting can save your life. But if a clot forms inside one of your blood vessels, it can block an artery in your heart or brain, causing a heart attack or stroke. If you remember, I talked about a test that measures fibrin in the previous chapter. A fibrinogen blood test lets you know whether you have too much of this protein or not. The antidote to too much fibrin was found by accident, like many medical discoveries.

Back in 1980, Dr. Hiroyuki Sumi, who had been researching enzymes and blood clots for many years, made a remarkable discovery. After testing nearly 200 foods for clot-busting properties, he found one that actually dissolved blood clots in just eighteen hours. It was the most potent clot-busting enzyme he had ever seen. And it had been hiding right under his nose in a popular Japanese food that he knew all his life—natto. Dr. Sumi dubbed the enzyme "nattokinase" and began studying it more thoroughly.

Dr. Martin Milner, a naturopath at the Center for Natural Medicine in Portland, Oregon, found that nattokinase both dissolves fibrin and helps the body make more plasmin and other blood clot-busting substances. "In some ways, nattokinase is actually superior to conventional clot-dissolving drugs," he says.

There have been many studies on nattokinase over the past two decades that show it can be effective in the prevention and treatment of stroke, chest pain (angina), fatigue, fibromyalgia, blood clots in the eye, atherosclerosis, diabetes, and deep vein thrombosis (DVT).

SECRET #364 Buy only good-quality nattokinase.

Not all nattokinase is alike. To make it, you need to add particular bacteria to boiled soybeans and ferment it. The bacterium in nattokinase is popularly called *Bacillus natto*. Actually, it's one of a number of strains of *Bacillus subtilis*. Herein lies the problem.

I'm particularly concerned about this bacteria. As I said in Chapter 2, some strains of *B. subtilis* are safe and some are not. Some are antibiotic resistant. Others can cause immune problems if your own immune system is already compromised. Since it's not easy for anyone to tell the difference between various strains of *B. subtilis*, I suggest you only buy nattokinase supplements from trusted companies.

One of my favorite companies that sells nattokinase is WobenzymUSA. This company makes superior digestive enzymes that I've recommended to my patients for decades. WobenzymUSA also makes Rutozym, a nattokinase enzyme formula, and sells it at a terrific price. See the Resources section for more information.

SECRET #365 Make sure nattokinase is working for you. Occasionally, it doesn't.

Nattokinase doesn't always work. It does, frequently, but each of the three doctors I interviewed who had used nattokinase to reduce fibrinogen found that there were instances when it was ineffective. In fact, they reported situations where fibrinogen levels actually increased! I know this all too well, because I was one of those people.

Nattokinase has many valuable qualities. It suppresses the thickening in arteries after a vascular injury. It also appears to heal blood vessels. Basically, we think that nattokinase works like Coumadin—but with additional benefits.

SECRET #366 Take this clot-busting formula before flying any long distances to prevent thrombosis in your legs.

If you have high fibrinogen levels and are taking nattokinase enzymes, you should be fine when you fly for long distances. But if you don't know whether or not you have blood clots, you may want to take this extra nutritional insurance.

You see, if you're taking an overseas plane flight, you're at risk for DVT. Here's what you can do to protect yourself. Move your legs. Whether you do this in your seat or walk up and down the aisles doesn't matter. But keep blood flowing by moving. Don't cross your legs. This cuts back on blood flow. In addition, you may want to take a product I found called FliteTabs.

FliteTabs is a proprietary blend of 150 mg of pycnogenol and nattokinase.

Pycnogenol is a powerful anti-inflammatory bioflavonoid that reduces swelling and strengthens the walls of capillaries. In an independent study, nearly 100 people took two capsules before flying, and two capsules six hours later. They had less swelling and pain than the controls. You can get FliteTabs in some health-food stores or pharmacies. See the Resources section for other options.

SECRET #367 Who should not take nattokinase.

It's obvious, but nevertheless an important reminder. Nattokinase thins the blood and breaks up blood clots, so you shouldn't take it if you have any type of bleeding disorder. This includes ulcers and hemorrhoids. If you've ever had intracranial bleeding or a stroke, avoid this supplement. And don't take it right before or after surgery.

Avoid nattokinase if you're on any blood-thinning medications unless you have your doctor's okay and are being closely monitored. Perhaps your doctor would allow you to take this natural supplement, which has excellent safety studies, rather than aspirin or other blood thinners. But don't make this decision on your own or take nattokinase under this situation without supervision, please.

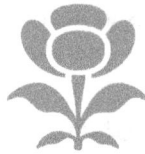

CHAPTER 43

How to Lower Your Blood Pressure Naturally

I'm constantly surprised to find that most of my female patients are more concerned about osteoporosis than high blood pressure and heart disease. They simply don't realize that heart disease is the leading cause of death for postmenopausal women in this country. Since 1984, deaths among women from heart disease have exceeded those in men. Hypertension is an important part of the picture. Presently, 60 percent of caucasian women and 79 percent of African-American women over the age of forty-five have high blood pressure.

Hypertension can often be prevented. When your blood pressure is normal, your risk for serious health problems drops significantly. I know it's not easy. We live in a stressful world where fast foods are low in fruits and vegetables and high in fats, sodium, and sugar. We're in a hurry to do everything we need to in a day that's packed with too many tasks.

Eating fast foods, junk foods, and some of the less healthful foods we grew up with and love to taste are fine every once in a while. But if you want to keep your blood pressure low and reduce your risk for heart disease and other problems, concentrate on a healthy diet along with stress reduction and regular exercise.

Some women believe that hormone replacement therapy reduces the risk for heart disease. They are hoping a quick fix will work equally as well as changing lifelong habits. This is wishful thinking. Now we're finding out that hormone therapy may not prevent heart disease.

If your blood pressure is high and your doctor has put you on medications, you could be taking them for the rest of your life. They're not only expensive, but also they can have side effects like fatigue, nausea, headaches, abdominal cramping, congestive heart failure, depression, and poor memory. Prescription and OTC drugs should be reserved for situations after all else fails.

Fortunately, there are several ways you can safely lower your blood pressure without spending your life's savings on drugs—even if your hypertension is genetic. Read about them, discuss them with your doctor, and give them a three-month trial. Then have your doctor monitor you and tell you how to get off your medications safely.

The first step is to *prevent* hypertension. If your blood pressure is already elevated, then you can look to some natural solutions.

You're going to have to make changes either to prevent hypertension or to control it, so you might as well prevent it. And as you'd suspect, it's much easier to prevent one of the risk factors for hypertension than to control it. In any case, you just can't escape the fact that you're going to have to make some important lifestyle changes. So the question is, what do you have to do and where should you start?

SECRET #368 High blood pressure strains your heart.

Let's begin by understanding just what high blood pressure, or hypertension, means. As you know, your heart pumps blood through your blood vessels and into your tissues. The force of this blood pressing against the walls of your arteries is known as blood pressure. The two numbers used to analyze your blood pressure are called "systolic" (the first or top number) and "diastolic" (the second or bottom number). Systolic blood pressure measures the force used by your heart to circulate through your blood vessels. Diastolic blood pressure measures the resistance to that force. The combination indicates how hard your heart has to work to circulate your blood.

If you have high blood pressure, it means that your heart is working harder than it should and your blood vessels may eventually become weaker. Then you're at an increased risk for cardiovascular disease, stroke, an aneurysm, congestive heart failure, kidney failure, and peripheral vascular diseases including phlebitis.

SECRET #369 Even a 5 percent weight loss can reduce your blood pressure.

Obesity is a risk factor for hypertension, as well as one of a number of other conditions that can lead to heart disease, congestive heart failure, and stroke. I've counseled many obese women during the more than twenty years I've been in practice as a nutritionist and I know how difficult it is to lose weight. But even a 5 to 10 percent weight loss can reduce blood pressure if it's high. It can also reduce hypertension by 20 to 50 percent if your blood pressure isn't very high.

Here's what I've found works best:

A positive, determined attitude: I know it's not so easy, but it really does help. You need to decide you *will* find a way to lose weight and keep it off, and you *won't* stop until you do, no matter how discouraged you may become at any moment. A defeatist attitude won't work. Become a warrior on your own behalf and face it with all your heart and might.

Address your emotional and physiological cravings: Find other ways to reward yourself, such as putting off unpleasant tasks or feeding an emotional void with food. Use emotional answers to emotional problems. Food is only a temporary fix.

Control your portions: Learn the difference between feeling stuffed and eating until you are no longer hungry. Use smaller plates and bowls. Chew your food well. Reduce your portions and wait fifteen minutes before taking seconds. If you are not hungry after eating less, stop. If you're still hungry, eat a little more.

Change your diet: Eat more dense foods that turn to sugar slowly, like beans, fish, and chicken. Concentrate on eating some protein (including beans and tofu) with each meal. Eat lots of vegetables. Drink water throughout the day.

Exercise more: Even if you don't lose any weight, half an hour of mild to moderate aerobic exercise done for three to six days a week can lower your blood pressure. A brisk walk is enough. When the weather is bad, try walking through a local shopping mall. Do your half-hour walk first, and then, after you've exercised, take time for any shopping or window-shopping.

Watch your alcohol intake: Limit your alcohol consumption to 5 ounces of wine, 12 ounces of beer, or 1 ounce of hard liquor a day at most. If you're overweight, consider drinking even less. These are empty calories. Instead, if you must drink, have a smaller drink or limit yourself to one drink a day on weekends. Of all alcohol, red wine is still the most beneficial alcoholic beverage in protecting you against heart disease because of the antioxidants it contains. But if you don't drink, don't start.

SECRET #370 These two vitamins can relax your blood vessels.

A study published in the journal *Hypertension* found that vitamins C and E reduced high blood pressure in rats. The theory behind this is that these antioxidants may protect nitric oxide in the body. Nitric oxide is a molecule that relaxes blood vessels, making them more pliable. The scientists who conducted this study caused oxidative stress in the rats and their nitric oxide levels decreased as their blood pressure rose. When vitamins C and E were added to their diets, their blood pressure dropped to normal.

What does this mean for you? A diet to prevent hypertension should include whole foods with plenty of fresh fruits and vegetables, along with a good multivitamin/mineral supplement. This should give you enough vitamins C and E. Don't depend only on supplements. Vitamin C is found in fruits and vegetables that also contain plenty of potassium. Begin by eating more of them. Vitamin E is plentiful in nuts, seeds, soy, and cold-pressed vegetable oils.

SECRET #371 **Lower your sodium intake and increase potassium to lower your blood pressure.**

You want to eat a diet higher in potassium than sodium, and many people eat the reverse. Reducing sodium lowers blood pressure in some people, but not everyone. One reason could be a sodium/potassium imbalance. You may need more potassium in addition to less sodium. You don't need a lot of salt to be healthy because your body conserves it so well. You do, however, need a lot of potassium.

In more than 100 people with high blood pressure, a diet low in sodium and high in potassium worked better than just lowering salt intake. We know from past studies that when our potassium is low, our blood pressure tends to rise.

There's more sodium in foods than you might think. Cow's milk and cheese may not taste salty, but they're high in sodium. Keep your dairy intake low. Read labels on all processed and canned foods. They tend to be high, as well. When you reduce your sodium intake to 2.5 grams a day (2,500 mg) or less, you are reducing your risk for hypertension—especially if you're over the age of sixty. Even a small reduction in salt can decrease blood pressure in people whose blood pressure is normal.

Supplemental potassium may be helpful in preventing and reducing high blood pressure, but only take them if your health practitioner advises it. Potatoes, sweet potatoes, beet greens, and avocados are all high in potassium. Most fruits and vegetables contain potassium. Eat fresh vegetables twice a day and fruit at least once a day, to give you enough potassium with very little sodium.

SECRET #372 **Magnesium helps regulate sodium and potassium.**

Low magnesium is a hidden risk for high blood pressure. The reason is connected to your need for potassium. Even a mild magnesium deficiency causes your body to excrete more potassium. A high magnesium intake is associated with lower blood pressure. This may be because magnesium activates a cellular membrane pump that pumps out sodium from the cells as it pumps potassium into them.

Don't just increase your consumption of potassium-rich foods. You need sufficient magnesium before potassium can be raised. Fortunately, many foods that are high in potassium are also high in magnesium. They include nuts, green leafy vegetables, and beans. Eat some of them every day. Your diet, and supplements, should be high in magnesium.

Consider increasing your magnesium supplementation as well. There's no fixed amount of magnesium that each of us needs. It can vary from 200 to 1,000 mg a day. Your body knows how to keep you from taking too much magnesium. It's called "bowel tolerance." Take as much magnesium as your bowels can tolerate.

Add 100 mg of magnesium in addition to your nutritional supplements, and increase it by 100 mg every few days until your stools are soft, but not uncomfortably loose.

Some women become hypertensive after their fifth month of pregnancy. When this hypertension is accompanied by edema and protein in the urine (proteinuria), it can cause pre-eclampsia, a condition that can lead to convulsions (eclampsia). While magnesium has not been found to reduce high blood pressure alone, studies have found it reduces both pre-eclampsia and eclampsia and is not at all harmful to the fetus. It stands to reason, that if magnesium can help lower pregnancy-induced high blood pressure, it should be featured in your preventive diet and supplement program. A higher ratio of potassium to sodium is also helpful in controlling pregnancy-related high blood pressure.

SECRET #373 Switch from drinking coffee to drinking tea.

Tea is the beverage of choice for most of the world, and for good reason. It is high in antioxidants and its flavonoids fight hypertension. When more than 200 women over the age of seventy drank a single cup of black tea a day, they lowered their blood pressure. Drinking two or three cups lowered it even more.

In another study, over 1,500 people with no history of hypertension were studied. Some drank at least half a cup of green or oolong tea a day while others drank it only occasionally, if at all. The tea drinkers had a 46 percent decreased risk for developing hypertension. The more tea they drank, the more protection it offered them. Those who drank $2\frac{1}{2}$ cups of tea a day had a whopping 65 percent decreased risk.

The caffeine content of tea has nothing to do with its blood pressure-lowering ability. Drink either regular or decaffeinated tea. If you insist on drinking coffee, have one cup in the morning and switch to green or black tea afterwards. I mix the two kinds of tea to give me a hearty morning blend that works for me as a substitute for coffee.

SECRET #374 Drink hard water, not soft water.

Lots of people buy water softeners. They like the way soft water cleans their clothes and hair. The problem is, soft water leaches heavy metals like lead out of pipes and faucets.

Calcium and magnesium make water hard. Your body needs both of them. Why put toxic metals into your body when you could put essential minerals in it instead? Drinking hard water is associated with lower blood pressure, possibly because of its magnesium content. The toxins in soft water like cadmium and lead can contribute to high blood pressure. If you have a water softener, buy bottled water for cooking and drinking.

SECRET #375 When all else fails, try a temporary vegetarian diet.

Trust me. It's not so bad. I've been eating a vegetarian diet for more than thirty years, and it doesn't contain a lot of weird stuff. Plenty of whole grains, beans, vegetables, and some fruit will give you a lot of nutrients needed to keep hypertension at bay.

Vegetarians have one-third to one-half less hypertension than non-vegetarians. When you look at the list of foods high in potassium, you can see why. I'm not suggesting you stop eating meat forever. But if your blood pressure stays high after trying everything else, you may want to go on a vegetarian diet temporarily. You could conceivably lower your blood pressure 5 to 10 mm Hg if you stop eating animal products.

Fish have beneficial essential fats that can help lower blood pressure. You can include fish in an otherwise vegetarian diet. I talked about ways to eat fish without building up pesticide and mercury residues in your body in Chapter 40. Please re-read that chapter if you're going to include fish in your blood-pressure-lowering program.

Give this diet a three-month trial. Need help? Read *The New Becoming Vegetarian* book by Vesanto Melina, M.S., R.D. and Brenda Davis, R.D. It contains simple and tasty meatless recipes along with lots of helpful information to make this diet work.

For more information on natural solutions to hypertension, pick up *The High Blood Pressure Solution* by Richard D. Moore, M.D., Ph.D. It's packed with more detailed information not only for you, but for your doctor as well.

SECRET #376 Don't forget to manage your stress every day.

Stress is not the primary cause of hypertension, but as anyone with normal blood pressure knows, your blood pressure can climb in stressful situations. If you are at the doctor's office waiting for a report on an exam, your blood pressure could be abnormally high, even when it is usually normal or low.

Chronic stress is, of course, the most harmful, because it's not a temporary condition. To prevent both stress-related high blood pressure and heart disease you need to set time aside to use some form of daily stress reduction like breathing from the diaphragm, meditation, or prayer. I'm not talking about dashing off a quick note to God to ask for calmness as you rush out the door. I'm talking about taking from ten to thirty minutes a day to do some form of active stress reduction.

In the 1960s and 1970s, researchers expected heart disease rates to climb among women as they began climbing corporate ladders. That didn't happen. The explanation for this surprise is that the increased personal satisfaction and higher levels of self-esteem that come with professional success appear to mitigate female stress. The type of stress experienced determines whether or not it will lead to high blood pressure and heart disease.

Feelings of frustration and powerlessness have been identified as a cause of higher heart-disease rates. A few years ago, the *Journal of the American Medical Association* published the results of a Duke University five-year study that concluded mental stress is more dangerous to the heart than physical stress.

If you find yourself frequently feeling frustrated, anxious, tense, edgy, restless, overwhelmed, or powerless, these feelings of stress may be increasing your heart disease risk. You may be able to lower heart-disease risk, however, with stress reduction techniques.

SECRET #377 Meditation lowers stress and has nothing to do with your religious beliefs.

The ultimate stress-reduction technique may be meditation. In 1978, researcher and physiologist R. Keith Wallace of the University of California at Los Angeles discovered that a group of meditation practitioners experienced 80 percent less heart disease (and over 50 percent less cancer) than those in a control group.

The simplest way to meditate is to find a quiet place to sit comfortably, close your eyes, and direct your attention to your breathing. Repeat one word, such as "calm," "peace," or "God" slowly and continually. As thoughts come into your mind, let them go. Do this fifteen minutes or longer. The goal is to be still, physically and mentally, until you feel extremely relaxed and peaceful. After stopping, try to keep the relaxed feeling with you. Some people find it helpful initially to receive more formal meditation instruction. Numerous meditation groups across the country offer this. Or pick up a copy of *How To Meditate* by Lawrence Leshan. All forms of meditation work, even when you aren't sure initially whether they're working.

SECRET #378 Don't forget these six ways to reduce stress. They're simple, and they work.

Don't limit yourself to these suggestions, but do something on a regular basis to lower your stress. You may have some lesser-known favorites of your own, such as listening to music or relaxation tapes, dancing, soaking in the tub, or just getting away by yourself for a while. For best results, use the combination of techniques that works best for you:

Laughter: Have you ever laughed so hard you nearly fell out of your chair? Do you remember the ultra-relaxed feeling you had afterward? Laughter is a powerful stress-relief tool. This probably explains in large part why prime-time TV is dominated by sit-coms—they help us unwind and de-stress. Other tools for regular laughter include funny movies, books, and looking at the humorous side of things, even in the midst of a tragedy. Medical research has confirmed the healing power of laughter and includes many reports of persons actually healing themselves with intensive laughter therapy.

Take a night out: A Swedish study found that people who regularly attended cultural activities—movies, concerts, plays, artistic events, and even sporting events—were half as likely to die as people in a control group who didn't. The lead researcher of this 12,000-person study even speculated that such activities have a stronger influence on longevity than income, physical activity, and even smoking by eliciting strong positive and healing emotions that, like simple laughter, boost the immune system's ability to fight stress.

Togetherness: Sexual arousal and orgasm boosts your resistance to stress. So does just being with others. Numerous studies show that people with the strongest ties to family, friends, church, and other community groups enjoy significantly greater longevity. Strained, unpleasant, and abusive relations with others create stress. Spend time with your friends, even if it's just by phone.

A positive, proactive approach: If you're prone to negativity, a little mindfulness and looking at the bright side can go a long way in helping you overcome it. The reward? Your stress resistance, effectiveness as an individual, and your enjoyment of life will soar. If necessary, get professional help to overcome excessive negativity or fatalism.

Get regular exercise: I'm not talking about a stroll around the mall or walking to and from your car or the grocery store. I mean doing some kind of aerobic exercise five times a week. No time, you say? Then how will you find time to recover from heart disease? Do you have time to spend sitting in doctors' offices waiting for appointments, tests, and prescriptions for medication?

Begin exercising slowly. Start today by exercising for ten minutes. Tomorrow, meditate or play a tape with a guided meditation or relaxation technique on it. Do this for ten minutes. Each day, do one or the other for ten minutes. At the end of a week or two, increase to fifteen minutes. When you are up to twenty minutes a day, do ten minutes of exercise and ten of meditation. Eventually, get your exercise up to twenty to thirty minutes five times a week. Walks with friends count. So does housework and gardening. Get active. Make your heart work a little harder at times. And open it up more with meditation, relaxation exercises, and prayer. It can change your health and change your life.

CHAPTER 44

Nutrients to Keep
Your Heart Healthy

You already know that a good diet is important to your health in general, but I'd like you to take a look at particular foods that have a direct effect on your heart. One of them is at the center of a huge controversy. I'm talking about soy, the foundation for many vegetarian diets. Experts are at war over soy's safety. Some say it's beneficial to the heart and protective against cancer. Others say it will damage your thyroid and contribute to cancer. After you read this chapter, you'll have a better idea of whether or not soy is safe for you.

Then there's the confusing subject of nutritional supplements. Many nutrients offer good comprehensive coverage, while other specifically support a healthy heart. A few key nutrients can make the difference between a strong heart and one heading for trouble. If you have any heart disease, or if it runs in your family, it's time to take out additional health insurance by making a few small but important adjustments to your supplement regime.

When all else fails, you may want to consider chelation therapy. But not just any chelation will work. Don't waste your time and money on a program that offers false hope at best. Invest in a program that has the best chance of succeeding.

SECRET #379 Heart-healthy fats raise your HDL (healthy) cholesterol and lower your LDL (harmful) cholesterol.

Fats: Your best diet for preventing heart disease is one low in saturated fats found in animal protein. Monounsaturated and polyunsaturated fatty acids, found in vegetable oils, reduce your risk for heart disease. Keep all fats below 30 percent of your diet. And 20 percent is better still, even if current fad diets tell you to eat more. When your fat intake is greater than 30 percent of your total calories, it will not help prevent heart disease. Don't eat a very low-fat diet or a fat-free diet, because while they will lower your harmful LDLs, they'll also lower your helpful HDLs. And low HDL levels put you at a higher risk for heart disease. In addition:

The best animal protein for heart protection is fatty cold-water fish containing high amounts of omega-3 fatty acids. However, cold-water fish, like salmon, which are farmed and not fed their usual diet of sea vegetation, are not high in these protective fatty acids. Make sure the fish you eat come from the ocean. When in doubt, ask.

Nuts and seeds: Include raw nuts or seeds in your diet as well. One study of Seventh-Day Adventists found that those who ate a handful of nuts a few times a week had significantly less heart disease than those who didn't eat them. Some nuts contain omega-3 fatty acids, and pecans and walnuts are two of the richest sources. Omega-6 and omega-3 are those essential fatty acids your body needs and can't manufacture—they must come from an outside source.

SECRET #380 Your sugar intake does more harm to your heart than feed inflammation.

Sugar: Keep your refined-sugar consumption low. In some people, it promotes atherosclerosis. In others, it raises cholesterol while lowering HDL. If you limit refined sugar to 10 percent of your caloric intake, you can still enjoy an occasional dessert, cookie, or muffin and have a healthy heart.

SECRET #381 These beverages lower cholesterol.

Green tea: Green tea, which is high in beneficial antioxidants, helps decrease total cholesterol, harmful LDL cholesterol, and triglycerides. It also appears to increase the beneficial HDL cholesterol. If you like it, you might want to incorporate two or three cups of green tea into your daily program. Because of all the current research on the benefits of green tea, this beverage is now widely available in most supermarkets.

Alcohol: If you can handle just a little alcohol and want to include it in your diet, limit yourself to one glass of red wine a day. It contains resveratrol, an antioxidant found to be helpful for the heart. If you have any liver disease, past or present, don't drink. Carefully weigh the data and make your choice a wise one.

The Great Soy Controversy

Soy is an ingredient in many health foods and nutritional supplements, yet there are experts who say it's not safe. If you've heard some of these objections, you may have cut back on soy. Or eliminated it from your diet completely. This would be unfortunate, because some of the objections to soy are based on half-truths.

SECRET #382 Soy protects against heart disease.

Soy is one of the most heavily studied foods of all times. It has been found to reduce hot flashes, lower cholesterol and risk of heart disease, prevent breast cancer, relieve vaginal dryness, and strengthen bones. In fact, the FDA has ruled that food manufacturers can say that soy protein (not its isolated isoflavones that are found in supplements) helps lower cholesterol and protect against heart disease. The balance of nutrients in soy foods is different from some of its components used in dietary supplements. In this chapter, I'm talking primarily about soy in various foods—not soy isoflavone supplements. Soy foods have many uses. Protecting against heart disease is just one that has been recognized as being both safe and effective.

SECRET #383 The allegations that soy is harmful have not been proven.

Several studies linking tofu intake to brain aging and atrophy, thyroid problems, and even the growth of breast tissue have sent out signals of alarm. The media, as usual, ran with the scary headlines. After all, it sells newspapers, magazines, and advertising space on radio and TV. But Elizabeth A. Yeatley, Ph.D., lead nutrition scientist at the Food and Drug Administrations (FDA) Center for Food Safety and Applied Nutrition (CFSAN) commented, "Every dietary health claim that has ever been published has had controversy."

So what's the real story about soy? I spoke with some of the experts on the subject to better understand what people are saying, why they're saying it, and what's behind the statements alleging that soy causes more problems than it solves.

It's truly difficult to get a clear picture since not all the studies cited to back up any particular point are as good as we'd like them to be. In fact, some are seriously flawed. People and organizations with vested interests often heavily influence the slant of articles both pro and con. Meanwhile, some scientists are concerned about soy's safety based on preliminary studies and it will be years before we get more studies to either back up these opinions or refute them. I'm convinced that some people don't tolerate soy well, but that doesn't mean soy is harmful to everyone. Let's look at just some of the allegations, and take a peek behind them at the "other" side.

SECRET #384 The assertion that eating tofu causes your brain to atrophy was based on an observational study and has never been proven to be true.

It made headlines for a while when Lon White, M.D., senior neuroepidemiologist at Pacific Health Research Institute and professor at the University of Hawaii School of Nursing, conducted a Hawaiian study on soy. His study concluded that Japanese men and their wives who ate the most tofu for twenty years between the ages of forty-five and sixty-five had the greatest loss of cognitive function after age seventy-five. In addition, their brains appeared to shrink and atrophy.

But Mark Messina, Ph.D., chairman of the Third International Symposium on the Role of Soy in Preventing and Treating Chronic Disease, noted that Alzheimer's disease has typically been found to be more prevalent among Japanese men living in Hawaii than those living in Japan. Dr. White's study proved nothing.

In fact, Dr. White's study was never designed to show a relationship between brain size and function and its possible cause. This study was filled with variables. Soy could have been one factor in a lifestyle that leads to lower cognitive function. Or the aluminum content of tofu could have been the culprit.

Aluminum is suspected of being implicated in Alzheimer's disease. William Harris, M.D., of Honolulu had sixteen samples of soy products tested for aluminum at the University of Hawaii. Some of the tofu was high in aluminum, and it was found that the aluminum content of soy is increased when it is cooked in aluminum pots. We don't know about the aluminum content of the tofu ingested by the people Dr. White found had decreased brain function. We do know that a two-year study of Japanese women living in Seattle did not show an association between tofu intake and cognitive decline.

Vesanto Melina, M.S., R.D., pointed out that, "The Hawaii study's research design was seriously flawed in a number of respects, including not quantifying the amounts of soy consumed. It is a single study, is not more widely reflected, and clearly factors other than soy could be responsible for the findings."

In fact, Dr. White agreed that it's too early to jump to any conclusions connecting soy with brain atrophy. He told me that only one other study had ever investigated this question, and it was a poor study. His study, he claimed, is about as good a trial as it gets so far. "But it is still an observational study," he said, adding, "Bottom-line is that we have too little information to attach significant importance to such comparisons beyond just saying they are interesting."

SECRET #385 Soy shouldn't harm your thyroid if you have enough of this mineral.

Some thyroid experts are down on soy. They say it produces goiters and leads to low thyroid function. In fact, as far back as the 1930s, studies have suggested that soy produced goiters in laboratory animals. But the key to these thyroid problems appears to be iodine. A goiter is an enlargement of the thyroid caused by an iodine deficiency or hypothyroidism (low thyroid function). A small number of babies who were fed soy formulas without added iodine also developed goiters.

Today's formulas contain iodine, which appears to have eliminated the problem. In addition, when soy is heated, the properties that lead to goiters are reduced. Dr. Messina points out that there have been no studies that have been designed to study the effects of soy formula on thyroid function.

There may be a connection between some soy products and thyroid problems. Researchers at the National Center for Toxicology Research (NCTR), who looked at laboratory (not human or animal) cell studies, proposed that isoflavones from soy, and other flavonoids, could lead to goiters. At the same time, they emphasized that this is most likely to occur in people with low iodine intake. It appears that low iodine is more of a problem than a high-soy diet!

A recent study out of the University of California School of Medicine indicates that including soy in your diet could actually protect you against thyroid cancer. More than 500 women were interviewed over a six-year period, and their diets were assessed for traditional soy foods (tofu and tempeh) and some of the newer foods on the market made with soy protein and soy flour (protein powder and veggie burgers). The traditional soy foods, highest in phytoestrogens like diadzen and genistein, were most protective against thyroid cancer.

In the first study designed to look at the effects of isoflavone supplements on thyroid function, researchers found no problems. The supplements didn't affect thyroid function in any of the participants over a period of six months. All of the women in this study had also been taking a multivitamin containing 150 mcg of iodine. Now, if you've read the latest data on iodine in Chapter 1, you know that this amount of iodine is very small. Still, it appears it was enough to prevent any damage from soy. By the way, the amount of isoflavones used in this study was two to three times the amount consumed by Japanese women through their diet. Other studies using soy protein in much higher quantities than are found in a typical Japanese diet came to the same conclusions. See Chapter 1 for more information on iodine testing and supplementation.

SECRET #386 The bad press on soy and thyroid comes from one flawed study.

Only one study has found adverse effects from soy. This is the study that's most often cited by opponents to soy. The difference between this study and the others is that the soy that was eaten was in the form of roasted soybeans, which were pickled and stored in vinegar. This is very different from soy protein or tofu, the soy products eaten in the United States and Japan.

There are several problems with this study. First, the amount of soybeans eaten was only equal to half the amount of soy found in a typical Japanese diet. This means that the women ingested half the amount of isoflavones as people on a traditional Japanese diet. Second, the participants in this study had an unusually high amount of gastrointestinal problems. In those studies with positive outcomes, there were few digestive problems. What caused them in this study? Possibly the pickling of the soybeans and their storage in rice vinegar. Based on all of the other studies, the gastrointestinal problems didn't come from soy.

SECRET #387 Soy food appear to be protective against breast cancer. Isoflavone supplements may or may not be.

Soy contains plant-based chemicals called isoflavones that have a weak, estrogenic effect. One of the isoflavones in soy, genistein, has been found in studies to slightly stimulate estrogen-receptor-positive breast cells. If you're taking isoflavone supplements, you could be placing yourself at risk. But higher amounts of genistein inhibit both estrogen-receptor-positive *and* estrogen-receptor-negative cell growth. So once again, it's possible that you're protecting your breasts. We don't know.

Let's complicate this situation by pointing out that the studies that came to these conclusions were done in vitro (in laboratories) not in vivo (in humans). Animal studies, which are better than in vitro studies, show soy actually *inhibits* chemically induced tumors. And there are no studies I've found that show soy foods increase the risk for breast cancer. Everything I've seen indicates the opposite is true.

The American Dietetic Association has suggested that women who are taking tamoxifen to prevent a recurrence of breast cancer avoid soy. But Dr. Messina reports an animal study that found the combination of miso with tamoxifen inhibited the development of chemically induced breast tumors by 50 percent. Tamoxifen alone had no inhibitory effect. Soy foods appear to be protective. While some oncologists actually use high amounts of isoflavones to help shrink breast cancer tumors, it might be wise, if you've had breast cancer, to avoid soy isoflavones in supplement form unless your doctor says otherwise.

Whether you're eating a diet high in soy, taking soy supplements, or taking cancer-fighting drugs alone or in combination with either of these, have your progress monitored. Perhaps the best, least invasive way to do this is through breast thermography. You can read more about this diagnostic tool in Chapter 46.

SECRET #388 Soy is safe . . . if you have sufficient iodine.

We need more long-range, double-blind, placebo-controlled studies or other well-designed studies with a large number of participants. Meanwhile, look at both sides of the soy picture. Consider this: The Japanese have eaten large quantities of soy for centuries and have a low incidence of heart disease. They also get plenty of iodine in their diet and get little breast cancer or thyroid problems. This says to me that eating soy daily is quite safe.

Still, it's important to realize that not all foods are good or safe for everyone, and that too much of a good thing may turn it into a harmful substance. A diet heavily weighted in soy will undoubtedly lead to negative side effects in some people, although the same amount may be safe for someone else. Clearly, there are other forms of protein than soy, even in vegetarian diets. If soy is your main source of protein, you may want to include other legumes (beans).

Some of the negative allegations about soy have come from two scientists at the FDA. The FDA responded by saying that the benefits of soy outweigh any potential problems, and that soy contains healthy substances and is safe to consume.

SECRET #389 How much soy do the experts eat?

The FDA has announced that 25 grams of soy protein a day along with a diet low in saturated fat and cholesterol may reduce the risk of heart disease. One cup of cooked soybeans (like edamame) contains 28.5 grams of protein, while half a cup of tofu has 17–20 grams. One veggie burger or soy hot dog has 9–13 grams of protein.

How much do some soy experts eat?

James W. Anderson, M.D., does soy research on people at the University of Kentucky. He believes that soy is more beneficial to our health than any other food we could eat. He eats two or more servings of soy a day, beginning with 20–25 grams of soy protein for breakfast. He also eats soybean chili, soy nut snacks, and includes tofu in stir-fry twice a week.

Mark Messina, Ph.D., has about ten servings of soy a week, and estimates he's eating from 10 to 40 grams a day. He says, "A healthy adult with adequate iodide intake can keep enjoying soy without reservation. It offers so much in terms of nutrients and health benefits—some of which are only now being discovered."

As for me, I add a little soymilk to my breakfast cereal. Then I choose from edamame, tofu, and an occasional veggie burger or soy dog for another meal on most days. I do eat many other legumes, as well, and that's what I recommend you do, too.

Supplements for a Healthy Heart

There are dozens of supplements you can use to support good heart health. You probably don't need all of them. The first category of nutrients to consider is antioxidants. They can keep your cholesterol from oxidizing, or spoiling.

SECRET #390 The issue isn't whether or not antioxidants protect against heart disease. It's whether or not they protect against disease.

Most antioxidant studies either have been conducted with men or have not differentiated between responses in each gender.

So while I have seen many scientific studies that link antioxidants to protection against heart disease, I'd like to focus on those that specifically mention their effectiveness with women.

An interesting fourteen-year-long study published in the *American Journal of Epidemiology* indicated that women did benefit from high intakes of vitamin E, vitamin C, and carotenoids. The best-known carotenoid is beta-carotene, but the family of carotenoids includes others, as well. What is of great interest is that all of these antioxidants were not only beneficial in reducing the risk of death from heart disease in men and women, but also *women had almost twice the protection as men.* This tells me that antioxidants in diet and supplementation are especially important for women. Fruits and vegetables contain the highest amount of these nutrients and may also contain additional protective factors (such as phytochemicals) that were not studied. The whole food is always better than any pill, although a combined approach may offer the most protection.

In the Nurses' Health Study, women who took 100 international units (IU) or more of vitamin E and multivitamin supplements had less major coronary heart disease than women who had a low intake of this vitamin. Long-term use of vitamin E seems to have a protective effect on atherosclerosis by reducing the LDL cholesterol (the sticky kind). The multivitamins also contained other antioxidants like vitamins A and C. If you are going to add vitamin E to your diet, use a dry form of d-alpha or mixed tocopherols. Dry or water-soluble vitamin E is better absorbed than the oil-based variety, and both d-alpha and mixed tocopherols are better utilized than the synthetic dl-alpha tocopherol.

SECRET #391 Magnesium is the most important nutrient you can take for your heart.

Your doctor may be telling you to take more calcium, but I disagree. Studies indicate that the mineral we need most is magnesium. Without enough magnesium, the calcium you take will not be absorbed. This doesn't mean it's harmless, either. Unabsorbed calcium that is not excreted (and most isn't) gets into your joints where it becomes arthritis or in your arteries where it becomes atherosclerosis. According to a review of magnesium done back in the 1970s, taking more magnesium can prevent your blood vessels from calcifying and developing into atherosclerosis.

But it's not just hardening of the arteries that magnesium helps prevent through its natural chelating action. Magnesium helps your heart relax. You need enough of it to produce the energy to contract. And that's what your heart does—contract and relax. Magnesium keeps excessive sodium out of your heart. Sodium attracts water, so a magnesium deficiency can contribute to edema (swelling) in your heart or lungs. You also need magnesium to keep your arteries contracting and dilating, allowing blood to flow through them easily. You can see some reasons why a magnesium deficiency is associated with a higher risk for heart attacks, cardiac arrhythmias, hypertension, and unexpected cardiac death.

According to Alan Gaby M.D., most of the people he sees in his practice have low levels of magnesium. A government survey shows the average American diet provides about 40 percent of the magnesium we need each day—based on the low recommended dietary allowance (RDA) levels. Approximately 75 percent of U.S. females are magnesium deficient. And most doctors still don't check magnesium levels in sick or dying patients in hospitals who are showing signs of magnesium deficiency (cardiac arrhythmia, muscle spasms, depression, and hypertension). Jean Durlach, M.D., president of the International Society for the Development of Magnesium Research, found that throughout the world, higher amounts of magnesium in drinking water correlated with lower death rates from heart disease.

It's not easy to know if you are low in magnesium. Most blood tests are inaccurate. Red blood cell–magnesium levels are better to check than the regular serum magnesium, according to Guy Abraham, M.D., a pioneer in the area of magnesium, PMS, and osteoporosis-reversal. If you prefer, you can just begin taking extra magnesium—up to 1,000 mg per day. Side effects from taking more than you need are loose stools. You can take the amount that will cause your stools to be loose without being runny. And you may be protecting yourself against heart disease as well as osteoporosis, stress, and other conditions.

That's magnesium, in general. What about magnesium, women, and heart disease? As usual, few studies are on women only, but in a study of about 100 menopausal women with mild or moderate hypertension, none of whom were taking medication, the high blood pressures of those who took magnesium for six months dropped significantly over those who did not take magnesium. High blood pressure leads to stroke. Other studies are not gender-specific, but indicate the broad necessity of including magnesium in the dietary and supplemental programs of all people at risk for heart disease.

Mildred Seelig, M.D., was considered by many to be the world's authority on magnesium. She strongly suggested that magnesium be given intravenously as soon as a person has a heart attack. In the ambulance, if possible. The bottom-line is don't wait until you're magnesium-deficient. Begin by increasing magnesium in your diet (whole grains and beans of all kinds are high in this mineral) and make sure any vitamin/mineral supplement you take has at least as much magnesium as calcium—and more magnesium if your bowels can take a bit more.

SECRET #392 It's oily fish, not just any fish, that helps your heart.

It's no secret that fish is included in a healthy heart diet. But not all fish are alike. Fish oils are the ingredients in fish that benefit your heart. They contain properties that cool down inflammation, keep your cholesterol and blood pressure low, and make beneficial HDL cholesterol. But not all fish are fatty, and many fatty fish are not popular. Salmon, herring, and mackerel are high in fats. When was the last time you had a heaping plateful of herring or mackerel?

You eat salmon, you say? It has plenty of good fats if it was caught in the wild. But if the salmon was farmed, it's low in these essential fats. I'll bet you're not eating wild salmon every day. If this is the case, consider fish-oil capsules, or essential fatty acid capsules that include fish oils. To make sure the fish and fish oils you're taking are not contaminated with pesticides or mercury, refer to Chapter 40.

SECRET #393 Your heart uses a lot of CoQ_{10} every day, but it makes less of it as you age.

CoQ_{10} is a waxy fat-soluble nutrient made in our bodies and used in large quantities by our hearts. The problem is, as we age our hearts make less CoQ_{10}. This is just when we need more of it. And it's the time of life when we start experiencing signs of CoQ_{10} deficiency: angina and arrhythmias. There are some dietary sources of CoQ_{10}: beef hearts and oily fish. It's just not practical to eat huge amounts of them every day. Supplementation is a better option.

More than 100 studies back up the use of CoQ_{10} for angina. In one of them, patients took 150 mg of CoQ_{10} a day for four weeks. Their pain was reduced by 53 percent. But there are other reasons to take CoQ_{10}. It reduces arrhythmias in many people. It reduces secondary heart attacks in people who have had an episode. And it reduces mortality from heart attacks. When you combine CoQ_{10} with vitamin E, it helps prevent your harmful LDL cholesterol from oxidizing (see Chapter 39 for more information).

You don't have to wait for a problem to occur before taking this valuable nutrient. In fact, it's better if you don't. Doses vary greatly from 100 to 400 mg, depending on your body's needs. You may want to start with a protective dose of 30 mg, three times a day, or 50 mg, once or twice a day. Since it's a fat-soluble nutrient, take it when you're eating an oily food like nut butter or oily fish, suggests Michael Janson, M.D. Or in a supplement that includes lecithin or other fats.

If you're already taking medications for your heart, be aware that statin drugs have a side effect that's rarely discussed. They lower your body's levels of CoQ_{10} —the nutrient your heart needs the most! Be sure to take CoQ_{10} if you're on statins. (For more information on this subject, see Chapter 39.)

SECRET #394 Hawthorn is the number one herb to consider for your heart.

Hawthorn (*Crataegus oxyacantha*) is the first herb I think of for heart conditions.

It is a hedge that contains powerful antioxidants in its leaves and flowers. This herb supports your heart by reducing inflammation and acting as a heart tonic.

The New York Heart Association has been running several trials using hawthorn with people who have congestive heart failure. Some of the symptoms of this disease include weakness, breathlessness, and swollen legs. Each trial was two months long and used different amounts of hawthorn extract containing 2.2% flavonoids. Each trial showed that hawthorn worked.

There were small improvements in heart function, the ability to exercise, and general well-being in participants who took 300 mg of hawthorn. But the improvements were significantly improved in the trials where participants took twice this amount. When people took 900 mg of hawthorn a day (300 mg, three times daily) their results were as good as for people who used pharmaceutical drugs like Captopril. The largest trial using 900 mg of hawthorn showed a reduction of symptoms by 66 percent.

Before taking hawthorn, talk with your physician, especially if you're taking digoxin—a cardiac drug that has a narrow safety margin. Hawthorn is safe for long-term use, but never self-medicate when you have a serious condition. And always tell your doctor about the herbs you're taking in case there are interactions you're not aware of. When treating a condition as serious as angina or heart disease with alternative and/or complementary medicine, it's always a good idea to work closely with a naturopathic doctor, or other healthcare professional who is knowledgeable about alternative treatments and can track your progress with the appropriate tests.

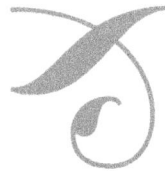

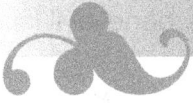

PART 9

NEW BREAKTHROUGHS to PREVENT and FIGHT CANCER

We're losing the battle for cancer in spite of all the surgeries, chemotherapy, diets, herbs, and supplements. Whether it's due to increased environmental pollutants or other factors, we need to look beyond known therapies. At the same time, we have to be cautious and not jump into any program that just sounds good or that happened to work for someone else.

Each of us is different, and there are many forms of cancers with different causes. We get positive results when we can match our needs to the right therapy. As you know, this isn't an easy task. Oncologists (cancer doctors) look at traditional medical approaches. The doctors of integrative medicine I know call their approach "slash and burn" because they either perform surgery or use chemotherapy drugs. Or both. I don't mean to suggest that surgery and chemotherapy don't have their place. They do. But without the right nutrients to help detoxify and support your body while you use traditional therapies, even the most appropriate program can fail.

There are new therapies you may not know about. They've been tested in scientific studies and found to be beneficial in many cases. They're also affordable and available. I'll tell you about some of them, as well as explain why breast thermography is one of the most exciting diagnostic techniques available. It can identify precancerous conditions years before a tumor forms. As you know, it's much easier to prevent a problem than to correct it.

I've found cancer salves that can be used to remove skin cancers, and an impressive substance that keeps cancer cells from clustering and forming tumors. But before I talk about them, let's explore ways to guard against cancer.

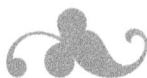

CHAPTER 45

Simple Steps to Guard Against Cancer

The most dramatic breakthroughs in cancer came over the last decade—and practically no one noticed!

Why? Because these breakthroughs had nothing to do with chemotherapy, surgery, or any other high-tech cures. Rather, these breakthroughs were all about prevention.

Yes, prevention. It is estimated that up to 90 percent of all cancers can be prevented—using knowledge that is already available!

While these breakthroughs are available, you still may not know about them. Or their importance in preventing cancer. I've found that the two most important steps you can take to protect yourself to prevent cancer are to limit your exposure to cancer-promoting substances and to increase your antioxidant intake with food and supplements.

SECRET #395 Limit your exposure to these dietary carcinogens.

Sounds obvious and simple, but it's not. Substances that promote cancer are everywhere. From heavy metals like mercury and lead to pesticides in fish, food dyes, and hormones, there's no way to escape cancer-promoting substances. You can, however, limit your exposure both by eating more organic foods and limiting your intake of processed foods. Make lifestyle and diet changes that include avoiding cigarettes and synthetic estrogens. Drink alcohol only in moderation—one or two glasses of wine a day—if at all.

Don't eat trans fats. Trans fats, like margarine and other solid man-made shortenings, have been linked to breast cancer. The recent government diet guideline, the *Dietary Guidelines for Americans* 2005, advises we limit our trans fats. That's misleading. No amount is safe. Trans fats are prevalant in many crackers, cookies, and snack foods. They don't have to be. Take the ever-popular Oreo Cookie by Kraft Foods as one example. Oreos contain trans fats; yet the organic alternative by Newman's Own called Newman-O's don't. It's obvious that the same products can be made with safer fats than trans fats. Kraft Foods has another solution to the trans fats problem. They've decided to change the focus of their Oreo ads and not target children. This is easier than changing the ingredients, but no safer.

Red food dyes have been linked to cancer. Read labels to see where they're hidden. You'll find them in candies and processed foods. You certainly don't need them or other foods with artificial coloring.

Avoid deep-fried foods. This is extremely important. Foods that have been commercially deep-fried like donuts and French fries have been fried in rancid oils. Once you reheat an oil, or it reaches a high temperature, it becomes rancid and carcinogenic. This is a good reason to not reheat oils at home. My mother used to save bacon grease and use it to fry potatoes or other foods. They tasted good, but they were filled with carcinogens.

Pan-frying damages all oils, although olive oil, macadamia nut oil, and coconut oil are more stable at higher temperatures than other oils. Use any of these oils with a medium flame, not a high one, to sauté your vegetables. Damaged oils are filled with harmful free radicals.

SECRET #396 Some free radicals are made by cancer cells; antioxidants stop them.

A tremendous amount of evidence suggests that damage by free radicals is, in part, responsible for the development of cancer, as well as other chronic diseases such as heart disease and diseases associated with aging. Researchers think that cancer cells may generate a surplus of oxidants, which then send signals that promote uncontrolled cell growth. Antioxidant nutrients may block these signals.

Oxygen-free radicals or oxidants are highly unstable molecules that can damage cell membranes and scramble the genetic information (DNA) in cells. This damage can start a chain reaction that could lead to cancer. They are produced in the body during normal cell metabolism, from tissue injury, and also as a result of exposure to tobacco smoke, sunlight, x-rays, and other environmental sources.

Vitamins A, beta-carotene, C, and E, and the mineral selenium function as antioxidants, agents with the ability to deactivate these free radicals. Other substances in foods also have antioxidant activity, and the body produces its own antioxidants. But for a good cancer-preventing diet, you'll want to eat plenty of fresh fruits and vegetables, and add supplemental antioxidants to your program.

SECRET #397 When you eat more foods high in antioxidants, you eat fewer foods that promote cancer.

From time to time, we hear about a study that says fruits and vegetables have no effect on preventing cancer. This is nonsense. We have plenty of good studies that found antioxidants offer powerful protection, and fruits and vegetables are packed with antioxidants. A research review conducted by the World Cancer Research Fund and the American Institute for Cancer Research reports that, "eating 5 to 10 servings of fruits and vegetables per day is one of the easiest things you can do to prevent cancer."

This review estimated that "diets high in vegetables and fruits (more than 14 ounces a day) could prevent at least 20 percent of all cancer incidence." Another review of the benefits of plant-based foods in the *European Journal of Cancer* concludes that in seventeen studies, women who consumed the most vegetables faced a 25 percent lower risk of breast cancer than those who ate the least.

Antioxidants stop the biochemical changes that cause cancer in their tracks. Also, their fiber is filling, so if you eat plenty of fresh produce you won't have room for a lot of junk foods. Unfortunately, the typical American diet is low in fruits and vegetables, and is thus low in antioxidants. It's also high in refined sugar and saturated fats—foods that promote cancer. It's no coincidence that the Standard American Diet is referred to as the SAD Diet. Truly, it's both disease promoting and a sad commentary on our lifestyle.

It's easy to eat the suggested 5–10 servings of fresh produce a day that these studies suggest. One serving is just one cup. This means that a salad entree could easily provide four to six servings at one meal. A side salad is around two cups.

An article in the *Journal of the National Cancer Institute* also reported that breast-cancer risk was cut in half for premenopausal women who ate the highest amounts of vegetables. Fruits did not reduce their risk. No single dietary factor explained why breast-cancer risks decreased so much when women ate more veggies. Perhaps it was the high sugar content of fruits that cancelled out the beneficial antioxidants.

Vegetables high in beta-carotene and vitamin C seem to offer some of the best protection, but vegetables contain thousands of natural phytochemicals that work in many different ways to combat cancer. One such group of chemicals, called indoles, is found in cruciferous vegetables like broccoli and cauliflower. The indoles seem to boost enzymes that make estrogen less effective at promoting breast cancer. In fact, the National Cancer Institute is studying indole-3-carbinol, the active ingredient in broccoli and other cruciferous vegetables, as a cancer-preventing nutrient. Here are some of your best choices for a cancer-prevention diet:

- Cabbage-family vegetables (cabbage, broccoli, cauliflower, kale, brussels sprouts, bok choy, and napa cabbage)
- Dried beans and legumes (rich in lignans and fiber)
- Tomatoes
- Citrus fruits

- Deep yellow-orange vegetables and fruits (sweet potatoes, yams, carrots, squash, apricots)

- Blueberries and cherries

- Dried fruits (prunes, raisins, etc.)

SECRET #398 Free radicals are beneficial if you don't have too many of them.

In spite of all the bad press they get, free radicals aren't all bad. Nature put them in our bodies for a good reason. They fight disease by helping white cells destroy bacteria and other foreign invaders. Problems occur when the production of free radicals overwhelms your body's ability to contain them. As with most things, balance is the key, and it is generally believed that a proper balance between free radicals and antioxidants is essential to good health. That's why the body's anti-oxidants try to gobble up excessive amounts of free radicals before they can cause damage.

SECRET #399 Antioxidants in your supplements are not enough.

Observational studies suggest that foods high in vitamin E, beta-carotene, and vita-min C provide strong preventive effects against a wide range of cancers. The few studies that have been conducted using single nutrients in supplement form have not shown the same across-the-board benefit. Some of these studies concluded that single antioxidants may have promoted disease. These studies were seriously flawed and misinterpreted. Other studies have shown protective effects against spe-cific cancers. It may be that a combination of nutrients—as found in natural dietary sources like fruits and vegetables—provides the greatest benefit. I wouldn't de-pend on getting all my antioxidants from food, however. Here are some supple-ments with science to back their effectiveness in preventing cancer.

Of the nutrients in supplement form, vitamin E, selenium, and multivitamin/min-eral formulations appear to be the most effective cancer preventives. Other vitamins and minerals believed to possess some degree of cancer-preventive effects include folate, vitamin D, calcium, and molybdenum.

SECRET #400 Vitamin E protects against many cancers, but especially those along the digestive tract.

Vitamin E (tocopherol), a potent fat-soluble antioxidant, shows strong cancer-pre-ventive evidence among supplemental nutrients. Scientists think vitamin E may defend cell membranes and DNA against damage caused by oxygen-free radicals.

Vitamin E also appears to bolster the immune system, which may play a significant role in cancer prevention. But this vitamin does its best work when it's combined with other nutrients. Vitamin E, vitamin C, beta-carotene, and selenium appear to work as a team.

Vitamin E in supplement form appears to significantly lower the risk of prostate cancer, as well as to protect against cancers of the colon, mouth, and throat. Consumption of vitamin-E rich foods is associated with a lower risk for cancers of the colon, stomach, mouth, throat, esophagus (food tube), liver, and breast (hereditary).

Another supplement study found supplemental vitamin E even more effective. Researchers at the Fred Hutchinson Cancer Research Center in Seattle determined that supplemental vitamin E (200 IU or more daily) cut colon cancer risk by 57 percent compared to those not taking vitamins. Interestingly, a daily multivitamin supplement lowered the risk by almost as much—51 percent The risk was also lowered in people taking supplements of vitamins A, C, folate, and calcium, but not as much. An analysis of the Iowa Women's Health Study Cohort found that foods high in vitamin E significantly reduced the risk of colon cancer in women under age sixty-five.

This effort was part of a larger study of breast cancer funded by the National Cancer Institute. The study of 35,215 women ages fifty-five to sixty-nine found that those with the highest dietary intake of vitamin E had the greatest protection. However, this protective effect was marginal for women over age sixty-five. Results broke down like this: Women ages fifty-five to fifty-nine showed the greatest benefit—an 84 percent lower risk; women ages sixty to sixty-four had a 63 percent lower risk; and women ages sixty-five to sixty-nine had a 7 percent lower risk. Women under age fifty-five were not studied. *Suggestion:* Take 400 IU of vitamin E a day.

SECRET #401 This mineral lowers different cancers in supplements than in food. You need both sources.

Selenium is a trace mineral that functions chiefly as a component of glutathione peroxidase, an antioxidant enzyme that works with vitamin E to help protect cell membranes from free-radical damage. Although most people get enough selenium from their diet, the soil in some areas of the country are low in this mineral.

Evidence suggests that selenium supplements may protect against some forms of cancer. Selenium in supplement form has been associated with a lower risk of cancers of the prostate, colon, and lung, as well as with a substantial reduction in cancer deaths. Dietary sources of selenium are associated with a lower risk for cancers of the esophagus and stomach.

After reviewing the cancer research on selenium, the Food and Nutrition Board's Committee on Diet and Health stated that "Low selenium intakes or decreased selenium concentrations in the blood are associated with increased risk of cancer in humans." The National Research Council said, "A large accumulation of evidence indicates that supplementation of the diet or drinking water with selenium protects against tumors induced by a wide variety of chemical carcinogens."

Selenium shows promise in preventing prostate, lung, colon, and rectal cancers. In a large intervention trial, people who took supplemental selenium had a 37 percent decrease in prostate, colorectal, and lung cancers as well as a 50 percent reduction in cancer deaths. That was the unexpected discovery of this ten-year trial on prevention of skin cancer, as reported in the *Journal of the American Medical Association*. As an intervention trial, this study carries more weight than uncontrolled observational trials.

The study was originally designed to see if selenium supplementation could lower the recurrence of basal cell and squamous cell cancers, the most common skin cancers, as two smaller studies had suggested. But researchers were pleased with the unexpected good tidings of a significant reduction in total cancer mortality. Subjects took 200 micrograms (mcg) tablets of selenium daily as brewer's yeast or a placebo. No cases of selenium toxicity occurred. The news of a reduction of cancer deaths was so good that the blinded phase of the trial, was stopped early to allow all participants to take selenium. *Suggestion:* Take 200 mcg of selenium a day.

SECRET #402 Beta-carotene may be bad for people who smoke, but it's not been found to be harmful to anyone else.

Beta-carotene, a carotenoid that serves as a "provitamin" or precursor of vitamin A, has gotten a lot of bad press. Bad enough to frighten some people off. This is unfortunate, because both beta-carotene and vitamin A are beneficial in protecting against cancer.

A Finnish study of male smokers found that beta-carotene increased the incidents of lung cancer and led to a higher death rate than in smokers who didn't take the supplement. What wasn't explained was that the men who had the most adverse effects drank one alcoholic drink a day in addition to smoking. This variable could explain the negative outcome. Also, the public panicked and never read the rest of the study. You see, when smokers took both beta-carotene and vitamin E there was no increased lung cancer or death. In fact, the incidents of prostate cancer dropped in supplemented men. Partial information can be dangerous.

Another study with women smokers who taook both beta-carotene and vitamin E found similar results. But other research with participants who didn't smoke and never smoked showed no increased incidence of lung cancer or death from other causes.

SECRET #403 Beta-carotene has been shown to prevent cancer.

Much of our intake of beta-carotene comes from eating plant foods, and our bodies convert about one-sixth of dietary beta-carotene to vitamin A. Beta-carotene is one of the pigments that gives vegetables like carrots and sweet potatoes their deep orange color. Beta-carotene in foods is completely safe. In fact, beta-carotene and other carotenoids function as antioxidants to neutralize free radicals and prevent the tissue damage they cause. Their antioxidant activity may counter the cell and DNA damage that leads to initiation of the cancer process. In addition, carotenoids promote enzymes that inhibit carcinogens and enhance white blood cell function.

In the early 1980s, a review of the epidemiological (population) studies clearly showed that people who ate diets of fruits and vegetables high in beta-carotene had significant protection against cancer. The risk for several cancers was lowered, including lung cancer by as much as 70 percent, as well as cancers of the stomach, esophagus, lung, oral cavity and pharynx (throat), endometrium, pancreas, and colon. Additionally, beta-carotene in supplement form appeared to substantially lower cancer risk in animal studies. *Suggestion:* Instead of taking beta-carotene supplements, take supplements containing 10,000 mg of mixed carotenoids. Mixed carotenoids contain a balance of pro-vitamin A substances that are more like those found in foods. You could also take vitamin A itself. Either will give you the benefits of beta-carotene.

SECRET #404 This antioxidant stops cancer-causing substances found in common foods.

Vitamin C (ascorbic acid) helps counter harmful effects of environmental contaminants and toxic chemicals, and inhibits the formation of cancer-causing nitrosamine compounds. Nitrosamines are formed in the stomach after we eat nitrates and nitrites. These chemicals are used in the curing of meats such as bacon, hot dogs, and ham. They're also a preservative in processed luncheon meats. If you've been eating any of these foods, it's time to stop. They don't belong in a cancer-preventive diet. Still, it's good to know that vitamin C can help counteract some of the effects of these toxins. These actions have led researchers to examine whether the evidence is better for foods containing vitamin C than for vitamin C supplements.

Studies suggest that consuming foods high in vitamin C has a preventive effect against several cancers. These include cancers of the stomach, bladder, breast, cervix, colon and rectum, salivary gland, esophagus, larynx, pancreas, prostate, and lung, as well as cancers of the blood and bone marrow, and lymph system.

SECRET #405 Vitamin C supplementation has strong anti-cancer effects.

Nearly 100 studies have found vitamin C protects against pancreatic, stomach, esophageal, cervical, breast, lung, and colon cancers. In one study, more than 11,000 men and women in a retirement community who never had cancer were given vitamin C supplements. Over an eight-year period, those who took the most vitamin C had the least amount of bladder and colon cancer. But what's best, foods or supplements? And if supplements, should you take vitamin C by itself or with other antioxidants? The answer appears to be both.

A combination of supplemental vitamin C and vitamin E appears to help protect against sunburn, which may indirectly prevent future skin cancer. In fact, vitamin C complements the action of vitamin E, and research suggests that a combination of antioxidants has an enhanced effect. Vitamin C is a water-soluble vitamin. You'll have more of it in your bloodstream if you take it throughout the day. Include fresh fruits and vegetables, and take a multivitamin supplement. Doses that have given positive results range from 200 to 1,000 mg taken four times a day. *Suggestion:* Take 500–1,000 mg from two to four times a day.

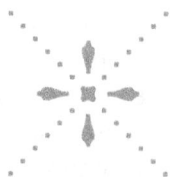

CHAPTER 46

The Newest Breakthrough in Detecting and Preventing Breast Cancer

If there was a way to find and remove cancers in the breast that are so tiny they don't even appear on a mammogram, more lives would be saved. If it were possible to detect cells that are just starting to become malignant and remove them before a tumor formed, even more lives would be saved. The good news is this is now possible. The bad news is, although women are relying on mammograms, they are often not enough.

Mammograms have their limitations when breasts are dense, when women are nursing, and when women are on hormone replacement therapy (HRT). If you have breast implants, mammograms may not be accurate.

I'm not saying that mammograms don't save lives. They do. But even though more women than ever before are having mammograms, deaths from breast cancer haven't decreased over the past forty years. Mammograms are finding cancers that breast examinations may miss, but they're not finding minute cancers or precancerous conditions.

We need a better system of early detection without the risks associated with mammograms. Fortunately, there's an excellent diagnostic tool that fits the bill. When it's combined with mammography, I believe it will save thousands of women's lives. It's called infrared imaging, or breast thermography.

Until recently, mammograms have been the best option to screen for breast cancer. All of us know some of its shortcomings: having our breasts squeezed so hard that cancer cells can spread, and being exposed to "just a little" radiation. Now there is an option for those women who refuse to have mammograms, or who can't have them because of their lifetime exposure to radiation. For the rest of the population, breast thermography is mammography's best partner.

SECRET #406 How mammograms contribute to breast cancer in some women.

Mary Helen Barcellos-Hoff, a cell biologist at the Lawrence Berkeley National Laboratory (Berkeley Lab), has found an association between low-level radiation and breast cancer. Berkeley Lab is a U.S. Department of Energy National Laboratory located in Berkeley, California. It conducts unclassified scientific research and is managed by the University of California.

Barcellos-Hoff and her research team noticed that exposure to radiation can cause breast cancer by damaging tissues that surround a breast cell. This surrounding tissue normally keeps cells from becoming cancerous. But when they're damaged, they have the opposite effect. When breasts are exposed to low doses of radiation, like from the small amount used in mammograms, tissues send out signals that can keep cancers from forming. But with greater exposure—like with multiple mammograms—the wrong signals get transmitted, and cancer can result.

Not all women have the same sensitivity to radiation. While many women may get mammograms, dental x-rays, and CT (computed tomography) scans that increase their exposure to radiation with no ill effects, others could end up with breast cancer. The decision to have mammograms is a personal one that you should make by evaluating your own risks. While mammography is now big business, studies are currently concluding that it doesn't save as many lives as we're being told. In my opinion, thermography offers a safer method of evaluating breast tissue for abnormalities way before cancer begins—in time to change the inner environment and prevent breast cancer.

SECRET #407 These three limitations of mammograms have sent women shopping for alternatives.

If you're sixty years old or older, your body has at least one type of dormant cancer. These cancer cells are harmless as long as they remain inactive. For the past twenty-five years, I've said that mammograms are not as safe as they are purported to be. Here are three reasons why. Any one of them is responsible for some women opting for other screening methods.

1. Mammography squeezes the breast so hard that encapsulated cancer cells occasionally rupture, causing the dormant cancer to become active and grow.

2. Mammograms are limited in what they can find. They can find tumors, not cancer cells, tiny tumors, or precancerous tissues. Physiological changes occur before a tumor is formed that can indicate malignancy is imminent, but mammography doesn't detect them. Preventing a disease is much more effective—and easier—than curing it or putting it into remission.

3. Mammograms "read" the breast via radiation. A high lifetime exposure to radiation is a known risk factor for cancer. Although modern mammogram machines emit much lower amounts of radiation than ever before, if you have regular mammograms and dental x-rays, your exposure to radiation increases every year. Add to this any chest x-rays to rule out pneumonia, and your lifelong accumulation of radiation increases.

Dr. John Gofman is a physician as well as a doctor of nuclear and physical medicine. In his book *X-Rays: Health Effects of Common Exams,* he explains that each mammogram increases your risk of breast cancer more than the last. Over the years, most of us have had yearly dental x-rays. When we fly in planes, we're exposed to environmental x-rays. If you've ever sprained or broken a bone, you've been x-rayed. Some of you may remember the little machines in shoe stores when we were children that showed the bones of our feet. I loved playing with them and did so as often as I could. These were x-rays, also. High amounts of radiation, in fact. Fortunately, not all breast diagnostic tools use radiation. Thermography uses a camera that detects heat.

SECRET #408 Thermography detects angiogenesis— a sign that cancer cells may be starting to form tumors.

The concept behind thermography is simple and sensible. Thermography, which is actually infrared imaging, works by identifying and measuring changes in heat in the body. These heat patterns are then translated into images. When the breast is cool, the amount of blood that flows into it is reduced.

Even before cells become malignant, the tissues surrounding precancerous cells and the area around breast cancers open up existing blood vessels and produce new ones. This is called angiogenesis. These extra blood vessels, and blood vessels with increased capacity, are needed to carry nutrients into hungry cancer cells. The new blood vessels, and the increased blood flow through them, create minute quantities of heat. Thermography can detect these slight variations in temperature, finding breast cancers and precancerous tissues long before they can be detected through mammography. It does this without compressing the breasts, without radiation, and without any other risks. A thermogram can detect mastitis (an inflammation in the breast), fibrocystic breasts, or benign tumors as well as cancer or precancerous tissues.

Today, thermography uses very sensitive infrared cameras along with state-of-the-art computers that produce high-resolution pictures of these variations in temperature. If thermography is performed with good-quality equipment, using strict protocols, and is read by board-certified doctors with experience in breast imaging, the results are excellent.

If you are monitoring your breast health, as you should, especially if you have a family history of breast cancer, in my opinion, the safest test you can get every year is a thermogram. If the results show any abnormality, you can get a mammogram to rule out breast cancer. Studies show thermography can indicate a cancer may be forming up to twelve years before any other test can detect any problem. It gives you early warnings long before a tumor forms. If you get an abnormal reading and no tumor is present, you can monitor that area carefully with breast self-exams, doctor's exams, and follow-up thermograms to catch any progressive changes. Meanwhile, you can take positive actions to improve your breast health by making changes in your diet and lifestyle to minimize any future problems.

SECRET #409 The combination of mammography and thermography is best.

When you combine mammography with thermography you get the very best, most accurate information in detecting the earliest cancers. Together, these diagnostic tools provide the widest possible coverage in cancer detection. Here's why. Mammography examines the anatomy. It looks at shadows on film for cellular change—like tumors—and pinpoints exactly where the problem is located. Thermography examines the physiology (cellular and chemical changes), like heat from blood vessels, the recruitment of blood vessels, and metabolic changes that occur before a mass grows and when a mass is present.

Thermography is excellent in finding precancerous conditions, but it isn't as accurate in locating some of the slow-growing tumors or those few tumors that don't have increased blood vessel activity. It also can't tell doctors exactly where the problem is located. Mammography locates some of these slow-growing tumors that thermography misses and can tell doctors just where any masses are located. But it can't identify precancerous conditions. Together, these two diagnostic tools locate 95 percent of troublesome changes in breast tissue.

SECRET #410 Thermography may have saved my life.

I frequently feel protected by some unseen force that pushes me in the right direction. That's what happened when I was asked to research and write an article on the subject of breast thermography. I found an excellent center several hours away from where I lived, and was invited to tour the facility and experience a thermogram. When I accepted, I began a three-week journey that was both difficult and rewarding. It was a journey that may have saved my life.

On a sunny, crisp California day, I drove down to Redwood City to visit PCRC Infrared Imaging Center, run at that time by Drs. William Amalu and Robert Kane. I wanted to see firsthand how thermograms were done and report about what the procedure was like. Not all centers use state-of-the-art equipment with stringent protocols. And not all thermograms are interpreted by board-certified thermologists. This one was, which was why I chose to visit it.

I never liked being exposed to radiation or having my breasts mashed, so I am one of the thousands of women who has not had regular mammograms. I do not advocate this. I'm just being honest with you. Between eating a healthy diet, taking good-quality nutritional supplements, not taking estrogen, and using regular stress reduction techniques—combined with breast self-exams, I felt I was doing enough. But I decided to have a thermogram because it was non-invasive and could give me some good information about my breast health. I was astonished to find that my thermogram was abnormal. I was also grateful, since it may have saved my life. But before I tell you what I did to reverse this abnormality, let me share with you what it's like to get a thermogram.

SECRET #411 Thermography simply takes a picture of your breasts . . . in a cold room.

The protocol for thermograms is pretty much the same no matter where you get them. I began by completing a one-page history that would help evaluate my risk for breast cancer. It's generally accepted, although not known for certain, that lifetime exposure to estrogens puts a woman at the greatest risk factor for breast cancer. Although I haven't had any children, I considered myself to be at low risk. The only other risk I noted on my history form was that my maternal grandmother had breast cancer. My ninety-three-year-old mother had none, nor had any other blood relatives. My diet has been an anticancer diet for the past thirty years or more, and I manage my stress as it comes along, not allowing it to get out of hand. So I was convinced my results would be negative. After completing the history, I had my thermogram.

The most discomfort from getting a thermogram is being a little chilly. Because this technology is based on reading heat in the breast, you need to be acclimated in a very cool room—between 68 and 73°F—for about fifteen minutes before the pictures are taken. Otherwise, the images are not accurate.

Before my breast images were taken, I disrobed from the waist up and sat with my arms on the armrests of a chair. Then the thermography technician had me move from side to side to look for any visible signs of abnormalities. There were none. Next, I lay on my back for fifteen minutes with my hands behind my head so that the heat from my arms and hands would not interfere with the heat in my breasts. Actually, it seemed more like I waited for half an hour! At first, I was comfortable and warm enough since I was lying down and my back was warm. But by the time the technician came into the room, I was a little colder than I like to be.

The technician had me stand in front of a camera and took pictures of various views of my breasts that were captured on a computer monitor. The procedure felt completely comfortable, both physically and emotionally. It was different from getting an x-ray or getting a mammogram. Nothing potentially harmful was coming out of the camera. It was simply taking a picture of my breasts.

Occasionally, another procedure is added that enhances the detection of increased blood-vessel activity if the doctor interpreting the thermogram thinks it's indicated. It's called a cold challenge and it causes blood vessels to constrict, giving the thermogram reader a better view of blood-vessel activity. To give me the full-thermography experience, I submerged my hands in ice water. The idea is to keep your hands in the ice water for forty-five to sixty seconds, or as long as you can, to allow blood vessels to get smaller. I lasted just twenty seconds—long enough, I was told. After I removed my hands from the water, additional pictures of my breasts were taken.

SECRET #412 An abnormal thermogram can be caused by too much estrogen in your breasts, even if your total blood estrogen levels are low.

I was surprised to find that my thermogram showed increased heat in both breasts. Was this a precancerous condition? The doctor who read my images believed the heat that was present in my thermogram was due, at least in part, to excess estrogen and insufficient progesterone in my breasts. I was shocked. I had been postmenopausal for more than a decade, and the previous year I had extensive blood and urine tests to assay my hormone levels. Both estrogen and progesterone levels were low. Now I was told I had too much estrogen. What was happening?

There's a difference between blood levels and breast levels of estrogen. Blood levels show the amount of hormones circulating in your blood. But fatty breast tissues produce estrogen, and even if your blood levels are low, you may, like me, have too much estrogen in your breast tissues. My thermogram was a powerful warning sign to get a mammogram, see my doctor, and closely watch that area.

Since I hadn't had a mammogram for a number of years, Dr. Amalu suggested that I get one, and have a follow-up thermogram in three months. When anything out of the ordinary shows on a thermogram and more information is needed, a mammogram is usually the next step. It would give me a baseline for comparison and could rule out a problem or locate the precise place where a tumor exists. Remember, the combination of thermography and mammography is 95 percent accurate in locating early stage cancers.

I must admit that I was surprised to find from Dr. Amalu that I was not as low risk for breast cancer as I had assumed. My grandmother's breast cancer, my not having children, and my failure to use natural progesterone all put me at a higher risk for breast cancer than I had thought.

SECRET #413 The first step in dealing with any abnormality is to calm down.

Although I've been a healthcare practitioner for more than twenty-five years and have a tremendous amount of knowledge, I was frightened to hear that my thermogram showed any signs of abnormality at all. My emotions and my rational mind, which usually travel along parallel paths, suddenly diverged. My mind told me that there was a sign of increased blood-vessel activity that might eventually lead to breast cancer years down the road. I had time to get more information and take steps to change this condition. But my emotions and my imagination were getting the best of me.

So instead of worrying, I went to a movie to take my mind off my immediate concern. Next, I took some kava to reduce my anxiety. The following morning, I called my doctor. My doctor, osteopath Terri Turner, is one of the most compassionate and knowledgeable people I know. Together, we planned dietary and supplement changes. The most important step for me to take was to apply progesterone cream directly to my breasts.

Getting a warning sign, or any bad news, feels like an inner earthquake. At times I was able to work, at other times, my mind shifted to dozens of "what ifs." I decided not to talk about my thermogram to anyone who did not have a possible part of my solution. So I didn't tell many of my close friends or my family. What I didn't want to hear was "you'll be all right" until I knew that this, in fact, was true.

To handle my ever-changing emotions, I meditated more, took kava extract to take the edge off my anxiety, and asked friends who use prayer in their daily lives to pray for me. I worked when I could and took time off when I couldn't. I was gentle with myself.

My doctor, who is a woman, was concerned about my emotional state and addressed it. None of the three male doctors I spoke with during these first three weeks ever asked me how I was feeling about this news. I was surprised at this, because I know that they are all deeply caring men. I sounded fine, so in their minds, perhaps, I was. Fear of getting breast cancer is a deep one shared by just about every woman I have met. In addition to information, I wanted and needed compassion.

Once I had a plan I could follow, along with the assurance of my doctors that my condition was reversible, my mind and emotions were once again on the same track. I went on an expanded supplement program that was designed to turn off estrogen receptors and boost my immune system so my body could take a different path—one of healing itself. It worked for me, but everyone's situation is a little different. The best approach is to work with a naturopathic doctor or a physician who uses integrative medicine.

You may ask why I didn't design my nutritional program myself. I turned to my superb medical doctors to be my partners because I wasn't convinced I could see my whole picture as clearly as they could. And I wanted the benefit of their experiences.

SECRET #414 Lifestyle changes can reverse an abnormal thermogram.

My patterns showed I was at moderate risk for developing cancer in the future, so I immediately took action and reviewed my diet, supplements, and lifestyle. Five months later, my thermogram showed a great improvement. In this time, I changed from a "potentially dangerous" to "watchful" condition. I'd like to share with you what worked for me. There's no way to know what caused my improvements. But past studies indicated that it was most likely a combination of many or all of these.

SECRET #415 Consider progesterone cream for estrogen dominance in breast tissues.

Progesterone cream: I wasn't taking any hormones at all. While my blood estrogen level was low, my thermogram showed I had too much estrogen in my breast tissues. At the same time, I had no progesterone to keep it in check. Unopposed estrogen is a huge risk factor for breast cancer.

I began applying one-quarter to one-half teaspoon of natural progesterone cream directly to my breasts morning and evening. Some doctors say you can rub the cream into any sensitive tissues like the inside of the thighs or arms, but in researching the subject, I found that more progesterone is absorbed into breast tissues when it's applied to them directly, and that's where I wanted most of the progesterone to go.

Not all progesterone creams are alike. I found a progesterone cream called PureGest that wasn't greasy, had no added ingredients, and was quickly absorbed. (See the Resources section for information on where to buy this product.) If I had not used this product, I would have had my doctor order a pure progesterone cream from a natural compounding pharmacy.

SECRET #416 Stress can contribute to breast cancer.

Stress and exercise: Stress causes your adrenal glands to make more cortisol, a hormone originally produced only during emergencies. Exercise helps lower cortisol levels. Unfortunately, many of us react to daily emergencies, causing too much cortisol to be produced. Excessive cortisol can lead to cancer by binding to proges-terone and blocking its utilization. Low progesterone and high estrogen is an envi-ronment that lends itself to breast cancer. This explains the link between stress, breast cancer, and lower-life expectancy.

It's important to not allow stress to "get" to you and cause anxiety. This just encourages your adrenal glands to keep pumping cortisol. I use meditation to help me relax and to bring down my anxiety. When I'm very anxious, I use a tincture of kava. After my initial thermogram, I relied heavily on both. Now I just meditate.

Exercise is an effective method for reducing cortisol. Unfortunately, I would rather read than move. But a long, healthy life is more important to me than my old, comfortable patterns. After my thermogram, I began walking five to six times a week. I also kayaked once or twice a week in good weather and used light hand weights every other day to tone and strengthen my arms. Breathing deeply while using weights is an effective way to lower stress and cortisol production.

A year after my thermogram, I took another giant step forward toward better health. I joined a gym. Not only did I join it, I go to it four to five times every sin-gle week. I exercise for at least an hour doing both cardiovascular exercises (tread-mill, bike, elliptical machine, etc.) and weight training. I can feel my stress melt away halfway through my cardiovascular exercises.

SECRET #417 Modifying your diet and supplements is key in reversing a positive thermogram.

Diet. My diet had been good, but it got better. I happen to be a vegetarian who eats some dairy and eggs, but I relied heavily on soy. In fact, I frequently ate soy prod-ucts two or three times every day. There's a controversy about soy, estrogen pro-duction, and how much soy is both safe and beneficial for postmenopausal women. In fact, a recent study found that the more soy foods a group of postmenopausal women ate, the lower their incidents of endometrial cancer. (For more on the latest research about soy, see Chapters 31 and 33.)

I think soy is very safe, but I still decided to lower my soy intake to once a day or less and eat more lentils, beans, and eggs. It was a more balanced diet, and bal-ance is always the best approach. I changed from adding soy protein powder to my cereal or breakfast smoothies to a rice protein powder. I still don't eat much dairy, but occasionally have a little goat cheese or non-fat yogurt.

I ate vegetables every day, but I had gotten lazy and ate fewer of them. Now I eat a good quantity of fresh, organic vegetables twice a day. This increases my fiber and antioxidant levels, lowering my risk for breast cancer.

Supplements: I don't believe I would have the same positive results from my thermograms without taking extra supplements. These are the ones I added to my basic nutrient schedule: an anti-inflammatory formula, calcium D-glucarate, indole 3-carbinol, folic acid, and medicinal mushrooms. Let me tell you why I chose each of them. You can find where to get them in the Resources section at the end of this book.

SECRET #418 Angiogenesis is an inflammatory process. You want a powerful anti-inflammatory supplement.

Anti-inflammatory: My thermogram pattern showed increased activity in blood vessels, which includes an inflammatory process. I found a formula that is more powerful than any I could locate in health-food stores. It's InflaThera from ProThera. I took one capsule twice a day. If you take a supplement like Zyflamend, available in health-food stores, you may want to increase the suggested dosage.

Calcium D-glucarate is a nutrient shown over a period of twenty years of studies to remove carcinogenic substances by increasing detoxification. I'll talk about it in more detail in Chapter 49. For now, know that this increased detoxification lasts for about five hours, so it's best to take calcium D-glucarate two or three times a day. I took 500 mg twice daily. I think this is one of the most helpful anticancer supplements available. You should be able to find it in most natural-food stores.

Indole 3-carbinol (I3C) is a nutrient from broccoli, cabbage, and other cruciferous vegetables that has been found to reduce breast cancer in numerous studies. I ate more broccoli, but I also took 200 mg twice a day of indole 3-carbinol. Just eating more cruciferous vegetables could be sufficient if you do this on a regular basis. But if you just eat them once or twice a week, I'd suggest taking a supplement until your thermogram is negative and remains so for six months. Lately, there have been some questions about the safety of I3C. It appears that another chemical in cruciferous vegetables, diindolylmethane (DIM), may be a better choice. Still, the safest form of each of these substances can be found in the vegetables themselves. Eat more broccoli, cabbage, and other cruciferous vegetables.

Folic acid is one of the B vitamins that seems to increase cell damage. This damage can lead to breast cancer. Because several large studies showed that taking supplemental folic acid is protective against breast cancer, my doctor suggested I take five grams a day. This is a very high (and safe) amount, not easily found in supplement form. However, Folazin, an oral rinse product made by ProThera, contains 5 grams in each capful. It's an inexpensive protection I chose to add.

Medicinal mushrooms support immunity, and cancer thrives in a poor immune system. I wouldn't be without mushrooms. I credit them with preventing colds and flu for the past five years. In the past, I was prone to catching colds that progressed to pneumonia from childhood. My favorite combination is MycoPhyto Complex.

See Chapter 3 for more complete information on medicinal mushrooms as well as this particular formula. I took two capsules of mushroom formula twice a day. By strengthening my immune system, I reduce my risk for all cancers. Other medicinal mushroom formulas should work, also. I prefer this one because the mushrooms are grown on immune-enhancing herbs. I get double protection with the herbs that are absorbed into the mushrooms, and from the mushrooms themselves.

SECRET #419 Use thermography to move beyond your fears and identify a potential problem before it develops into a disease.

Remember, the increased presence of blood vessels can be a sign that cancer is beginning to appear. Breast thermography can detect these abnormalities years before any tumor forms. Sometime, a slightly abnormal thermogram will resolve itself. An abnormal thermogram could be due to a mild infection or other temporary condition. A follow-up thermogram will let you know if this is the case. By using this sensitive diagnostic tool, you may be able to either prevent cancer or catch it before it would be visible through any other tests.

Thermography gave me an opportunity to learn more about my body and how to care for it. It helped me break through illusions and showed me that even though early signs of a problem bring up fears, they are less frightening than finding a more serious condition. We all have to face our changing health and look carefully at our options. We need to choose them based on the input from doctors and other health practitioners we trust. And in this process, hopefully, we will each see that your journey and mine are not so different. As we look at this connection, we can see and feel a tremendous amount of support and caring that is unique with women.

SECRET #420 Thermography is a valuable diagnostic tool for tracking the effectiveness of any breast cancer therapy.

What if you could know before having surgery whether or not the chemotherapy treatment for your breast cancer was working?

What if you could also monitor the effectiveness of complementary therapies like modified citrus pectin (MCP), calcium D-glucarate, or progesterone?

Well, John Keyserlingk, a medical doctor in Canada, completed a study showing that breast thermography can tell just how well chemotherapy is working. If it can follow the results of chemotherapy, thermography can be used to monitor other treatments as well. And if your treatment is working, surgery and additional medications may be totally unnecessary.

Dr. Keyserlingk is a surgical oncologist at the Ville Marie Medical Center in Canada. He wanted to know whether or not surgery was necessary for women with breast cancer who were on chemotherapy. He headed a team of M.D.s who selected a group of women with locally advanced breast cancer. These women would ordinarily be given chemotherapy before having their cancers removed surgically. Dr. Keyserlingk wanted to see if thermography could follow this treatment without the risks from radiation or other invasive monitoring tools.

He recruited twenty women with advanced breast cancer and took thermograms of their breasts before and after their chemotherapy treatments for three to six months. They then removed these women's breasts. I know. It was a pretty radical treatment. But the women consented, of course, and the results were so carefully monitored that we now know more about what thermography can do.

All of the women originally had abnormal readings in the area of their tumors and all of their tumors decreased by the end of the treatment. Thermograms indicated that four of them had no detectible cancer. But these breasts were removed, also. All of the breasts were then biopsied, and the results paralleled those seen on the thermograms. The women who showed no activity on their thermograms had no breast cancer. Those who had indications of an improvement had smaller tumors.

But the implications for using thermography as a monitoring tool goes way beyond chemotherapy. It could be effective in monitoring natural therapies, as well. In fact, breast thermography should be particularly effective in helping to determine how well any therapies that reduce angiogenesis are working. This way, if your treatment isn't working, your doctor can suggest another one.

SECRET #421 Finding a good thermography center may not be easy.

Now that I've shared my excitement with you about thermography, I have bad news. Thermography is not as widely available as mammography. What's even more disappointing is that insurance companies are not reimbursing for them yet. I still think it's worth the $175 to $225 charged for this test. But make sure you only go to a reputable center.

Not all places that do thermograms use accurate equipment and adhere to the strict protocols necessary to get the excellent results I've talked about. Most good clinics are on the west coast. But they're starting to appear in other parts of the country as well. Hopefully, if you think thermograms are as valuable as I do, you can tell your doctor you want this technology available to you.

If you have access to a computer, you can find clinics that meet the stringent qualifications for accurate breast thermography on the following website: www. breastthermography.com. If you do not have a computer, go to the Appendix for more information.

SECRET #422 Thermography can be extremely accurate . . . if you choose a reputable center.

Clearly, breast thermography is giving us more information than other more invasive techniques like mammograms and needle biopsies. Not only can it detect suspicious activity that may be . . . or may lead to . . . breast cancer, now we know it can also give us immediate feedback on whether or not a particular therapy is working.

THE BEST THERMOGRAPHY CENTERS HAVE THESE FEATURES:

- New cameras that produce excellent images.
- Computer software that allows images to be sent to more than one site so you can get a second opinion if you like.
- Images read by board-certified clinical thermologists.
- Reports that are signed by the thermologist who read the images, so you and your doctor know who to contact with any questions.
- Thermologists who are willing to talk with you.

Breast thermography is not new, but its technology and interpretations are light-years ahead of where they were only a handful of years ago. So if your doctor pooh-poohs it, tell him or her that you understand. Today's thermography isn't anything like it was in the past. Cameras are better and many of the people who interpret thermograms are highly trained. In Appendix A on page 370, you can find a list of thermography centers I've checked out and found to be reliable.

It's true that in the past some thermography equipment was substandard. And even now, some centers use older equipment. What's worse, some thermograms are read by people who lack the training necessary to write these reports.

If you decide to go to a lab that's not identified in Appendix A, be sure the following conditions are present:

- The temperature of the room is between 68 and 73°F.

- You have been acclimated for at least fifteen minutes after disrobing.

- There is no draft of cold air on your body.

- The background color on your thermogram is black. Any other color means the room is too warm.

- Your thermogram is read—and signed—only by a board-certified healthcare provider who is licensed to diagnose, trained in breast imaging, and certified by a legitimate organization, such as the International Academy of Clinical Thermology, International Thermographic Society, American Academy of Medical Infrared Imaging, or the American Academy of Thermology. If your analysis is not signed, do not accept it.

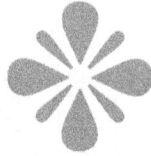

CHAPTER 47

When the Diagnosis Is Cancer—What to Do and What Not to Do

Once you've been diagnosed with cancer, everyone begins to tell you what you should do. Your doctors will suggest the therapies they know best. These may be best for you, or not. Friends will tell you about miracle cures they've seen or heard about. It's tempting to rush into whatever sounds the best and will end your panic. This is the opposite of what you should do.

None of us is exactly alike. Our genetic predispositions differ. You may have a gene that puts you at a higher risk for cancer that prevents a particular approach from working. Also, our immune systems differ. Yours may be strong and able to support a therapy that would overwhelm someone with suppressed immunity. As tempting as it may be to jump into the first therapy that seems to make sense, it's time to take stock first.

Cancer is big business. There are new chemotherapy drugs and more sophisticated surgical procedures. Nutritional supplement companies are making strong claims for products they say will reverse your condition. And alternative therapies bombard all of us with stories that suggest they truly have some answers. Don't make snap decisions. Take your time to look at your situation and talk it over with the doctor who will be your primary physician.

SECRET #423 As tempting as it may be, don't rush into any treatment.

A medical-doctor friend of mine who specializes in treating cancers and immune problems taught me this important lesson. It's one he passes on to each of his patients. He tells them not to rush into anything. There's usually enough time to evaluate their condition and start making some decisions. It's not a time to panic or rush into the first, or second, therapy that sounds good.

Occasionally, a cancer is aggressive. In this case, decisions need to be made quickly and treatment should begin immediately. That's rare. Usually, there's time to step back, take some deep breaths, and begin to do some research and better understand your specific condition.

SECRET #424 Learn what your lump means.

Just because you have a lump in your breast doesn't mean you have cancer. Here are some possibilities.

Pseudo lump: This is breast tissue approaching one inch in diameter that has formed into a lump, such as a pocket of dead fat or scar tissue that resulted from trauma caused by surgery or injury. It can also include pieces of silicone. Your lump may be the result of the deterioration of silicone breast implants, or from saline implants which are encapsulated in plastic.

Lumpiness: This condition consists of little lumps that are approximately an eighth of an inch in diameter. Some doctors still needlessly alarm patients by diagnosing general lumpiness as fibrocystic breast disease. In reality it is harmless, perfectly natural, and has not been linked to later development of breast cancer.

Cyst: These lumps are fluid-filled sacs that are most common in women between thirty and fifty-five. Cysts feel squishy near the surface. Those that are more deeply embedded in breast tissue feel harder because overlying tissue obscures the squishiness.

Fibroadenoma or fibroid: This is a lump ranging from approximately half an inch to two and a half inches or larger in diameter. A rare cancer, called cystosarcoma phyllodes, occurs in about 1 percent of all fibroadenoma lumps (usually the larger ones). This type of cancer is relatively harmless because it doesn't spread. You've got plenty of time to look at all of your options.

Cancer lump: By the time a cancerous lump is large enough for you to feel, it has usually grown to about half an inch in diameter. If a cancerous lump is much smaller, you won't feel it. This is because in the early stages, a lump of cancerous cells feels like normal tissue. Once this lump of cells has grown big enough for the body to react to it, scar tissue will form around it that makes it detectable by touch. In this way, a cancer lump can appear suddenly. It will not change with menstrual cycles and is rarely painful.

Unless the type of cancer you have is extremely aggressive, you still have time to get more information and examine your options.

SECRET #425 Get the best research available for your condition.

There's a lot of money to be made in cancer therapies. Some have studies to back up their effectiveness. Place a lot of weight on these. Some have good track records—excellent doctors with real data of remissions, or beating the odds in length of survival and quality of life. Give them some serious consideration. Others, on the other hand, are just ways to get you to trade your money for hope and base their information on testimonials. I would discount these until they can back the testimonials with studies.

To complicate matters, cancer therapy is a highly individual issue. Not all cancers are alike. And people differ tremendously in their biochemical makeup. This makes it easy to get confused when you hear about the results others have gotten with various treatments. Just because something worked for someone else doesn't mean it will work for you.

Fortunately, there are people who do nothing but research different types of cancers, talk with scientists and doctors around the world, and prepare reports on your specific kind of cancer. These reports range from twenty to forty pages, are packed with information and suggestions, and can help take a lot of the guesswork out of selecting a course of treatment.

SECRET #426 The Moss Report is one of the best sources of effective cancer treatments you'll find.

Ralph Moss, Ph.D., one of the most highly regarded cancer treatment researchers, writes the *Moss Report* and numerous books on alternative cancer therapies. He is the first American to become an honorary member of Germany's Society of Oncology and is on the National Institutes of Health Cancer Advisory Panel. Dr. Moss worked in the public affairs department of Memorial Sloan-Kettering's cancer hospital, and was fired after he refused to cover up research data on the benefits of laetrile. This man is one smart cookie. He's constantly following up on new research and updating his database and reports.

For $297, Ralph Moss sends you a lengthy report on treatments for your specific diagnosis. He updates his reports whenever new information is available, and includes scientific studies that back them up. The fee includes follow-up sessions with Dr. Moss' assistant, Anne Beattie, who speaks daily with Moss and gives out his replies to your questions or concerns. How long can you use this service without paying anything more? Indefinitely, says Beattie, who encourages people to ask questions and understand their condition and options.

SECRET #427 CANHELP can also help you get a different view of your condition and options.

Another highly respected cancer treatment report comes from the late cancer researcher Patrick McGrady, Jr., who initiated a service called CANHELP out of Port Ludlow, Washington. An expert staff, headed by Madeleen Herreshoff, has taken over this service. This report isn't cheap; it costs $350–450 depending on how quickly you need it. Opt for the less expensive price. You'll get the same report in seven to ten business days rather than in two to three. This fee includes one year's worth of personalized phone consultations. You get a lot of personal attention and information for your money.

With a CANHELP report, you're paying for expert recommendations and evaluation, not just a listing of people throughout the world who deal with your kind of cancer. Your report is tailored to your diagnosis, age, history, stage of cancer, and any complicating factors. It also will give you information on fad cures and scams that can cost you a lot of money and precious time.

I looked at reports from Ralph Moss and CANHELP on the subject of ovarian cancer. Each report had different information that was valuable. Both reports are skewed toward alternative therapies that are frequently not covered by health insurance policies. But then, many effective treatments aren't covered by insurance.

Still, it's often preferable to pay out-of-pocket for the therapy of your choice, especially if it looks like it will be your most effective choice. Insurance coverage can still be valuable for what it does cover, especially expensive diagnostic tests. Many individuals choose complementary courses of treatment—those that combine alternative and traditional therapies—in which case traditional therapies are covered by insurance and alternative therapies usually aren't.

SECRET #428 Here are some of the best books on cancer therapies.

Nothing beats personal attention in the area of alternative cancer therapies. Still, numerous books on the subject also have a lot to offer.

Perhaps the most important book for every cancer patient to read is *Questioning Chemotherapy* by Ralph Moss. This book gives a lot of information on specific chemotherapy agents and which ones might be appropriate for you to consider. It also serves as an excellent companion to your doctor's suggestions and brings you face to face with the hard reality that in many (but not all) cases chemotherapy simply doesn't work. This is especially true with advanced cancers. Dr. John Cairns of the Harvard University School of Public Health has said that only about 5 percent of cancer patients are helped by chemotherapy. Perhaps this is because the toxic substances used to destroy cancer also destroy the immune system.

Herbs, however, can both destroy cancer cells and support the immune system and Moss has a second book on this topic. *Herbs Against Cancer* gives you an easily understood overview of numerous herbs from around the world used in cancer treatment, including Essiac tea, the Hoxey formula, and Hulda Clark's protocol. Instead of running off and trying every herbal therapy you hear about, you may want to take a look at this book first for guidance.

A final cancer therapy essential is good nutrition. If you need help in putting together tasty, nutritious meals, you may want the *Cancer Survivor's Nutrition & Health Guide* by Gene Spiller, Ph.D., and Bonnie Bruce, R.D. In addition to giving plenty of easy-to-prepare recipes, this book contains valuable information on what to do if you have difficulty swallowing or chewing, if you lose weight, or if foods don't have much taste.

Whatever your method is, take the time to find your own way and make your best decisions.

Most important, find a health practitioner who's experienced in working with cancer patients, and who'll assist you in decision making (including making time to discuss issues of concern to you), and then monitor your program and your progress. Don't skip around and try everything you hear about. You won't always know what's working. Stick with one or two treatments over a longer period of time to get results. Choose therapies that have good science behind them. Some don't.

SECRET #429 The Zapper is a cancer therapy that lacks solid research studies and seems to be based on a false premise.

Naturopath Hulda Clark, author of *The Cure for All Cancers,* speaks with authority about how all people with cancer have a liver fluke parasite called *Fasciolopsis buskii (F. buskii).* She claims that propyl alcohol, a substance used in cosmetics, hair sprays, rubbing alcohol, decaffeinated coffee, white sugar, and other products, renders the body's immune system helpless against destroying these flukes. This has caused thousands of people to avoid contact with propyl alcohol, and to buy Clark's Zapper, a machine that allegedly destroys these parasites. The deluxe model of this unproven device with no science behind it will set you back $169 or more.

When the Centers for Disease Control (CDC) looked for parasites in stool samples of more than 200,000 people, only one had *F. buskii.* Clark claims that everyone who has cancer or is about to get cancer, and most who have had it in the past, has this parasite. Statistics don't prove her right.

SECRET #430 Sharks don't get cancer because sharks and humans are different.

Some years ago, a book called *Sharks Don't Get Cancer* appeared in bookstores. The premise was that shark cartilage prevented them from getting any cancers. But a 1997 study sponsored by the company that manufactures shark cartilage and published by the American Society of Clinical Oncology showed there was no anti-cancer activity in the product. Shark cartilage may prevent cancer in sharks, but it doesn't seem to have the same effect on humans.

Judah Folkman, M.D., of Harvard is a researcher who experimented with shark cartilage. He used more than one ton of shark cartilage to get a few millionths of a gram of the protein that supposedly has anticancer properties. He found the protein was too large to get into the bloodstream. There are no good clinical trials with shark cartilage, according to Folkman, and no reason, other than hearsay, to spend money on it.

SECRET #431 Cancer needs sugar, not oxygen, to thrive.

When there's not enough oxygen in your blood, the stage is set for cancer to develop.

Normal cells need oxygen. Cancer cells do not. They need sugar more than oxygen to thrive. In fact, cancer only flourishes in the *absence* of oxygen. This means if you introduce plenty of oxygen into the cells, you will reverse the growth of the cancer by suffocating the tumor. Dr. Otto Warburg, two-time Nobel Laureate said, "the primary cause of cancer is the replacement of normal oxygen respiration of body cells by anaerobic cell respiration." (Anaerobic means without oxygen.) Dr. Warburg received the Nobel prize in 1931 for his work on anaerobic cancer metabolism. He was the first to spell out the nature of how cancer cells thrive and spread, not in an oxygenated state but instead by fermentation of sugars.

The wholesale destruction of our forests, especially the rain forests, have decreased the level of oxygen in our atmosphere from 38 percent to below 20 percent! Our bodies are not designed for low-level oxygen consumptions. "All normal cells have an absolute requirement for oxygen, but cancer cells can live without oxygen—a rule without exception," says Dr. Warburg, "Deprive a cell of 35 percent of its oxygen for forty-eight hours and it may become cancerous."

He should know. Dr. Warburg was the first person to propose that a lack of oxygen was the culprit in the development of cancer. He showed that embryonic cells that were healthy adopted the fermentation form of respiration when oxygen levels were low. He suggested that by normalizing the metabolism of cancer cells, the cancer could be treated effectively and also in a way that is far less toxic than chemotherapy and safer than radiation. The way to do this is oxygen therapy.

SECRET #432 This oxygen therapy can snuff out cancer.

Oxygen therapy is a standard practice in many of the alternative clinics that specialize in the treatment of cancer. When you withhold sugar and flood the tissues with oxygen you will starve or suffocate the cancer. Hyperbaric oxygen therapy (HBOT) is one way of flooding your tissues with oxygen.

In hyperbaric oxygen therapy (HBOT), you are placed inside a pressurized chamber that delivers 100 percent oxygen at a pressure greater than sea-level atmospheric pressure. As you breathe, oxygen has to move from outside air, with a pressure tension of 150 mm, to a cellular oxygen tension of not much more than 1 percent of that! It's easy to see how and why we're so dependent on an uninterrupted supply of oxygen every second of our lives. It is a long and arduous path for oxygen to travel from the outside air to the deep recesses of the body. This is made even more difficult when you have heart disease. Then, blood vessel obstructions slow down the flow of red blood cells.

In addition, your red blood cells have a diameter actually larger than the diameter of the capillaries. This means they need to be flexible to bend in its passage through the capillaries. A poor diet and obstructions in blood vessels contribute to red blood cell inflexibility. With hyperbaric oxygen, you bypass the problems found within the red blood cells. HBOT alters body physics allowing it to manage oxygenation of compromised tissues *totally independently* of red blood cells.

Good hyperbaric oxygen chambers are expensive, so you'll find them in the hands of doctors of integrative medicine and in clinics of alternative medicine. Since HBOT can be used for wound repair, after stroke, and for many other purposes, make sure any doctor you see for this therapy is well versed in its application for cancer.

It's important to always take good quantities of antioxidants if you are using any oxygen therapies to protect against oxidative stress. Oxygen is necessary for cellular respiration and energy production, but it must be carefully handled within the cell or the mitochondria will be damaged due to oxidative changes.

SECRET #433 This simple addition to your supplement regime can help your skin heal after radiation treatment.

If you've had radiation treatments for breast, head, neck, or other cancers, you know that the exposed skin tissues that lie just beneath the skin become thicker and more fibrous. A study published in the *Journal of Clinical Oncology* showed that a combined treatment of 1,000 IU daily of vitamin E, along with the drug pentoxifylline (Trental, 800 mg daily), used for at least six months, significantly improved the affected tissues. Pentoxifylline thins the blood and increases blood flow, enhancing tissue oxygenation. Historically, it has been used for peripheral vascular disease. Vitamin E is also a blood thinner.

The study compared the combined therapy with either single therapy. The combination of vitamin E with pentoxifylline was considerably more effective. If you have changes in your tissues due to radiation therapy, or if you're planning on having radiation, you may want to bring this study to the attention of your doctor to see if it's appropriate for you. See the Bibliography for more information on this study.

CHAPTER 48

This Little-Known Nutrient Can Stop Cancer in Its Tracks

I'm very excited about this supplement. It's one of a small handful of nutrients that can change the lives of everyone who has cancer or has had it in the past, or who is at high risk. There are a number of substances that can help you fight cancer, but none of them stops cancer from progressing like modified citrus pectin.

Not every citrus pectin product will work. I'm talking here specifically about a modified citrus pectin (MCP) product called PectaSol, the product used in all of the scientific studies. I've seen it work wonders in patients with breast and prostate cancers. It's the first supplement I suggest for any new cancer patient. It can't hurt you and it could give you remarkable results.

We might not know about MCP if it wasn't for a chance remark made to a young boy more than thirty years ago. The story of how modified pectin came into use still gives me goosebumps.

SECRET #434 A series of "coincidences" led to the discovery of modified citrus pectin.

Let me begin by saying that I don't believe in coincidences. To me, they're "miracles of perfect timing." Recently, a series of these little miracles put me in contact with a substance found in oranges that stops cancer metastasis (the spread of cancer). These little miracles sat me right next to the doctor who developed it and brought it to this country. They had my book publisher ask me to write a small book on this nutrient. They placed every bit of research in my lap, and they even allowed me to see for myself how well it worked on people in my community.

This doctor, Isaac Eliaz, M.D., has since become a close personal friend and colleague because of his vision, compassion, and knowledge. The story of how he helped develop this cancer-stopping substance is filled with more little miracles.

As I said, it began over thirty years ago when Isaac was a young boy living in Israel. Like many children, he enjoyed visiting his neighbors. Drs. Ruth and Leo

Cohen both had Ph.D.s in organic chemistry and were pioneers in the burgeoning citrus industry. Leo's specialty was citrus pectin, a substance found in the skins of oranges.

One day Ruth made a chance remark that changed Isaac's life and the lives of many cancer patients forever. Seemingly out of the blue, she said to him, "Isaac, one day they will find out that there's a cure for cancer in the peel of the orange." Her remark was quickly forgotten. Thirty years later, Isaac Eliaz had become a medical doctor practicing in the United States with a specialty in integrative medicine. He was determined to find cancer-fighting nutrients in foods that could help stop and reverse cancers.

SECRET #435 When pectin is modified, its properties are enhanced.

In 1995, Isaac read an impressive paper on the use of citrus pectin to prevent prostate cancer from spreading. Suddenly, he remembered Ruth's comment. He picked up the phone and dialed the Cohen's old phone number in Israel. Remarkably, their phone number was the same and Ruth answered.

"Ruth, do you remember what you told me so many years ago?" Isaac asked, excitedly. "You were right!"

The Cohens put Isaac in touch with the world's foremost authorities on citrus pectin. They helped him develop a modified citrus pectin product with molecules small enough to get into the bloodstream. You see, the molecules of ordinary pectin are too large to move through the intestinal walls.

You may be familiar with using pectin to stop diarrhea or to end constipation. It works well as a soluble fiber and bulking agent. But pectin and MCP have very different properties. Don't mistake one for the other. Modifying pectin enhances its capabilities tremendously. By reducing pectin's molecular size and weight, Isaac found it could travel into the bloodstream and target cancer cells. Although MCP has been most widely studied with prostate cancer, studies show it works with other cancers as well. "There's a particularly close relationship between breast and prostate cancers," says Stephen Strum, M.D., an oncologist who specializes in prostate cancer. "The treatment that works for one frequently works for another," he said.

SECRET #436 Not only does sugar feed cancer cells, it helps them form tumors.

Cancer cells have more of a particular type of sticky protein called galectins than healthy cells. Galectins love sugars. They attach themselves to sugar molecules on the surface of cells. This helps cells hold onto one another and communicate. Cancer cells have more galectins than healthy cells, making it easier for them to grab onto one another and form tumors. These clusters can also invade neighboring tissues and spread to other sites.

Of all the galectins, the one that has been studied the most and seems to play a key role in cancer metastasis is called galectin-3. Galectin-3 helps cancer cells stick together so they can travel through the blood to other sites. It helps groups of cancer cells attach to these sites and form tumors. And it stimulates the growth of blood vessels, the food source for cancer cells. MCP attaches itself to the same sites. Prostate and breast cancer are very similar types of cancer, as both are very high in galectin-3 molecules.

It's beautifully simple. Cancer cells can't live alone. They have to cluster together or die. Modified citrus pectin attaches itself to cancer cells so they can't hold on to one another. By preventing cancer cells from clustering, MCP stops cancer from spreading.

MCP also stops new blood vessels—which deliver cancer's food supply—from forming. Without food, cancer cells starve to death.

SECRET #437 For MCP to have anticancer-clustering properties, it has to be "just right."

It reminds me of the three bears and their porridge. Before citrus pectin can stop cancer—even when it's been modified—its particles can't be too large or too small. They have to be just the right size and weight.

Not all modified citrus pectins are alike. Some don't work very well. Others don't work at all. The size of the pectin's molecules determines where they can go, what they can do, and how well they can stop cancer tumors from forming.

Regular apple or citrus pectins have a molecular weight between 50,000 and 150,000 daltons. These molecules are so large that they can travel only within the intestines. This explains why ordinary pectin is a good bulking agent, but won't stop breast cancer. It could stop colon cancer, but that's all.

A high-quality MCP has uniform molecules between 10,000 and 20,000 daltons. This smaller size allows modified citrus pectins to be absorbed through the intestines and get into the bloodstream. Unless MCP can get through your intestines, it can't fight cancer. Dr. Eliaz conducted some cell-culture studies with pectins with various molecular weights. He found that the pectins with smaller or larger molecular weights were less effective than those between 10,000 and 20,000 daltons. Pectins with large molecules couldn't get into the bloodstream, and those with a smaller molecular weight broke down too quickly and were excreted before they could work.

The structure of MCP, or its degree of esterification, varies in products as well. Esterification determines whether or not sugar molecules are the right size to allow galectins to grab onto them. The higher the degree of esterification, the larger the sugar molecules are, and the more difficult it is for MCP to attach itself to cancer cells. If MCP can't grab onto malignant cells, other cancer cells will. This is how tumors are formed.

The only form of MCP that was found to work in clinical studies has a low degree of esterification—10 percent or less. And the only product that meets all of these specifications is the MCP developed by Dr. Eliaz and his researchers called PectaSol. All others fall into a category of "the great unknown." There's no evidence at all that they work.

SECRET #438 Five reasons to use MCP as part of your cancer treatment.

1. To reduce the size or growth of primary tumors

2. To prevent or slow metastasis

3. To prevent or slow angiogenesis

4. For detoxification; to reduce heavy metal load

5. To reduce the chance of metastasis before a biopsy when cancer is suspected

SECRET #439 How and when to take MCP for best results.

You may want to consider using MCP if you have had cancer and are concerned about having a relapse. It not only stops renegade cancer cells from spreading to other sites, but it can also stop tumors from growing and reduces them in many cases. You can use MCP safely along with other cancer treatments, including chemotherapy. There are no known contraindications.

If breast or colon cancer runs in your family, or if cancer is prevalent in an area where you live, consider using MCP. If you live in an area that's heavily sprayed with pesticides and insecticides, you can protect yourself against the many environmental pollutants that have been associated with cancer by taking MCP.

The amount of MCP found in studies to be effective for serious conditions like cancer is 5 grams, three times a day. For prevention, or for long-time exposure to toxins like heavy metals or environmental pollutants, Dr. Eliaz suggests beginning with the full amount and then reducing it to 3–5 grams a day after the first month.

It's best to take MCP in divided doses and not just once a day to keep it circulating in your bloodstream. To save money, get the powder rather than capsules. It's less expensive, dissolves well in water, and tastes just fine. Use the capsules for convenience when you travel.

I've seen PectaSol work in some of my patients, and have read every study that has been done on MCP. In my opinion, it's one of the first lines of defense for anyone who has cancer or who has had it in the past. Read the book I've written, and decide for yourself.

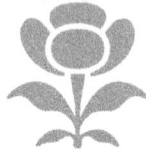

CHAPTER 49

Super Nutrients
to Battle Cancer

Obviously, I can't cover all the various supplements here that are being used to fight cancer. If I did it would be too confusing. Instead, I'd like to discuss a handful of nutrients that are backed by enough scientific data for you to seriously consider including one or more in your supplement program. You may be familiar with a few of them, but perhaps not as anticancer nutrients.

They bring up additional questions. For instance, we know that antioxidants can help prevent and fight free radicals that can lead to cancer. But should you take them if you're on chemotherapy? I've researched this subject for you and the answer might be surprising. Finally, is there anything you can do other than surgery if you have skin cancer? There may be. But don't use this method without being monitored closely by a good dermatologist. And make sure that your condition is mild enough to give you the time to explore other options.

SECRET #440 Antioxidants could be helpful if you're on chemotherapy drugs.

We know that some antioxidants like vitamins A, C, and E inhibit the growth of cancer cells. It happens that they also enhance the effects of chemotherapy, radiation, and interferon. In fact, a review of seventy scientific papers on antioxidants and chemotherapy found that taking antioxidants makes chemotherapy treatments more effective.

In two studies—one a randomized, controlled trial, and the other a laboratory study—vitamin E was found to protect against nerve damage from cisplatin, a common chemotherapy drug. In addition to being protective, vitamin E didn't reduce cisplatin's effectiveness.

In a one and a half year trial, patients on cisplatin, who also took 300 IU of vitamin E a day right before their chemotherapy treatment and continued taking it for three months after their treatments ended, had less nerve damage than those on cisplatin alone. Nerve damage occurred in 85.7 percent of people on chemo alone, but only in 30.7 percent of people on both chemo and vitamin E. Not only was there a lower incidence of nerve damage, but also it was less severe in patients taking this antioxidant.

Cisplatin falls into the category of chemotherapy agents called alkylating agents. Some cancer specialists believe this type of drug has a weaker effect when antioxidants are taken at the same time. Alkylating agents are thought to work by producing free radicals in cancer cells and, in theory, antioxidants would interfere with this action. But they don't.

This study looked only at vitamin E's activity with chemotherapy. Hopefully, there will be studies using chemotherapy with other antioxidants like selenium and vitamins A and C. I predict the results will find that drug therapy with antioxidants is more effective and less toxic than the chemotherapy alone.

Ralph Moss, Ph.D., an expert in the field of alternative therapies for cancer treatment and the author of numerous books on cancer (see Chapter 47), agrees. He points out that using antioxidants as part of cancer therapy has been given a bad rap. Within the field of oncology, he says, there's still a debate over whether or not chemotherapy has any benefits. That said, if you're on chemotherapy or radiation therapy, you may very well want to add an antioxidant formula to your regime. It could enhance the effects of your chemotherapy.

SECRET #441 The amount of antioxidants you take during treatments determines whether they help you.

Antioxidants are strange substances. Their effects on tumors depend on the doses being used. For instance, a study published in *Cancer Research Review* points out that a high dose of an antioxidant prevents cancer cells from growing without affecting normal cells. What's a high dose, you ask? Up to 10 grams of vitamin C, 1,000 IU of vitamin E, 10,000 IU of vitamin A, and 60 mg of natural beta-carotene a day.

These high doses are protective *only* if you take them before, during, and after radiation. Lower amounts—between the recommended dietary allowance (RDA) and these high amounts—could reduce radiation's effectiveness.

A mixture of antioxidants appears to work better than using single nutrients. This is why it's important to use antioxidants during radiation and chemotherapy only under the direction of trained healthcare professionals. Your safest course would be to eat plenty of fresh fruits and vegetables. They contain mixtures of antioxidants and won't interfere with your treatments.

SECRET #442 CoQ$_{10}$ not only supports your heart and brain, but it also helps fight cancer.

Coenzyme Q$_{10}$ (CoQ$_{10}$) is a fat-soluble vitamin (vitamin Q$_{10}$) like vitamins A and

E. Since the largest concentrations are in the brain and heart, you may be familiar with its role in supporting the health of these organs. But CoQ_{10} is found in all cells, and while your heart and brain are very dependent on this nutrient, so, it seems, is breast tissue.

CoQ_{10} has been found to be low in people with cancer, but particularly breast cancer. Breast-tumor tissues contain lower levels of CoQ_{10} than healthy breast tissue. Researchers found that malignant cells use more CoQ_{10} than healthy cells, and this affects antioxidant enzyme levels. It appears that the more CoQ_{10} you have in your bloodstream, the more likely you are to survive breast cancer—if you even get it.

SECRET #443 This vitamin has reversed serious cases of breast cancer.

There has been a dramatic decrease in CoQ_{10} levels in cancers with a bad prognosis.

In fact, doctors can fairly reliably determine if you will survive breast cancer by the CoQ_{10} levels in your body! The higher your blood levels, the better your chance of survival.

Karl Folkers, Ph.D., of the University of Texas, Austin, reported on six breast-cancer cases that were treated with CoQ_{10}. The findings were nothing short of amazing: "The overt survival for five to fifteen years of six cancer patients, without evidence of cancer, and the complete regression of cancer in five cases, and now a regression of metastases in the liver, are extraordinary. . . ."

Once cancer moves into the liver "it's a prelude to eminent death," said one researcher involved in the study. So the fact that CoQ_{10} was able to eliminate cancer in the liver is, indeed, a miracle.

This same researcher, Knud Lockwood, M.D., said: "Although in the past, the ethical treatment of breast cancer was based on mastectomy, x-ray treatment, and anticancer drugs, this overall treatment rarely, if ever, caused highly significant regressions of the primary tumor and metastases in the liver." He then concluded: "Therefore, our recording of the disappearance of liver metastases in even one patient having breast cancer is extraordinarily salient. . . ."

Although these patients had breast cancer, there is no reason to believe that CoQ_{10} won't work in other cancers. However, there is still a lot of work to be done in regard to cancer treatment with CoQ_{10}. We're a long way from having this research done.

Since CoQ_{10} is a fat-soluble vitamin, it requires fatty acids to be taken along with it for best absorption. Some CoQ_{10} products have no fatty acids added to them. If they don't, you will want to take them with a meal that contains some fats. Other products have fatty acids added, and are well absorbed at any time.

SECRET #444 A substance found in produce detoxifies toxins from pesticides and other sources.

Everything has a cause. Cancer often begins with exposure to a variety of toxic substances that encourage tumor production. Your risk for this and other diseases accelerates when your body can't remove enough toxins fast enough. Many of these carcinogenic (cancer-causing) or mutagenic (causing cell mutation) agents originate in our diet and environment.

Devra Lee Davis, Ph.D., a professor at Carnegie Mellon University, found Canadian and Danish studies that showed high levels of carcinogenic toxins in women appearing years before their cancer was diagnosed. These toxins, found in cured meat, red meat, plastic wrap, synthetic pesticides, cigarette smoke, and car exhaust are the same cancer-inducing agents that are removed by the body naturally through a detoxification process called glucuronidation. You may not be able to escape exposure to these toxins, but you can do something to increase the rate at which they're removed.

Calcium D-glucarate is a natural substance that is found in fruits and vegetables that actually helps your liver remove carcinogenic chemicals by increasing glucuronidation.

Caffeine, cigarettes, and marijuana contain toxins and also slow down glucaronidation. The more coffee or colas you drink and the more cigarettes you smoke, the more toxins you accumulate and the more glucaric acid you lose. Exposure to dietary and environmental toxins, and a family history of cancer, are two reasons to increase your intake of fruits and cruciferous vegetables (foods high in glucaric acid), and to think about adding calcium D-glucarate to your supplement regime.

SECRET #445 Calcium D-glucarate is a patented form of glucaric acid that promotes detoxification through glucuronidation.

Glucuronidation is a chemical reaction that occurs in your liver where a water-soluble substance combines with a toxin and removes it from your cells. This is a major pathway of detoxification that occurs naturally in our bodies. Many of these toxins are known to be carcinogenic like those found in some molds, or nitrosamines (found in cured meat like ham and lunch meats). Other tumor promoters, like steroid hormones (too much estrogen, for example), can contribute to cancer and are removed through glucuronidation as well.

You may remember hearing that "every action has an opposite reaction." Well, this is true with glucuronidation, also. Along with promoting detoxification, your body also produces an enzyme called beta-glucoronidase that *stops* it. Calcium D-glucarate blocks this antidetox substance, beta-glucuronidase, promoting greater detoxification. I believe that many people who get cancer, Parkinson's disease, and other chronic health problems have reduced glucuronidation. This means that their bodies accumulate toxins at a greater rate than they can be eliminated. Doesn't this make sense? If your body can get rid of harmful substances, they can't stay around and contribute to causing a disease.

SECRET #446 When glucarate is attached to calcium, it stays in your body and detoxifies longer.

Glucarate, D-glucarate or DGA (for its active ingredient, D-glucaric acid) is a natural substance found in many fruits and vegetables. High levels are found in apples, grapefruit, bean sprouts, broccoli, cauliflower, and cabbage. Glucarate binds itself to some harmful environmental pollutants and other toxins in foods, beverages, and cigarette smoke, and attaches itself to excessive estrogen, removing these unwanted materials. Calcium D-glucarate is glucarate attached to calcium. The calcium is a carrier that allows glucarate to be present much longer. Instead of having glucarate remain in your body for one hour, by binding it to calcium, calcium D-glucarate stays in your body for five hours!

SECRET #447 Calcium D-glucarate reduces dangerously high levels of estrogen.

Thomas Slaga, Ph.D., a cancer researcher, has done a great deal of research on glucarate over the past twenty years. I was fortunate to meet Dr. Slaga and talk with him for more an hour. I am very impressed with his work. In his book *D-Glucarate: A Nutrient Against Cancer,* Dr. Slaga explains how glucarate has protected against breast, lung, colon, liver, bladder, skin, and prostate cancers by enhancing this detoxification pathway. He reported results of a study on glucarate and breast cancer that showed estrogen levels decreased when calcium D-glucarate was taken. For women worried about having an increased risk for breast cancer from estrogen therapy, glucarate appears to offer a unique form of protection.

Now, it's important for you to realize that calcium D-glucarate will lower your estrogen no matter how low it is. However, if you read Chapter 46 on breast thermography, you know that your blood levels of estrogen may be low while the amount of estrogen in your breast tissues is high enough to promote cancer. This is why I used calcium D-glucarate as one of the anticancer nutrients that helped normalize my thermogram. You may want to do the same. Talk this point over with your doctor.

SECRET #448 The amount of calcium D-glucarate that's best for you can vary greatly depending on your genetics and lifestyle.

According to Dr. Slaga, 200–2,000 mg of glucarate gives a protective effect. But remember that calcium D-glucarate supports glucuronidation for about five hours. So eat a healthy diet and consider taking calcium D-glucarate supplements two or three times a day.

The amount of calcium D-glucarate you decide to take depends on your health, diet, lifestyle, and inherited strengths and weaknesses. If you want some added protection, eat well, don't smoke, and are not exposed to a lot of toxins, 200 mg two to three times a day may be fine. If you want more protection because of past indiscretions or a family history of cancer or Parkinson's disease, 500 mg twice a day makes sense. That's what I took, even though my diet was healthy and I live in the country where the air is relatively clean. However, for thirty years I lived in Southern California and was exposed to high amounts of air pollution, so I want to move any accumulated and stored toxins out of my body. Dr. Slaga has not seen any evidence of toxicity or any side effects with 10 grams (10,000 mg) of any form of glucarate.

D-GLUCARIC ACID IS NATURALLY FOUND IN THESE FOODS:

1 cup broccoli	530 mg
1/2 pink grapefruit	443 mg
1 cup Brussels sprouts	419 mg
Whole apple	311 mg

Source: D-Glucarate: A Nutrient Against Cancer, Thomas Slaga, (McGraw-Hill, 1999)

SECRET #449 Calcium D-glucarate does not fight cancer per se. It promotes detoxification of known and suspected carcinogens.

Products with glucarate are not being advertised as anticancer supplements, and for good reason. They're not. When I speak with oncologists who use nutrition in their practices, these doctors tell me: "There are two steps you need to take. Detoxify, and support the immune system. The body does the rest." Glucarate may be a key nutrient in helping us reduce our body's toxic burdens from everything from a lifetime exposure to toxic substances to a course or two of chemotherapy or other drugs.

Since calcium D-glucarate, or glucarate, is a patented nutrient, any supplement you find on the market with this name on it is the real thing. You can safely shop for quantity of the nutrient versus price and availability, and be sure you're getting the same quality ingredient. Are products with glucarate necessary? I don't know. But they do offer good protection, especially if you've ever been a heavy smoker, eaten processed meats, or drank a lot of caffeine. If you still smoke, you may want to take a more serious look at these products. Just remember that glucarate does not take the place of changing your lifestyle to a healthy one. And it doesn't promise to cure anything. But it could give your body the support it needs to remain healthier longer.

SECRET #450 A substance in grapes can stop cancer from starting and progressing.

Back in the 1920s, a naturopath named Johanna Brandt wrote a book claiming that grapes cured her cancer. In her book *The Grape Cure,* Dr. Brandt explains that a grape fast, eating only grapes, is the method she used to treat her disease. At one point, she was eating as many as four pounds of grapes a day!

Obviously, Dr. Brandt's cure hasn't hit the mainstream, but the principles of the grape cure are now being used by doctors of integrative medicine.

It started when *Science* magazine published an article from the University of Illinois, Chicago that stated, "Resveratrol can inhibit all three stages of chemical carcinogenesis—tumor initiation, promotion, and progression" (quoted from the *Lancet*).

SECRET #451 Resveratrol is found only in grapes that are being attacked by a fungus.

Grape plants produce resveratrol, a bioflavonoid, as a natural defense mechanism against fungus infection. But not all grape plants will produce this protective substance. It's only when the plant comes under the attack of a fungus that resveratrol is produced to fight off or kill the fungus. And it's this protective mechanism that has proved to be so beneficial in fighting off cancer. This means that resveratrol may be in short supply from vineyards that spray antifungals.

This specific class of bioflavonoids that has such powerful anticancer effects is also found in pine bark, lemon tree bark, hazel nut tree leaves, blueberries, cherries, cranberries, and others. But the most concentrated quantity is found in the skin of certain purple grapes (resveratrol is also found in the grape seeds, but in lower concentrations).

To find resveratrol, suppliers must travel throughout the world testing grape skins and seeds for their resveratrol content. Once they find a vineyard with a high content of resveratrol, they purchase the entire lot. The grapes are then transported to a facility where they undergo a natural process using water to make a high potency extract, which is then used in the supplements.

SECRET #452 Resveratrol is a natural COX inhibitor.

Resveratrol has been found to be an effective combatant against the latest cancer dragon called COX—cyclooxygenase. This enzyme stimulates tumor cell growth and suppresses "immune surveillance," the early warning system that signals your body to attack the dangerous cells that are going cancerous. COX can also activate some carcinogens. So we need "COX inhibitors" to fight this new-found enemy within.

Work done at the University of Illinois, Chicago, concluded that resveratrol in grape skins appears to be a powerful COX inhibitor. And it's worth repeating that resveratrol can inhibit *all three stages of chemical carcinogenesis,* an unusual phenomenon and highly significant in the treatment of cancer. In fact, resveratrol is the most significant molecule to challenge cancer, at least in the laboratory, in many decades and perhaps ever.

Resveratrol interferes with the development of cancer on several levels, such as growth inhibition of cancer cells and reversal of precancer cells to normal. As the *Lancet* put it: "Grapes are good for you, but leave the skins on." You'd have to drink a lot of wine to get an effective dose of resveratrol. The head of this study even went so far as to remind us that "eternal health is not to be found in the bottom of a wine bottle."

I don't suggest you go on a grape fast like Dr. Brandt. For one thing, it's too high in sugars. But you may want to take resveratrol—especially if cancer runs in your family. If you can't find a good brand at your local health-food store, or one you can trust, see the Resources section at the end of this book.

Resveratrol is nontoxic and there is essentially no known toxic dose. There was no toxicity to pregnant women, nursing mothers, or their babies. Stick to the recommended dosage on the label.

SECRET #453 There are topical ointments that can remove skin cancers.

Most people are unaware that there are salves that can draw malignant tumors out of the body, providing them with alternatives to surgery, radiation, and chemotherapy. Surgery is not the only method for excising tumors.

A few years ago, a friend who is familiar with medicinal herbs told me how she had used a salve to treat a malignant tumor on her dog's lip. This salve consisted of bloodroot, chaparral, and zinc chloride. Over a period of a month, the tumor slowly detached from the dog's lip, leaving a crater where blood vessels could be seen. Eventually, this crater healed. The tumor was gone.

Then I contacted an oncologist friend who was retired from private practice. He used to prescribe herbs and nutritional supplements for his patients and had a very high rate of success. He was familiar with both yellow and black salves for drawing out malignant tumors and had found them to be extremely effective. I read his detailed instructions on their use, along with their warnings, and decided these salves are nothing to play around with. If a tumor is being drawn out of the body, I want someone with a lot of knowledge to be able to monitor this treatment and to intervene if necessary. A dermatologist, other medical doctor, nurse practitioner, or healthcare specialist skilled in the use of cancer salves should administer them.

SECRET #454 This guidebook to cancer salves can help your doctor decide when they're appropriate and how to use them.

Ingrid Naiman, author of *Cancer Salves: A Botanical Approach to Treatment,* agrees. She has written a complete and well-researched guide to their history, formulations, and use. It is an excellent treatment guide for practitioners and offers explanations of various options open to cancer patients. In this book, Naiman has a quote from an unnamed doctor who has treated 10,000 patients with yellow and black salves successfully. This doctor was the oncologist friend I had contacted. Small world!

Cancer is known to have existed for thousands of years. Before surgery, caustic salves were used to remove tumors. In fact, cancer salves have been used for 2,500 years. In the twelfth century, Hildegard von Bingen, a German mystic, used a combination of violets, olive oil, and billy goat tallow successfully on cancerous tumors. Since then, numerous doctors have worked with various formulas, many of which originated with Native American tribes. Many of these salves contain zinc chloride and bloodroot (*Sanguinaria*). But more complicated formulas have been found useful, as well.

Naiman's book is divided into three sections: a historical overview of cancer salves; use of cancer salves (when they're appropriate and what to expect from using them); and various methods of treating cancer with salves, diet, and ingesting herbs. This fascinating book provides little-known information in an easy-to-read format. It does not suggest using any of these salves on your own, but instead to find a practitioner skilled in using them. Barring this feat—and Naiman admits that not many practitioners exist who do know a lot about them—the book can serve as a guide to any responsible medical practitioner who is willing to work with salves and monitor their patients closely.

SECRET #455 This is how caustic salves that burn away a tumor work.

Some cancer salves fall into a category called escharotic salves, which means they have caustic substances that cause itching and burning on tissues. They work by increasing circulation around the site of the tumor, which creates heat and blistering. This can be painful. Some people won't have any major reaction, while others will find the skin around the tumor gets red, blisters, and then changes color numerous times.

Eventually, a crust develops and the tumor, which hangs on by a thread, drops off leaving a crater that eventually repairs itself. There may be a discharge of a clear fluid or pus. Cancer salves can remove all traces of malignancy or just part of a tumor. You want every bit of cancer removed, not just some of it! This is another reason why you want a highly skilled health practitioner working with you. An untrained eye cannot tell whether or not any malignancy remains, and the choice of salve along with length of treatment is highly individualized. Don't attempt to use cancer salves on your own.

While some cancer salves work by burning and irritating, some work by destroying tumors or separating them from healthy skin. Still others draw tumors up and out of the skin. Then there are salves used to help heal the craters that have been left when tumors are excised. By reading Naiman's book, you and your doctor can choose an appropriate treatment plan.

SECRET #456 The combination of salves and surgery may be best.

Frederic Mohs, M.D., at the University of Wisconsin, developed a system for treating skin cancer with a paste of bloodroot, zinc chloride, and stibnite (made from ore of antimony). Both he and Ralph Moss, Ph.D., a cancer researcher I spoke about earlier in Chapter 47, claim a 99 percent success rate with all primary basal cell carcinomas. The technique used by Dr. Mohs is called chemosurgery, a combination of salves and surgery. He has used this technique on various types of cancer, and his method has been studied on tens of thousands of patients.

Drs. John Pattison, Eli Jones, and the more popular herbalist John Christopher all have different methods of removing cancers using salves, diet, homeopathics, and herbs. But you should remember that these doctors had years of experience treating patients and observing the changes that came from their treatment plans. While it may seem simple to think of putting a salve over a spot on your body and getting rid of the cancer beneath, a great deal of knowledge is needed to know what treatment to use and when to change it.

In this age of over-information, we're looking for "magic bullets"—quick fixes to our problems. By using a salve, an herb, or a nutritional supplement that eliminates our symptoms, we're ignoring the underlying problem that caused the symptoms. Ingrid Naiman knows this. She understands that we need to explore our emotional past and present, look at the way we view ourselves and the world, and change our lives to improve our health. Cancer salves are not "magic bullets." They may, however, be part of a treatment plan that not only eliminates tumors, but their cause(s).

Still, if you're going, to use salves, they must be used responsibly. Ingrid Naiman's book provides cancer patients and their health providers with the information they need to use them. It gives people an option that goes beyond surgery, radiation, and chemotherapy. This book should be in the library of every healthcare practitioner and physician interested in cancer therapies, whether or not they use them.

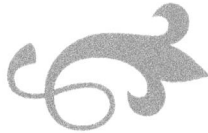

Conclusion

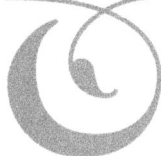

Information is power. You are now a much more powerful person than you were before you read this book. You also have more options and, hopefully, a greater understanding of your role in your own health care.

In the past, you may have put your health in the hands of your doctor. Now you know that it's possible to take a more active role and form a partnership with a skilled healthcare practitioner for the best possible care. In fact, you may bring this person information that they previously missed—information that can make the difference between your ability to heal or not.

As good as your doctor may be—and there are many good doctors out there—he or she is most likely not familiar with all of the current scientific data, products, and therapies. It takes a lot of time to read studies and separate the good ones from those that are biased or poorly designed. That's what I do as a Health Detective. And it's why I often have more and different information than doctors—even some excellent doctors of integrative medicine.

My goal in writing this book was to show you that there are literally hundreds of pertinent pieces of information you can use to make a difference in your life. They offer health secrets to help you get and stay well—no matter how sick you are.

I was not trying to write about comprehensive programs for various illnesses. Those books already exist. Instead, my concentration was on discovering little-known information that can have a profound effect on your health. You can implement some of them safely on your own. For others, it would be wiser to have a knowledgeable healthcare practitioner as your partner to monitor you.

You may be tempted to make a lot of changes all at once. I'd like to caution against this. Instead, begin slowly by making dietary changes. Then look at some of the diagnostic tests like breast thermography, fibrinogen, or the iodine-loading test. They can point to your next step: supplementation. Always remember that supplements cannot replace the nutrients in your diet. Diet first; supplements second.

Whatever you decide to do first, I hope you found *many* valuable suggestions in the preceding pages. While not every one of my "456 Most Powerful Healing Secrets" will be right for everyone, I'm sure that many of them will be helpful *to you*.

Of course, it's impossible for any book to be completely up to date. New discoveries are being made every day. That's why I'd like to suggest one of the very first things you do is to go to my website and sign up for the free Health Alerts I send out every week. That way you'll know about the latest health research, late-breaking discoveries, and other cutting-edge information long before others report on it.

You don't need to be a subscriber to my monthly newsletter, *Women's Health Letter,* to receive these Health Alerts. Simply go to my website, www.womenshealthletter.com, click on "Health Alerts," and type in your email address. We'll do the rest.

Please join the thousands of people who are taking control of their health, and getting *more* out of life.

Your voice of reason,
Nan Kathryn Fuchs, Ph.D.
Editor in Chief, *Women's Health Letter*

Thermography Centers

United States

Alaska

PhysioScan DITI
Michael Wedge, L.Ac.
808 S. Bailey, Suite 103
Palmer, AK 99645
(907) 745-7928

Arizona

Gail Research Lab
Robert LaBine, Provisional C.T.T.
Kent Hoppenworth, Provisional C.T.T.
14640 N. Tatum Blvd., Suite 6
Phoenix, AZ 85032
(602) 923-1075

Thermal Imaging of Arizona
Daniel Perry, C.T.T.
Jo Ann Nicolosi, Provisional C.T.T.
Bonnie Stout, Provisional C.T.T.
1921 S. Alma School Rd., Suite 315
Mesa, AZ 85210
(480) 768-1100
www.thermalimagingofaz.com

California

CCI-Thermal Imaging Center
Anand Chaudhry, D.C., C.T.T.
8465 Old Redwood Hwy.
Windsor, CA 94592
(707) 838-2146
www.breast-thermography.com

CLEAR Center of Health
Beth McDougall, M.D.
125 Throckmorton Ave.
Mill Valley, CA 94941
(415) 388-5520
www.clearcenterofhealth.com

Clinical Thermography Associates
George Chapman, D.C., D.A.B.C.T.,
    D.I.A.C.T., F.I.A.C.T.
298 Shasta St.
Chula Vista, CA 91910
(619) 422-3339
www.clinicalthermography.com

Core Care Imaging Center
Mark Weil, Cindy Crawford
3023 Filmore St.
San Francisco, CA 94123
(415) 928-5423

Health Medicine Institute
William J Kneebone, D.C.,
    D.I.A.C.T., D.C.C.T.
3799 Mount Diablo Blvd.
Lafayette, CA 94549
(925) 962-3799

HealthScan Thermal Imaging Center
William C. Amalu, D.C., D.A.B.C.T.,
    D.I.A.C.T., F.I.A.C.T.
Linda Hernandez, Provisional C.T.T.
621 Middlefield Rd.
Redwood City, CA 94063
(650) 361-8908
www.breastthermography.com
www.healthscanonline.com

Intrahealth
Petra Eggert, D.C., PT, Provisional C.T.T.
21020 Homestead Rd., Suite 2
Cupertino, CA 95014
(408) 530-0005

Pleasanton Infrared Imaging
James Sievers, D.C., Provisional C.T.T.
Beth Y. Gordon, Provisional C.T.T.
5737 Valley Ave., Suite D
Pleasanton, CA 94566
(925) 462-2633

Pro-Active Health Imaging
Jayne Rayner, C.T.T.
350 N. Lantana, Suite 225
Camarillo, CA 93010
(805) 641-0010
www.breastthermography.com

Trinity Health Club
Robert Rowen, M.D.
Terri Su, M.D.
2200 County Center Dr., Suite H
Santa Rosa, CA 95403
(707) 571-7560

William Cockburn, D.C., D.I.A.C.T.,
    F.I.A.C.T., F.A.B.F.E.
11695 National Blvd.
Los Angeles, CA 90064
(562) 699-7921 (Call for locations in
    Downey, CA and Glendora, CA)

Woodside Thermal Imaging
Robert Kane, D.C., D.A.B.C.T.,
    D.I.A.C.T., F.I.A.C.T.
950 Woodside Rd., Suite 5
Redwood City, CA 94061
(650) 568-9555

Colorado

The Thermogram Center
Tirza Derflinger, Provisional C.T.T.
315 S. Boulder Rd., Suite 110
Louisville, CO 80027
(866) 492-2174
www.thermogramcenter.com

Florida

**Spirit Mountain Thermal
    Imaging, Inc**
Nelly L. Yefet, Acupuncture Physician
21400 West Dixie Hwy.
Aventura, FL 33180
(305) 933-2360

Georgia

Charis Infrared Thermal Imaging, Inc.
Nina Rea
P.O. Box 5312
Athens, GA 30604
(706) 338-3611

Health-e-u
Monique Myrick
4017 Cinnamon Fern Lane
Woodstock, GA 30189
(770) 924-0650

Hawaii

Thermal Imaging Hawaii
Linda Fickes, D.C., C.C.T.
4821 Kaimoku Way
Honolulu, HI 96821
(808) 377-1811

Illinois

Beth Ann Connell, D.C., D.A.B.C.T.
N. Mill St.
Utica, IL 61373
(815) 667-4819

Infrared Thermal Imaging
Jan Crawford, R.N.
129 S. Phelps Ave., Suite 9
Rockford, IL
(815) 227-5454

Indiana

Priority 1 Medical
Charles Solano, D.C., D.A.B.C.T.
4082 Pendleton Way
Indianapolis, IN 46226
(317) 546-1915

Kentucky

Larry Payne, D.C., D.A.B.C.T.
7349 Burlington Pike
Florence, KY 41042
(859) 525-7443

Louisiana

**Elliot-Elliot-Head Breast Cancer
Research and Treatment Center**
Robert Elliot, M.D., Ph.D.
17050 Medical Center Dr., 4th Floor
Baton Rouge, LA 70816
(800) 762-5315

Thermology Associates of Louisiana
Tim Green, D.C.
205 E. Boundary St.
Farmerville, LA 71241
(318) 368-9348

Michigan

Michigan Institute for Thermography
120 State St.
Howell, MI 48843
(517) 546-3967

William Dudley, D.C., D.I.A.B.C.T.,
F.A.B.C.T.
1181 South Main St.
Plymouth, MI 48170
(734) 455-2145

Nebraska

Mark Osborn, D.C., D.A.B.C.T.
6001 S. 58th St., Suite F
Lincoln, NE 68516
402) 423-8226

Body Scan
Chris Driscoll, D.C., Provisional C.T.T.
13304 W. Center Rd., Suite 126
Omaha, NE 68144
(402) 334-5533
www.wescanu.com

West Holt Memorial Hospital
406 West Neely St.
Atkinson, NE 68713
(402) 925-2811
www.westholtmed.org

New Jersey

Thermographic Diagnostic Imaging
Philip Getson, D.O.
100 Brick Rd., Suite 206
Marlton, NJ 08053
(856) 596-5834

(Every three months, Dr. Getson goes to NYC to do thermograms. He will travel anywhere within his area for four or more appts.)

New Mexico

Medical Advantage Imaging, Inc.
Janet Greene, M.D., Dennis Kramer, N.D.
2019 Galisteo, Suite N4
Santa Fe, NM 87505
(505) 984-0700

New York

Global Wellness
Moshe Dekel, M.D.
373 Sunrise Hwy.
W. Babylon, NY 11704
(631) 422-2424

Ohio

Hal Blatman, M.D., D.A.A.P.M.
10653 Techwoods Circle, Suite 101
Cincinnati, OH 45242
(513) 956-3200
www.blatmanpainclinic.com

Pennsylvania

Gregory Johnson, D.C.
800 West Fourth St.
Park Place, Suite G-02
Williamsport, PA 17701
(570) 323-8961

Texas

Optimal Natural Health Center
Leilani Tejeda, C.T.T.
660 Preston Forest Center, Suite 330
Dallas, TX 75230
(888) 641-2547
www.optimalnaturalhealth.com

Wisconsin

Christian Medical Center
William Hobbins, M.D., F.A.C.S.,
    F.A.B.C.T.
5510 Medical Circle, Suite B
Madison, WI 53719
(608) 273-4274

Canada

**Ville Marie Medical and Womens
    Health Center**
John R. Keyserlingk, M.D., F.A.C.S.
1538, rue Sherbrooke Ouest, Suite 1000
Montreal, QC H3G 1I5
(514) 933-2778
www.villemariemed.com

John Keyserlingk, M.D., FACS
1538, rue Sherbrooke Ouest, Suite 1001
Montreal, QC H3G 1I5
(514) 933-9635

England

**Royal National Hospital for
    Rheumatic Diseases**
E.F.J. Ring, Ph.D.
Upper Borough Walls
Bath, BA1 1RL
United Kingdom
www.rnhrd.nhs.uk

France

**Louis Pasteur University School
    of Medicine**
Biomedical Thermology Laboratory
Michel Gautherie, Ph.D.
11, rue Humann
67085 Strasbourg Cedex
France

Resources

Chapter 1

De-chlorinating Shower and Bath Filters

Showerhead and bath balls from Rainshow'r: (800) 728-2288

Iodine-loading Test

Jorge Flechas, M.D., #80 Doctor's Drive, Suite 3, Hendersonville, NC 28792; www.helpmythyroid.com or (828) 684-3233
Price of test: $75 (includes shipping).

Iodine Studies

For copies of iodine studies, contact Dr. Guy E. Abraham at optimox@iname.com or (800) 223-1601
Available to healthcare practitioners only.

Seaweeds

Naturespirit Herbs, P.O. Box 150, Williams, OR 97544; www.naturespiritherbs.com or (541) 846-7995.
Clean, good-quality seaweeds, including capsules of powdered Fucus (best for the thyroid), as well as capsules of powdered green and red seaweeds.

Ocean Harvest Sea Vegetable Company, P.O. Box 1719, Mendocino, CA 95460; www.ohsv.net; e-mail ohveggies@pacific.net or (707) 937-0637
Sells a variety of seaweeds in 1-ounce packages. This is an inexpensive way to see which varieties you like. They also have a recipe booklet to help you integrate the different seaweeds into your diet.

Ryan Drum Island Herbs & Kelp, P.O. Box 25, Waldron Island, WA 98297; www.ryandrum.com
Various forms of seaweed are available, including powdered Bullwhip kelp and Fucus (bladder wrack). To schedule an appointment with Dr. Drum, e-mail him at RyanDrum2020@yahoo.com. (You will need a referral from a caregiver before he will make an appointment.)

Chapter 2

Books

The Probiotic Solution by Mark Brudnak (Dragon Door Publications, 2003)
Explains the differences between many of the popular formulas.

Probiotic Formulas

Advanced Probiotic Formula from Women's Preferred: www.womenspreferred.com
or (800) 728-2288
*A combination of strong probiotics that survive stomach acid and colonize in the
intestines for one-half to one-third the price of other excellent formulas.*

Dr. Ohhira's Probiotics 12-Plus from Healthy by Nature: www.probiotics12.com or
(877) 262-7843
Mention this book and they'll give you a discount.

Healthy Trinity from Natren: www.natren.com or (866) 462-8736
*This formula costs $59.95 for a one-month supply of thirty capsules and needs to be
refrigerated. Mention my* Women's Health Letter *and your price drops to $47.96 for
as long as you order this product from them.*

Chapter 3

Medicinal Mushroom Formulas

Pure *Cordyceps* from Eclectic Institute: www.eclecticherb.com or (800) 332-4372
Take two capsules after heavy exercise, or one to two capsules daily.

Trimyco-gen from Gourmet Mushrooms: www.mycopia.com or (800) 789-9121
*This formula contains equal amounts of reishi, shiitake, and Cordyceps. The least
expensive form is the powder, which has a mild, pleasant taste. Order two bottles
at once for a large savings. I use one-half teaspoon of this powder almost daily,
and especially after heavy physical activity.*

MycoPhyto Complex from Advanced Bionutritionals: www.advancedbionutritionals.
com or (800) 728-2288
*This strong immune formula contains Cordyceps, along with five other medicinal mush-
rooms—all grown on immune-enhancing herbs. I take two to three capsules every day.*

Usnea Tinctures

Usnea liquid extracts from Herb Pharm: www.herb-pharm.com or (800) 348-HERB
(4372)

Usnea extracts from Eclectic Institute: www.eclecticherb.com or (800) 332-4372

Chapter 4

Books

The Antibiotic Alternative by Cindy L.A. Jones, Ph.D. (Healing Arts Press, 2000)

Herbal Antibiotics by Stephen Harrod Buhner (Storey Books, 1999)

Chapter 5

Books

Padma: An Ancient Tibetan Herbal Formula by Nan Kathryn Fuchs, Ph.D. (Basic Health Publications, 2003)

Padma

EcoNugenics: www.econugenics.com or (800) 308-5518
For circulatory problems, begin with 2 tablets, three times a day, for two to four months. Reduce to 2 tablets, two times a day for a total of six months. As a maintenance dose, take 1 tablet, two times a day.
Women's Preferred: www.womenspreferred.com or (800) 728-2288

Chapter 6

Books

Brain Fitness by Robert Goldman, M.D., D.O., Ph.D. (Doubleday, 1999)

BrainRecovery.com by David Perlmutter, M.D. (Perlmutter Health Center, 2000)

Natural Hormone Balance for Women by Uzzi Reiss, M.D. (Atria, 2002)

The Memory Solution by Julian Whitaker, M.D. (Avery Publishing, 1999)

Supplements

Advanced Memory Formula from Women's Preferred: www.womenspreferred.com or (800) 728-2288

Quality pregnenolone (25 mg) and phosphatidyl serine (100 mg) from ProThera: www.protherainc.com or (888) 488-2488

Chapter 7

Supplements

Alpha-lipoic Acid Supplements and Fomulas

Alpha-lipoic acid (100 mg) from ProThera: www.protherainc.com or (888) 488-2488

Alpha-lipoic acid from Source Naturals (50–300 mg)

Available in most health-food stores.

Advanced Vision Formula from Women's Preferred: www.womenspreferred.com or (800) 728-2288

Chapter 8

Books

ConsumerLab.com's Guide to Buying Vitamins & Supplements by Tod Cooperman (ConsumerLab.com, 2003)

User's Guide to Calcium and Magnesium by Nan Kathryn Fuchs (Basic health Publications, 2002)

Multivitamin/Mineral Supplements

High-quality supplement suppliers that offer money-back guarantee. Ask them for catalogs or brochures.

ProThera: www.protherainc.com or (888) 488-2488

Rainbow Light: easily found in health-food stores

Source Naturals: easily found in health-food stores

Women's Preferred: www.womenspreferred.com or (800) 728-2288

Quality Herbal Formulas

HerbPharm: www.herb-pharm.com or 800-348-4372

Zand Herbals: (800) 232-4005

Quality PMS and Osteoporosis Formulas

Gynovite (for osteoporosis prevention) from Optimox: www.optimox.com or (800) 223-1601

Optivite (for PMS) from Optimox: www.optimox.com or (800) 223-1601

Tests to Assess Antioxidant and Nutritional Status

SpectraCell Laboratory: www.spectracell.com or (800) 227-5227
Many insurance companies reimburse for these tests. This lab accepts Medicare assignment. Call for specific information.

To Locate a Healthcare Practitioner in Your Area

American Association of Naturopathic Physicians (AANP): www.naturopathic.org or (866) 538-2267

American College for Advancement in Medicine (ACAM): www.acam.org or (800) 532-3688

American Holistic Health Association: www.ahha.org/ahhaprs.htm or (714) 799-6152

American Holistic Medical Association: www.holisticmedicine.org or (505) 292-7788

American Osteopathic Association: www.osteopathic.org or (800) 621-1773

International Society for Orthomolecular Medicine (ISOM): www.orthomed.org or (416) 733-2117

Chapter 9

Books

Why Stomach Acid is Good for You by Jonathan V. Wright, M.D. and Lane Lenard, Ph.D. (M. Evans and Company, 2001)

Probiotic Supplements

Advanced Probiotic Formula from Women's Preferred: www.womenspreferred.com or (800) 728-2288

A combination of strong probiotics that survive stomach acid and colonize in the intestines for one-half to one-third the price of other excellent formulas.

Dr. Ohhira's Probiotics 12-Plus from Healthy by Nature: www.probiotics12.com or (877) 262-7843
Mention this book and they'll give you a discount.

Healthy Trinity from Natren: www.natren.com or (866) 462-8736
This formula costs $59.95 for a one-month supply of thirty capsules and needs to be refrigerated. Mention my Women's Health Letter *and your price drops to $47.96 for as long as you order this product from them.*

Standardized Turmeric Capsules

Tea Garden Herbal Emporium: www.teagarden.com or (800) 288-4372

Chapter 10

Books

Healthy Digestion by David Hoffman, B.Sc. (Storey Books, 2000)

Chapter 11

Books

Dairy-Free & Delicious by Brenda Davis, R.D. (Book Publishing Company, 2001)

Digestive Wellness by Elizabeth Lipski, M.S., C.C.N. (3rd edition, McGraw-Hill, 2004)

The Yeast Connection and Women's Health by William G. Crook, M.D., Hyla Cass, M.D., and Elizabeth B. Crook (Professional Books, 2005)

Chapter 12

Candida Tests

Comprehensive Stool Analysis Candida Test from Genova Diagnostics: www.GDX.net or (800) 522-4762

Genetic Candida Test, contact Dr. Steven Witkin's team: switkin@med.cornell.edu or (212) 746-3165

Chapter 13

Books

Guess What Came to Dinner? by Ann Louise Gittleman, M.S., C.N.S. (Penguin/Putnam, 2001)

Ulcer Free! Nature's Safe and Effective Remedy for Ulcers by George Halpern, M.D. (Square One Publishing, 2004)

Diagnostic Tests

Intestinal Permeability Assessement Test from Genova Diagnostics: www.GDX.net or (800) 522-4762

Parasite Tests from Genova Diagnostics: www.GDX.net or (800) 522-4762

Uni Key Health Systems: www.unikeyhealth.com or (800) 888-4353/(208)762-6833

Chapter 14

Books

Natural Highs by Hyla Cass, M.D. and Patrick Holford (Avery Publishing, 2003)

Overcoming the Legacy of Overeating by Nan Kathryn, Fuchs, Ph.D. (Lowell House, 1999)

The Packard Weight Health Plan by Andrew Packard, M.D. (Ballantine Books, 2004)

Supplements

Advanced Diet Support from Women's Preferred: www.womenspreferred.com or (800) 728-2288

TheraSlim from ProThera: www.protherainc.com or (888) 488-2488

Chapter 15

Books

The Fast Track One-Day Detox Diet by Ann Louise Gittleman, M.S., C.N.S. (Morgan Road/Broadway Books, 2005)

The Fat Flush Plan by Ann Louise Gittleman, M.S., C.N.S. (McGraw-Hill, 2002)

Chapter 16

Books

Lick the Sugar Habit by Nancy Appleton (Avery Publishing, 1996)

Staying Healthy with Nutrition by Elson Haas (Celestial Arts, 1992)

The Stevia Cookbook by Ray Sahelian, M.D. and Donna Gates (Avery Publishing, 1999)

Stevia Dessert Cookbook by Kristen Younger (self-published; to order send $10 plus shipping to 1948 Pleasant Hill Road, Sebastopol, CA 95472)

Chapter 17

Products

Coconut crème (for cooking) from Botanical Preservation Corps: Box 1368, Sebastopol, CA 95473 or www.botanicalpreservationcorp.com

Chapter 18

Books

Overcoming the Legacy of Overeating by Nan Kathryn Fuchs, Ph.D. (Lowell House, 1999)

The Packard Weight Health Plan by Andrew Packard, M.D. (Ballantine Books, 2003)

Natural Highs by Hyla Cass, M.D. and Patrick Holford (Avery Publishing, 2003)

Smart Medicine for Your Skin by Jeanette Jacknin, M.D. (Avery Publishing, 2001)

User's Guide to Calcium and Magnesium by Nan Kathryn Fuchs, Ph.D. (Basic Health, 2002)

The Wrinkle-Free Zone by James Meschino, D.C, M.S. (Basic Health, 2004)

Gotu Kola and Horse Chestnut Extracts

HerbPharm: www.herb-pharm.com or call (800) 348-4372

Skin-Care Products

Z Mei skin-care products: http://zmei.net or call (800) 576-0232
Mention this book and receive 25 percent off your first order.

Chapter 19

Books

Before the Change by Ann Louise Gittleman, M.S., C.N.S. (HarperSanFrancisco, 2004)

Hormone Replacement Therapy: Yes or No? by Betty Kamen, Ph.D. (*Nutrition Encounter,* 2002)

Natural Hormone Balance for Women by Reiss Uzzi, M.D. (Atria, 2002)

The Cortisol Connection by Shawn Talbott, Ph.D. (Hunter House, 2002)

DHEA Supplements

ProThera: www.protherainc.com or (888) 488-2488

Natural Compounding Pharmacies

Belmar Pharmacy: www.belmarpharmacy.com or (800) 525-9473

Women's International Pharmacy: www.womensinternational.com or (800) 279-5708

Chapter 21

Books

Iodine: Why You Need It, Why You Can't Live Without It by David Brownstein, M.D. (Medical Alternatives Press, 2004)

St. John's Wort: Nature's Blues Buster by Hyla Cass, M.D. (Avery Publications, 1997)

Ways to Better Breathing by Carola Speads (Healing Arts Press, 1992)

Herbal Formulas

Usnea barbata from HerbPharm at www.herb-pharm.com or 800-348-4372

Rhodiola rosea from Planetary Formulas at 800-606-6226

Herbal Lung Formula

Clear Lung Plus from Pacific Health Sciences available through Dr. Brian Roeteger, D.G. www.pacifichealth.com or (310-457-1775)

Iodine Information for Doctors

Optimox, Inc.: www.optimox.com or (800-223-1601)
Dr. Abraham will send an information packet on iodine including a two-hour CD PowerPoint presentation, studies, reports, and information on Iodoral to any physician at no charge.

Iodine-loading Test

Jorge Flechas, M.D., #80 Doctor's Drive, Suite 3, Hendersonville, NC 28792; www.helpmythyroid.com or (828) 684-3233
Price of test: $75 (includes shipping).

Indoral (Supplemental Iodine/Iodide)

Belmar Pharmacy: www.belmarpharmacy.com or (800) 525-9473
Available to consumers without a test if you're not on thyroid medications; if you're on medications, talk with the pharmacists first about being monitored by your doctor.

Jorge Flechas, M.D.: For contact information, see "Iodine-loading Test" above.
Available after test determines a need a need for it.

Optimox, Inc.: www.optimox.com or (800) 223-1601
Available to physicians only.

Chapter 23

Ignatia 30C and books on homeopathy

Homeopathic Educational Services (Dana Ullman): www.homeopathic.com or (800) 359-9051

Chapter 25

Additional Information on Prolotherapy

Dr. Thomas Dorman: www.paracelsusclinic.com

Books

Prolo Your Pain Away: Curing Chronic Pain with Prolotherapy by Ross A. Hauser, M.D. (Beulah Land Press, 1998)

To locate a doctor using prolotherapy

American Association of Orthopedic Medicine (AAOM): www.aaomed.org; (800) 992-2063

American College for Advancement in Medicine (ACAM): www.acam.org; (800) 532-3688

American College of Osteopathic Pain Management and Sclerotherapeutic Pain Management (ACOPMS): www.acopms.com; (800) 471-6114

National web listing: www.getprolo.com

Chapter 26

Books

Why Am I Always So Tired? by Ann Louise, M.S., C.N.S. (HarperSanFrancisco, 2000)

What Your Doctor May Not Tell You About Migraines by Alexander Mauskop, M.D. (Warner Books, 2001)

Supplements

Rainbow Light's MigraSolve: www.rainbowlight.com or (800) 548-8686

Dr. Mauskop's MigreLief: www.migrahealth.org or (800) 758-8746

Chapter 27

Books

Reflexology: Health at Your Fingertips by Barbara and Kevin Kunz (DK Publishing, 2003)

Stretching by Bob Anderson (Shelter Publications, Inc., 2000)

Reflexology Charts

Small hand and foot reflexology charts are available from Reflexology Research, P.O. Box 35820, Albuquerque, NM 87176; (505) 344-9392: www.reflexology-research.com

Chapter 28

Books

User's Guide to Calcium and Magnesium by Nan Kathryn Fuchs, Ph.D. (Basic Health Publications, 2002)

Supplements

Cetyl Myristoleate Supplements

CM-Plus from Longevity Science: www.longevity-science.net or (800) 933-9440

Myristin from EHP Products: www.cetylmyristoleate.com or (888) 347-0100

Chapter 29

Books

Chronic Fatigue, Fibromyalgia and Lyme Disease by Burton Goldberg and Larry Trivieri, Jr., 2nd edition (Celestial Arts, 2004)

Chronic Fatigue Syndrome by Michael T, Murray, N.D. (Prima Publishing, 1994)

From Fatigued to Fantastic by Jacob Teitelbaum, M.D. (Avery Publishing, 2001)

User's Guide to Calcium and Magnesium by Nan Kathryn Fuchs, Ph.D. (Basic Health, 2002)

Supplements

Super Malic Plus from Optimox: www.optimox.com or (800) 223-1601

Magna-Calm from Longevity Science: www.longevity-science.net or (800) 933-9440
A well-tolerated powdered magnesium supplement.

Chapter 30

Topical Antivirals

Shingle Aid from Simplers Botanicals: www.simplers.com or (800) 652-7646
Available from Rosemary's Garden: www.rosemarysgarden.com or (707) 829-2539

Shingle-Eeze from Merix Health Care Products: www.viramedx.com or (800) 224-4024

Chapter 31

Books & Sites for Additional Information

Before the Change by Ann Louise Gittleman, M.S., C.N.S. (2nd edition, HarperSanFrancisco, 2004)

Hormone Replacement Therapy: Yes or No? by Kamen, Betty, Ph.D. (Nutrition Encounter, 2002)

Natural Hormone Balance for Women by Uzzi Reiss, M.D. (Pocket Books, 2001)

Natural Hormone Replacement for Women Over 45 by Jonathan V. Wright, M.D., and John Morgenthaler (Smart Publications, 1997)

Natural Progesterone Advisory Network: www.natural-progesterone-advisory-network.com

Preventing and Reversing Osteoporosis by Alan R. Gaby, M.D. (Prima Publishing, 1995)

Natural Compounding Pharmacies

Belmar Pharmacy: www.belmarpharmacy.com or (800) 525-9473

Women's International Pharmacy: www.womensinternational.com or (800) 279-5708

Progesterone Cream

PureGest from Kevala: www.kevalahealth.com or (800) 826-7225

Chapter 32

Books

Resetting the Clock: Five Anti-Aging Hormones That Improve and Extend Life by Elmer Cranton, M.D. and William Fryer (M. Evans and Co., Inc, 1997)

To Locate Doctor Who Uses HGH

American Academy of Anti-Aging Medicine: www.worldhealth.net or (773) 528-1000; in Florida: (561) 997-0112

Hormone Supplements

ProThera: www.protherainc.com or (888) 488-2488

Chapter 33

Books

Super Nutrition for Menopause by Ann Louise Gittleman, Ph.D., C.N.S. (revised edition, Bantam, 2004)

Women's Encyclopedia of Natural Medicine by Tori Hudson, N.D. (Keats Publishing, 1999)

Hot Flash Formulas

Hot Flash Formula from Women's Preferred: www.wwomenspreferred.com or (800) 728-2288

EstroThera from ProThera: www.protherainc.com or (888) 488-2488

Chapter 34

Books

The Myth of Osteoporosis by Gillian Sanson (MCD Century Publications, 2003)

Perfect Bones by Pamela Levin, R.N. (Celestial Arts, 2002)

User's Guide to Calcium and Magnesium by Nan Kathryn Fuchs, Ph.D. (Basic Health Publications, 2002)

Chapter 35

Books

Food and Our Bones by Annemarie Colbin (Plume, 1998)

Pilates on the Ball by Colleen Craig; includes book and DVD (Healing Arts Press, 2003)

DVDs and Videos

Pilates for Beginners by Gaiam (available on DVD only): www.gaiam.com or (877) 989-6321

Pilates Powerhouse DVD Collection by Gaiam (available on DVD only): www.gaiam.com or (877) 989-6321

Products

OsteoBall Bone Fitness Exerciser: www.bonefitness.com or (310) 458-1102

Chapter 36

Books

Tooth Fitness by Thomas McGuire, D.D.S. (St. Michael's Press, 1994)

Products

The Germ Terminator GT-100: www.germterminator.com or (800) 247-1000
Regularly $49.99, but mention this book and the price drops to $39.99!

Supplements

Resveratrol Plus from Women's Preferred: www.wwomenspreferred.com or
(800) 728-2288

Chapter 38

Books & Sites for Additional Information

American Federation for Aging Research. "The latest research on the role of
inflammation in heart disease," www.infoaging.org (accessed October 24, 2004)

The Heart Revolution by Kilmer S. McCully, M.D. (Harper, 2000)

The Inflammation Syndrome by Jack Challem (John Wiley & Sons, Inc., 2003)

Padma: An Ancient Tibetan Herbal Formula by Nan Kathryn Fuchs, Ph.D., (Basic
Health Publications, 2003)

Stopping Inflammation by Nancy Appleton, Ph.D. (Square One Press, 2005)

Why Your Toothbrush May Be Killing You by James Song (American Health
Conferences, Henderson, NV, 2004)

Fish Oils Guaranteed to Be Contaminant Free

Marine Fish Oil from ProThera: ProThera: www.protherainc.com or (888) 488-2488

Mixed Fatty Acids from Women's Preferred: www.womenspreferred.com or
(800) 728-2288

Super Omega-3 from Carlson Laboratories: www.carlsonlabs.com or (888) 234-5656
Easily found in health-food stores.

Herbal Anti-Inflammatories

InflaThera from ProThera: www.protherainc.com or (888) 488-2488
A one-month supply of this strong formula is $20/month.

Zyflamend from New Chapter: www.new-chapter.com or (800) 543-7279
Also available in many health-food stores. Price is around $28 for a two-month supply.

Padma Basic

EcoNugenics: www.econugenics.com or (800) 308-5518

Women's Preferred: www.womenspreferred.com or (800) 728-2288

Chapter 39

Books

An Alternative Medicine Guide to Heart Disease, Stroke & High Blood Pressure by Burton Goldberg (Future Medicine Publishing, 1998)

Modified Citrus Pectin (MCP) by Nan Kathryn Fuchs, PhD. (Basic Health, Publications, 2003)

Supplements

Resveratrol

Resveratrol Plus from Women's Preferred: www.womenspreferred.com or (800) 728-2288

Grape Extract with Resveratrol from ProThera: www.protherainc.com or (888) 488-2488

Grape Seed Extract from Source Naturals: available in health-food stores

Guggulipid and Policosinol

Advanced Cholesterol Formula from Women's Preferred: www.womenspreferred.com or (800) 728-2288

PectaSol (Modified Citrus Pectin)

EcoNugenics: www.econugenics.com or (800) 308-5518

Longevity Science: www.longevity-science.net or (800) 933-9440

Pure Encapsulations: www.purecaps.com or (800) 753-2277

Chapter 40

Books

Healthy Fats for Life by Lorna R. Vanderhaeghe, B.Sc. and Karlene Karst, B.Sc., R.D. (2nd edition, John Wiley & Sons, 2004)

Know Your Fats by Mary G. Enig, Ph.D. (Bethesda Press, 2000)

Safe Food: Eating Wisely in a Risky World by Michael F. Jacobson, Ph.D., et al. (reprint edition, Berkley Publishing Group, 1993)

Mercury- and Pesticide-Free Supplements

Mixed Fatty Acids from Women's Preferred: www.womenspreferred.com or (800) 728-2288

Super Omega-3 from Carlson Laboratories: www.carlsonlabs.com or (888) 234-5656
Easily found in health-food stores.

Marine Fish Oil from ProThera: www.protherainc.com or (888) 488-2488

Chapter 41

Books

An Alternative Medicine Guide to Heart Disease, Stroke & High Blood Pressure by Burton Goldberg, (Future Medicine Publishing, 1998)

Prescription Alternatives by Earl Mindell, R.Ph., Ph.D. (3rd edition, McGraw-Hill, 2003)

Chapter 42

Nattokinase Supplements

FliteTabs from ARC Nutrition: www.flitetabs.com or (877) 272-3508

Rutozym from WobenzymUSA: www.wobenzym.com or (888) 766-4406
Best price through www.wobenzym.com.

Chapter 43

Books

The High Blood Pressure Solution by Richard D. Moore, M.D., Ph.D. (2nd edition, Healing Arts Press, 2001)

How to Meditate by Lawrence LeShan (reissued, Little Brown, 1999)

The New Becoming Vegetarian by Vesanto Melina, M.S., R.D. and Brenda Davis, R.D. (Healthy Living Publications, 2003)

Overcoming the Legacy of Overeating by Nan Kathryn Fuchs, Ph.D. (3rd edition, Lowell House, 1999)

Chapter 44

Coenzyme Q_{10}

Chewable CoQ_{10} tablets made with lecithin from Women's Preferred: www.womenspreferred.com or (800) 728-2288

Books

User's Guide to Heart-Healthy Supplements by Michael Janson, M.D. (Basic Health Publications, 2004)

Chapter 46

Books

Life's Delicate Balance: Causes and Prevention of Breast Cancer by Janette D. Sherman, M.D. (Taylor & Francis, 2000)

Calcium D-Glucarate

ProThera: www.protherainc.com or (888) 488-2488

Thorne Research www.thorne.com or (800) 228-1966

Advanced Physicians' Products: www.nutritiononline.com or (800) 220-7687

Natrol: www.natrol.com or (800) 326-1520

Folic Acid

Folazin from ProThera: www.protherainc.com or (888) 488-2488

Herbal Anti-Inflammatory

InflaThera from ProThera: www.protherainc.com or (888) 488-2488

Indole 3-Carbinol

ProThera: www.protherainc.com or (888) 488-2488

Thorne Research: www.thorne.com or (800) 228-1966

Medicinal Mushroom Formula

MycoPhyto Complex from Advanced Bionutritionals:
www.advancedbionutritionals.com or (800) 728-2288

Progesterone Cream

PureGest from Kevala: www.kevalahealth.com or (800) 826-7225

Chapter 47

Books and Other Sources of Information

CANHELP: www.canhelp.com or (800) 565-1732

Cancer Survivor's Nutrition & Health Guide, by Gene Spiller, Ph.D., and Bruce, Bonnie, R.D. (Prima Publishing, 1996)

Herbs Against Cancer by Ralph Moss, Ph.D. (Equinox Press, 1998)

The Moss Reports by Ralph Moss, Ph.D.
Contain information on your specific cancer diagnosis. Reports can be downloaded from his website (www.cancerdecisions.com) or ordered by phone (800-980-1234). Sign up at his website for free Cancer Decisions e-mail newsletter.

Questioning Chemotherapy by Ralph Moss, Ph.D. (Equinox Press, 1995)

Chapter 48

Books

Modified Citrus Pectin: A Super Nutraceutical by Nan Kathryn Fuchs, Ph.D. (Basic Health Publications, 2003)

PectaSol

EcoNugenics: www.econugenics.com or (800) 308-5518
Dr. Eliaz's company provides technical support for healthcare practitioners.

Longevity Science: www.longevity-science.net or (800) 933-9440

Women's Preferred: www.womenspreferred.com or (800) 728-2288

Chapter 49

Books

Cancer Salves: A Botanical Approach to Treatment by Ingrid Naiman (Seventh Ray Press, 1999)

D-Glucarate: A Nutrient Against Cancer, by Thomas J. Slaga, Ph.D. and Judi Quilici-Timmcke, M.S. (Keats Publishing, 1999)

The Grape Cure by Johanna Brandt (Benedict Lust Publications, 1971)

Calcium D-Glucarate

Advanced Physicians' Products: www.nutritiononline.com or 800-220-7687

Natrol: www.natrol.com or (800) 326-1520

ProThera: www.protherainc.com or (888) 488-2488

Thorne Research: www.thorne.com or (800) 228-1966

Resveratrol

Resveratrol Plus from Women's Preferred: www.womenspreferred.com or (800) 728-2288

Grape Extract with Resveratrol from ProThera: www.protherainc.com or (888) 488-2488

Grape Seed Extract from Source Naturals: available in health-food stores

References

Chapter 1

Abraham, GE. "Iodine supplementation markedly increases urinary excretion of fluoride and bromide," *The Townsend Letter for Doctors,* May 2003: 105–06.

Abraham, GE. "The safe and effective implementation of orthoiodosupplementation in medical practice," Optimox Corporation, 2004. [report]

Abraham, GE, et al. "Orthoiodosupplementation: iodine sufficiency of the whole human body," *The Original Internist,* 2002; 9: 30–41.

Abraham, GE, JD Flechas, and JC Hakala. "Effect of daily ingestion of a tablet containing 5 mg iodine and 7.5 mg iodide as the potassium salt, for a period of three months, on the results of thyroid function tests and thyroid volume by ultrasonometry in 10 euthyroid caucasian women," Optimox Research Info, March 16, 2002. [report or study]

Brownstein, D. *Iodine: Why You Need It, Why You Can't Live Without It,* Medical Alternatives Press, 2004.

Drum, R. "Botanicals for thyroid function and dysfunction," Medicines from the Earth. Official proceedings, 3–5, June 2000.

Konno, N, et al. "Clinical evaluation of the iodide/creatinine ratio of casual urine samples as an index of daily iodide excretion in a population study," *Endocrine Journal,* 1993; 40: 163–69.

Persky, VW, et al. "Effect of soy protein on endogenous hormones in postmenopausal women," *American Journal of Clinical Nutrition,* 2002; 75(1): 145–53.

Chapter 2

Agerholm, JS, et al. "A preliminary study on the pathogenicity of *Bacillus licheniformis* bacteria in immunodepressed mice," *APMIS,* Jan 1997.

Banerjee, C, et al. "Bacillus infections in patients with cancer," *Arch Intern Med,* 1998; 148(8): 1769-74.

European Commission Health & Consumer Protection Directorate-General, "Opinion of the scientific committee on animal nutrition on the use of *Bacillus licheniformis* NCTC 13123 in feedstuffs for pigs," April 18, 2002. [report]

European Commission Health & Consumer Protection Directorate-General, "Opinion on the use of certain micro-organisms as additives to feedstuffs," Oct 17, 2002.

"Guidelines for the evaluation of probiotics in food." Report of a joint FAO/WHO Working Group on drafting guidelines for the evaluation of probiotics in food, London Ontario, Canada, Apr 30–May 1, 2002.

Hamilton-Miller, JMT. "Bacillus spp as probiotics," Professor of Medical Microbiology, Royal Free & University College Medical School, June 5, 2002). [report]

Hoa, NT, et al. "Characterization of *Bacillus species* used for oral bacteriotherapy and bacterioprophylaxis of gastrointestinal disorders," *Applied and Environmental Microbiology,* Dec 2000; 66(12): 5241-47.

Hoa, NT, et al. "Fate and dissemination of *Bacillus subtilis* spores in a murine model." *Applied and Environmental Microbiology,* Sept 2001; 67(9): 3819-23.

Kawakami, M, et al. "The influence of lactic acid bacteria (OM-X) on bone structure," *Journal of Applied Nutrition,* 2003; 53(1).

Oggioni, MR, et al. "Recurrent septicemia in an immunocompromised patient due to probiotic strains of *Bacillus subtilis,*" *Journal of Clinical Microbiology,* Jan 1998.

Ohhira, I. "Studies on Lactic Acid Bacteria Enterococcus faecalis TH10," Biobank Co, Ltd, Okayama, Japan, 2003. [report]

Salkinoja-Lalonen, MS., et al. "Toxigenic strains of Bacillus licheniformis related to food poisoning," *Applied and Environmental Microbiology,* Oct 1999; 65(10): 4637-45.

Turnbull, P. "Bacillus," Medmicro Chapter 15, Graduate School of Biomedical Sciences at the University of Texas Medical Branch. [Report]

Yance, Donald. *Herbal Medicine, Healing & Cancer,* Keats Publishing, 1999.

Chapter 3

Halpern, George M. *Cordyceps: China's Healing Mushroom,* Avery Publishing, 1999.

Hobbs, Christopher. *Medicinal Mushrooms,* Botanica Press, 1986.

Lieberman, Shari and Ken Babal. *Maitake: King of Mushrooms,* Keats Publishing, 1997.

Xu, R and X Peng. "Effects of *Cordyceps sinesis* on natural killer cell activity and formation of Lewis lung carcinoma colonies," *Bulletin Human Medicine Collectives,* 1988.

Yance, Donald. *Herbal Medicine, Healing & Cancer,* Keats Publishing, 1999.

Ying, J., et al. *Icons of Medicinal Fungi from China,* translated by X Yuehan, Beijing: Science Press, 1987

Zhu, D "Recent advances on the active components in Chinese medicine," *Abstracts of Chinese Medicines,* 1987; 1.

Chapter 4

Buhner, Stephen Harrod. *Herbal Antibiotics,* Storey Books, 1999.

Hickling, Lee. "Antibiotics for the birds: FDA moves to withdraw approval," drcoop.com Health News (accessed Nov 3, 2000).

Hickling, Lee. "New antibiotic recommended for FDA approval," drkoop.com Health News (accessed April 5, 2000).

Jones, Cindy. *The Antibiotic Alternative,* Healing Arts Press, 2000.

Ray, WA, et al. "Oral erythromycin and the risk of sudden death from cardiac causes," *New England Journal of Medicine,* Sept 9, 2004.

Chapter 5

Drabaek, H, et al. "A botanical compound, Padma 28, increases walking distance in stable intermittent claudication," *Angiology,* Nov 1993; 44(11): 863–67.

Feyerer, Gabriele. *Padma: Integrating Ancient Wisdom and Modern Research Using Traditional Tibetan Herbs for Today's Diseases,* Lotus Press, 2003.

Khalsa, DS. "Integrated medicine and the prevention and reversal of memory loss," *Alternative Therapies,* Nov 1998; 4(6): 39–40.

Panjwani, HK, and MD Priestley. "Clinical evaluation of Padma 28 in treatment of senility and other geriatric circulatory disorders: a pilot study," Study report/personal communication, New Jersey, 1986: 1–15.

Schrader, R, et al. "Effects of the Tibetan herbal preparation Padma 28 in intermittent claudication," *Schweiz Med Wochenschr,* June 1985; 115(22): 752–56.

Smulski, HS. "Treatment of chronic ischemia of the lower extremities with complex herbal preparation," *Ann Acad Med Stetin,* 1991; 37: 191–92.

Winther, K, et al. "Padma 28, a botanical compound, decreases the oxidative burst response of monocytes and improves fibrinolysis in patients with stable intermittent claudication," *Fibrinolysis* 1994; 8(suppl 2): 47–49.

Wojcicki, J and L Smaochowiec. "Controlled double-blind study of Padma 28 in angina pectoris," *Herba Polonica,* 1986; 32: 107–14.

Wojcicki, J, et al. "Effect of Padma 28 on experimental hyperlipidaemia and atherosclerosis induced by high-fat diet in rabbits," *Phytotherapy Research,* 1988; 2(3): 119–23.

Chapter 6

Goldman, Robert. *Brain Fitness,* Doubleday, 1999.

Perlmutter, David. *BrainRecovery.com,* Perlmutter Health Center, 2000.

Whitaker, Julian. *The Memory Solution,* Avery Publishing, 1999.

Chapter 7

Hagen, TM. "Alpha-lipoic acid," Linus Pauling Institute, 2002–2003. [report]

Head, K. "Natural therapies for ocular disorders, part two: cataracts and glaucoma," *Alternative Medicine Review,* 2001; 6(2).

Jacques, PF, et al. "Long-term nutrient intake and early age-related nuclear lens opacities," *Arch Ophthalmol,* July 2001; 119(7).

Kottler, UB, et al. "Is a cataract avoidable? Current status with special emphasis on the pathophysiology of oxidative lense damage, nutritional factors, and the ARED study," *Ophthalmologe,* Mar 2003; 100(3).

Maitra, I, et al. "Alpha-lipoic acid prevents buthionine sulfoximine-induced cataract formation in newborn rats," *Rad Biol Med,* Apr 1995; 18(4).

Oc, P, et al. "Thioctic (lipoic) acid: a therapeutic metal chelating antioxidant?" *Biochemical Pharmacology,* 1995; 50.

Chapter 8

Alberto, Susanne. "Navigating the sea of coral calcium," Health Products Business, March 2003. [report]

Boerner, Paula. "Functional intracellular analysis of nutritional and antioxidant status," *J of Amer Nutraceut Assn,* 2001; 4(1).

Cooperman, Tod. *Calcium Review,* www.consumerlab.com.

Dragland S, H Senoo, K Wake, et al. "Several culinary and medicinal herbs are important sources of dietary antioxidants," *J Nutr,* May 2003; 133(5): 1286–90.

Hudson, Tori. *Women's Encyclopedia of Natural Medicine,* Keats Publishing, 1999.

Chapter 9

Sleisenger, Marvin and John Fordtran. *Gastrointestinal Disease,* 3rd edition, W.B. Saunders Company, 1978.

Wright, Jonathan V. and Lane Lenard. *Why Stomach Acid is Good for You,* M. Evans and Company, 2001.

Chapter 10

Hoffman, David. *Healthy Digestion,* Storey Books, 2000.

Robbers, James and Varro Tyler. *Tyler's Herbs of Choice,* Haworth Herbal Press, 1999.

Chapter 11

Crook, William G, Hyla Cass, and Elizabeth Crook. *The Yeast Connection and Women's Health,* Professional Books, 2003.

Davis, Brenda. *Dairy-Free & Delicious,* Book Publishing Company, 2001.

Lipski, Elizabeth. *Digestive Wellness,* Keats Publishing, 1996.

Chapter 12

Collin, J. "Treating candidiasis without nystatin, ketoconazole, or diflucan," *Townsend Letter for Doctors,* Dec 1996; 161.

Lahorz, S. Colet. *Conquering Yeast Infections: The Non-Drug Solution,* Pentland Press, 1996.

Martin, Jeanne Marie and P. Rona Zoltan. *Complete Candida Yeast Guidebook,* Prima Publishing, 1996.

"The PDR Family Guide to Women's Health and Prescription Drugs," *Medical Economics*, Montvale, NJ, 1994.

Pini, Pia. "New candidaemia patterns emerge in the USA," *Lancet,* Aug 1996; 348: 395.

Truss, C. Orian. *The Missing Diagnosis,* Birmingham, AL, 1983.

Witkin, SS, et al, personal conversation.

Chapter 13

Ackerson, A and Corey Resnick. "The effects of l-glutamine, n-acetyl-d-glucosamine, gamma-linolenic acid, and gamma-oryzanol on intestinal permeability," Tyler Encapsulations, *Townsend Letter for Doctors,* Jan 1993.

Monograph, *"Plantago ovata* (psyllium)," *Alternative Medicine Review,* 2002; 7(7): 155–59.

Murray, Michael and Joseph Pizzorno. *Encyclopedia of Natural Medicine,* Prima Publishing, 1998.

Rogers, Sherry A. *Wellness Against All Odds,* Prestige Publishing, 1994.

Shrive, E, et al. "Glutamine in treatment of peptic ulcer," *Tex J Med,* 1957; 53: 840–43.

Svedlud, J, et al. "Upper gastrointestinal and mental symptoms in the irritable bowel syndrome," *Scand J Gastroenterol,* 1985; 20.

Chapter 14

Fuchs, Nan Kathryn. *Overcoming the Legacy of Overeating,* Lowell House, 1999.

Chapter 15

Atkins, Robert. *Dr. Atkins' Age-Defying Diet Revolution,* St. Martin's Press, 2000.

Cherniske, Stephen. *The Metabolic Plan,* Ballantine Books, 2003.

Gittleman, Ann Louise. *The Fat Flush Plan,* McGraw-Hill, 2002.

Smith, Timothy J. *Renewal: The Anti-Aging Revolution,* St. Martin's Press, 1998.

Williams, Roger J. *Biochemical Individuality,* John Wiley & Sons, Inc, 1959.

Wright, Jonathan V. "The 'original human diet' secret to erasing cancer, diabetes, obesity, and more," *Nutrition & Healing Newsletter,* Jan 2003.

Chapter 16

Appleton, Nancy. *Lick the Sugar Habit,* Avery Publishing, 1996.

Haas, Elson. *Staying Healthy with Nutrition,* Celestial Arts, 1992.

Gardana, C, et al. "Metabolism of stevioside and rebaudioside A from *Stevia rebaudiana* extracts by human microflora," *J Agric Food Chem,* Oct 22, 2003.

Geuns, JM. "Stevioside," *Phytochemistry,* Nov 2003.

Jeppesen, PB, et al. "Stevioside induces antihyperglycaemic, insulinotropic and glucagonostatic effects in vivo," *Phytomedicine,* Jan 2002.

Tallmadge, Katherine. "Do Net Carbs Add Up?" *Washington Post,* Feb 25, 2004.

Willet, Walter. Harvard University, personal communication.

Yale-New Haven Nutrition Advisor, www.ynhh.org/online/nutrition/advisor. "Thinking about going low-carb?"

Chapter 17

Bruce Fife. *Eat Fat, Look Thin,* HeartWise, 2002.

Byrnes, Stephen. "'I've got a lovely bunch of coconuts: coconut holds promise for immune-suppressed people," *Townsend Letter for Doctors,* April 2002.

Enig, Mary G. *Know Your Fats,* Bethesda Press, 2000.

Fife, Bruce. *The Healing Miracles of Coconut Oil,* Piccadilly Books, 2001.

Rogers, Sherry A. "Genetic engineering makes nightshades doubly damaging," *Dr. Sherry Rogers' Total Wellness,* Oct 2000.

Chapter 18

"Adding vitamins to the mix: skin care products that can benefit the skin," American Academy of Dermatology, March 2000. [report]

Atkins, Robert C. *Dr. Atkins' Age-Defying Diet Revolution,* St. Martin's Press, 2000.

Begoun, Paula. *The Beauty Bible,* 2nd edition, Beginning Press, 2002.

Cherniske, Stephen. *The Metabolic Plan,* Ballantine Books, 2003.

Fuchs, Nan Kathryn. *Overcoming the Legacy of Overeating,* Lowell House, 1999.

Gittleman, Ann Louise. *The Fat Flush Plan,* McGraw-Hill, 2002.

Gugliotta, Guy. "FDA red flags dietary supplement: 134 cases of death or serious illness linked to ephedra," *Washington Post,* March 19, 2000.

Sies, H and W Stahl. "Nutritional protection against skin damage from sunlight," *Annu Rev Nutr,* 2004.

Smith, Timothy J. *Renewal: The Anti-Aging Revolution,* St. Martin's Press, 1998.

Tavakkol, A, et al. "Delivery of vitamin E to the skin by a novel liquid skin cleanser: comparison of topical versus oral supplementation," *J Cosmet Sci,* Mar-Apr 2004.

Uehara, M, et al. "A trial of oolong tea in the management of recalcitrant atopic dermatitis," *Archives of Dermatology,* 2001; 137.

Walter Willet, Harvard University, personal communication.

Williams, Roger J. *Biochemical Individuality,* John Wiley & Sons, Inc, 1959.

Wright, Jonathan. "The 'original human diet' secret to erasing cancer, diabetes, obesity, and more," *Nutrition & Healing Newsletter,* January 2003.

Yale-New Haven Nutrition Advisor, www.ynhh.org/online/nutrition/advisor. "Yale-New Haven Hopital dermatologist offers solutions to wintertime dry skin," Jan 16, 2004. [news release]

Chapter 19

Barnhart, KT, E Freeman, JA Grisso, et al. "The effect of dehydroepiandrosterone supplementation to symptomatic perimenopausal women on serum endocrine profiles, lipid parameters, and health-related quality of life." *J Clin Endocrinol Metab*, 1999; 84: 3896–902.

Cranton, Elmer, and William Fryer. *Resetting the Clock: 5 Anti-Aging Hormones That Improve and Extend Life*, M. Evans and Company, Inc, New York, 1996.

Gittleman, Ann Louise. *Before the Change*, HarperSanFrancisco, 1998.

Helzlsouer, KJ, AJ Alberg, GB Gordon, et al. "Serum gonadotropins and steroidhormones and the development of ovarian cancer." *Journal of the American Medical Association*, 1995; 274: 1926–30.

Kamen, Betty. "Hormone Replacement Therapy: Yes or No?" *Nutrition Encounter*, 1997.

Lee, John R. *What Your Doctor May Not Tell You About Premenopause*, Time Warner, 1999.

Reiss, Uzzi. *Natural Hormone Balance for Women*, Pocket Books, 2001.

Wolf OT, O Neumann, DH Hellhammer, et al. "Effects of a two-week physiological dehydroepiandrosterone substitution on cognitive performance and well being in healthy elderly women and men." *J Clin Endocrinol Metab*, 1997; 82: 2363–67.

Zand, Janet, Allan Spreen, James LaValle. *Smart Medicine for Healthier Living*, Avery Publishing, 1999.

Chapter 20

Scheffer, Mechthild. *Bach Flower Therapy: Theory and Practice*, Thorsons Publishers, 1987.

Scheffer, Mechtild. *The Encyclopedia of Bach Flower Therapy*, Healing Arts Press, 2001.

Weeks, Nora. *The Medical Discoveries of Edward Bach*, C.W. Daniel Company, 1969.

Chapter 21

Abraham, GE. "The safe and effective implementation of orthoiodosupplementation in medical practice," Optimox Corporation, 2004. [report]

Blumenthal, Mark, et al. *The ABC Clinical Guide to Herbs*, American Botanical Council, 2003.

Brown, RP, et al. "*Rhodiola rosea*: a phytomedicinal overview," *HerbalGram*, 2002; 56.

Brownstein, David. *Iodine: Why You Need It; Why You Can't Live Without It*, Medical Alternatives Press, 2004.

Darbinyan, V, et al. "*Rhodiola rosea* in stress induced fatigue: a double blind cross-over study of a standardized extract SHR-5 with a repeated low-dose regimen on the mental performance of healthy physicians during night duty," *Phytomedicine*, 2000; 7(5).

Harer, G. "Hypericum and phototherapy," *Schweiz Rundsch Med Prax*, Dec 14, 2000. [article]

Manber, R., et al. "Alternative treatments for depression: empirical support and relevance to women," *J Clin Psychiatry*, Jul 2002.

"Monograph: *Rhodiola rosea,*" *Alternative Medicine Review,* 2002; 7(5).

Shevtsov, VA, et al. "A randomized trial of two different doses of a SHR-5 Rhodiola rosea extract versus placebo and control of capacity for mental work," *Phytomedicine,* Mar 2003.

Spasov, AA, et al. "A double-blind, placebo-controlled pilot study of the stimulating and adaptogenic effect of *Rhodiola rosea* by stress during an examination period with a repeated low-dose regimen," *Phytomedicine,* 2000; 7(2).

Werbach, Melvyn and Michael Murray. *Botanical Influences on Illness,* Third Line Press, 1994.

Zand, Janet, et al. *Smart Medicine for Healthier Living,* Avery Publishing, 1999.

Chapter 22

Harer, G. "Hypericum and phototherapy," *Schweiz Rundsch Med Prax,* Dec 14, 2000. [article]

Manber, R., et al. "Alternative treatments for depression: empirical support and relevance to women," *J Clin Psychiatry,* Jul 2002.

Zand, Janet, et al. *Smart Medicine for Healthier Living,* Avery Publishing, 1999.

Chapter 23

Chappell, Peter. *Emotional Healing with Homeopathy,* North Atlantic Books, 2003.

Chapter 24

Klein, Laura Cousino and Elizabeth Corwin. "Seeing the unexpected: how sex differences in stress responses may provide a new perspective on the manifestation of psychiatric disorders," *Current Psychiatry Reports,* 2002; 4: 441–48.

Taylor, Shelley, et al. "Behavioral responses to stress in females: tend-and-befriend, not fight-or-flight," *Psychological Review,* 2000; 107(3): 411–29.

Taylor, Shelley, et al. "Toward a biology of social support," *Handbook of Positive Psychology,* Oxford University Press, 2002.

Chapter 25

Dorman, Thomas. Paracelsus Clinic of Washington, 2505 S. 320th Street, Suite 100, Federal Way, WA 98003 (253-529-3050), e-mail: TD@Paracelsusclinic.com. [personal communication]

Hauser, Ross. Caring Medical and Rehabilitatin Services, 715 Lake Street, Suite 600, Oak Park, IL 60301 (708-848-7789) e-mail: drhauser@caringmedical.com. [personal communication]

Hauser, Ross and Marion Hauser. *Prolo Your Pain Away,* Beulah Land Press, 2000.

Kennedy, Ron. *The Thinking Person's Guide to Perfect Health,* Context Publications, 1996.

Ongley, MJ, RG Klein, TA Dorman, et al. "A new approach to the treatment of chronic low back pain." *Lancet,* Jul 1987; 2(8551): 143–146.

Reeves, KD and K Hassanein. "Randomized prospective double-blind placebo-controlled study of dextrose prolotherapy for knee osteoarthritis with or without ACL laxity," *Altern Ther Health Med,* Mar 2000; 6(2).

Tunick, Barbara. Article on prolotherapy, *Woman's World Magazine,* May 23, 2000.

Wood, Sylvia. Article on prolotherapy, *Albany Times Union,* 1998.

Chapter 26

Green, Steven. "Migraine," *The Townsend Letter for Doctors,* Nov 2000.

Hauser, Ross and Marion Hauser. *Prolo Your Headaches & Neck Pain Away,* Beulah Land Press, 2000.

Mauskop, Alexander. *What Your Doctor May Not Tell You About Migraines,* Warner Books, 2001.

Murphy, JJ, et al. "Randomised double-blind placebo-controlled trial of feverfew in migraine prevention," *The Lancet,* July 23, 1988.

Murray, Michael and Joseph, Pizzorno. *Encyclopedia of Natural Medicine,* 2nd edition, Prima Health, 1998.

Werbach, Melvyn. *Textbook of Nutritional Medicine,* Third Line Press, 1999.

Werbach, Melvyn and Michael Murray. *Botanical Influences on Illness,* Third Line Press, 1994.

Zand, Janet, et al. *Smart Medicine for Healthier Living,* Avery Publishing, 1999.

Chapter 27

Anderson, Bob. *Stretching,* Shelter Publications, Inc., 2000.

Kunz, Barbara and Kevin. *Reflexology: Health at Your Fingertips,* DK Publishing, 2003.

Chapter 28

Hesslink, R, et al. "Cetylated fatty acids improve knee function in patients with osteoarthritis," *J Rheumatol,* Aug 2002; 29(8): 1708–12.

Hunter, KW, et al. "Synthesis of cetyl myristoleate and evaluation of its therapeutic efficacy in a murine model of collagen-induced arthritis," *Pharmacology Research,* Jan 2003; 47(1): 43–47.

Reeves, KD. personal communication, December 19, 2004.

Rogers, Sherry A. *Pain Free in 6 Weeks,* Prestige Publishing, 2001.

Chapter 29

Abraham, GE and J Flechas. "Management of fibromyalgia: rationale for the use of magnesium and malic acid," *Journal of Nutritional Medicine,* 1992; 3: 49–59.

Rogers, Sherry A. *Wellness Against All Odds,* Prestige Publishing, 1994.

Russell, John, et al. "Treatment of fibromyalgia syndrome with Super Malic: a randomized, double blind, placebo controlled, crossover pilot study," *Journal of Rheumatology,* 1995; 22: 5.

Werbach, Melvyn. *Textbook of Nutritional Medicine,* Third Line Press, 1999.

Chapter 30

Cummings, Stephen and Dana Ullman. *Everybody's Guide to Homeopathic Medicines,* Jeremy P. Tarcher, 1984.

Jacknin, Jeanette. *Smart Medicine for Your Skin,* Avery Publishing, 2001.

Mindell, Earl. *Prescription Alternatives,* Keats Publishing, 1998.

Chapter 31

Gittleman, Ann Louise. *Before the Change.* HarperSanFrancisco, 1998.

Hudson, Tori. *Women's Encyclopedia of Natural Medicine,* Keats Publishing, 1999.

Kamen, Betty. "Hormone Replacement Therapy: Yes or No?," *Nutrition Encounter,* 1997.

Lee, John R. *What Your Doctor May Not Tell You About Premenopause.* Time Warner, 1999.

Lobbo, Rogerio A. "Menopause management for the millennium," *Women's Health Clinical Management,* 2001; 1.

Reiss, Uzzi. *Natural Hormone Balance for Women,* Pocket Books, 2001.

Zand, Janet, Allan Spreen, and James LaValle. *Smart Medicine for Healthier Living,* Avery Publishing, 1999.

Chapter 32

Barnhart, KT, E Freeman, JA Grisso, et al. "The effect of dehydroepiandrosterone supplementation to symptomatic perimenopausal women on serum endocrine profiles, lipid parameters, and health-related quality of life." *J Clin Endocrinol Metab.* 1999; 84: 3896–902.

Cranton, Elmer and William Fryer. *Resetting the Clock: Five Anti-Agining Hormones That Improve and Extend Life,* M. Evans and Co, Inc, 1996.

Helzlsouer, KJ, AJ Alberg, GB Gordon, et al. "Serum gonadotropins and steroidhormones and the development of ovarian cancer." *JAMA,* 1995; 274:1926–30.

Henson, Shari. "HerbClip," 010242–255, April 30, 2004. www.herbalgram.org.

Wolf OT, O Neumann, DH Hellhammer, et al. "Effects of a two-week physiological dehydroepiandrosterone substitution on cognitive performance and well being in healthy elderly women and men." *J Clin Endocrinol Metab,* 1997; 82:2363–67.

Chapter 33

Arici, A and O Bukulmez. "Phyto-oestrogens and the endometrium," *Lancet,* Dec 11, 2004.

Blumenthal, Mark. *Herbal Medicine: Expanded Commission E Monographs,* Integrative Medicine Communications, 2000.

Editorial: "HRT: what are women (and their doctors) to do?," *The Lancet,* Dec 11, 2004.

Gittleman, Ann Louise. *Super Nutrition for Menopause,* Avery Publishing, 1998.

Hudson, Tori. *Women's Encyclopedia of Natural Medicine,* Keats Publishing, 1999.

PDR for Nutritional Supplements, Medical Economics Co., 2001.

Robbers, James E, and Varro E. Tyler. *Tyler's Herbs of Choice*, Haworth Herbal Press, 1999.

Smith, CJ. "Non-hormonal control of vaso-motor flushing in menopausal patients," *Chic Med*, Mar 7, 1964.

Stage, Sarah. *Female Complaints: Lydia Pinkham and the Business of Women's Medicine*, W.W. Norton & Co., 1979.

Weed, Susun. *New Menopausal Years: The Wise Woman Way*, Ash Tree Publishing, 2002.

Werbach, Melvyn R. *Textbook of Nutritional Medicine*, Third Line Press, 1999.

Chapter 34

Levin, Pamela. *Perfect Bones*, Celestial Arts, 2002.

National Women's Health Network. *The Truth About Hormone Replacement Therapy*, Prima Publishing, 2002.

Sanson, Gillian. *The Myth of Osteoporosis*, MCD Century Publications, 2003.

Chapter 35

Liangzhi, Xu, et al. "Does dietary calcium have a protective effect on bone fractures in women? A meta-analysis of observational studies," *British Journal of Nutrition*, 2004.

Lieberman, Shari. *Dare to Lose*, Avery Publishing, 2002.

Rapuri, PB, et al. "Protein intake: effects on bone mineral density and the rate of bone loss in elderly women," *Amer J Clin Nutr*, Jun 2003; 77(6): 1517–25.

Stendig-Lindberg, G, et al. "Prolonged magnesium deficiency causes osteoporosis in the rat," *J Am Coll Nutr*, Dec 2004; 23(6): 704S-11S.

Turner, Lori W, et al. "Influence of yard work and weight training on bone mineral density among older U.S. women," *Journal of Women & Aging*, Mar–Apr 2002; 14.

Chapter 36

McGuire, Thomas. *Tooth Fitness*, St. Michael's Press, 1994.

Chapter 37

"Fosamax-type osteoporosis drugs noted to cause serious eye problems," www.mercola.com, 2002.

Hauselmann HJ and R Rizzoli. "A comprehensive review of treatments for postmenopausal osteoporosis," *Osteoporos Int*, Jan 2003; 14(1): 2–12.

Luckey, MM, N Gilchrist, HG Bone, et al. "Therapeutic equivalence of alendronate 35 milligrams once weekly and 5 milligrams daily in the prevention of postmenopausal osteoporosis." *Obstet Gynecol* 2003; 101(4): 711-21.

Chapter 38

Brzosko, WJ, et al. "Padma 28 in the treatment of chronic active hepatitis," *Biologische Medizin* 1986; 15(6): 300–305.

Challem, Jack. *The Inflammation Syndrome,* John Wiley & Sons, Inc., 2003.

Fox, Maggie. "Painkillers damage intestine, U.S. expert says," Reuters, Jan 3, 2005.

Gladysz, A, et al. "Influence of Padma 28 on patients with chronic active hepatitis type B," *Phytotherapy Research* 1993; 7: 244–47.

Heart Protection Study Collaborative Group. "MRC/BHF Heart Protection Study of cholesterol lowering with simvastatin in 20,536 high-risk individuals: a randomized placebo-controlled trial," *The Lancet,* Jul 6, 2002.

Ichihara, K and K Satoh. "Disparity between angiographic regression and clinical event rates with hydrophobic statins," *The Lancet,* June 22, 2002.

Jankowski, A, et al. "Treatment with Padma 28 of children with recurrent infections of the respiratory tract," *Therapiewoche Schweiz* 1986; 2(1): 25–32.

Shepherd, J. "Resource management in prevention of coronary heart disease: optimizing prescription of lipid-lowering drugs," *The Lancet,* June 29, 2002.

Chapter 39

Bliznakov, Emile G and Gerald L Hunt. *The Miracle Nutrient CoEnzymeQ$_{10}$,* Bantam Books, 1989.

Bruce, B., et al. "A diet high in whole and unrefined foods faborably alters lipids, antioxidant defenses and colon function," *J Am Coll Nutr,* 19(1), 2000.

Crespo, N, et al. "Comparative study of the efficacy and tolerability of policosanol and lovastatin in patients with hypercholesterolemia and noninsulin dependent diabetes mellitus," *Int J Clin Pharmacol Res,* 1999: 19(4).

Goldberg, Burton. *Alternative Medicine Guide: Heart Disease, Stroke & High Blood Pressure,* Future Medicine Publishing, 1998.

Haas, Elson M., MD. *Staying Healthy With Nutrition,* Celestial Arts, 1992.

Hendler, Sheldon Saul and David Rorvik. *PDR for Nutritional Supplements,* Medical Economics, 2001.

Lininger, Schuyler. *A-Z Guide to Drug-Herb-Vitamin Interactions,* Prima Health, 1999.

Chapter 40

ConsumerLab.com's Guide to Buying Vitamins & Supplements by Tod Cooperman, ConsumerLab.com, 2003.

Enig, Mary G. *Know Your Fats,* Bethesda Press, 2000.

Jacobson, Michael F, et al. *Safe Food: Eating Wisely in a Risky World,* Living Planet Press, 1991.

Simopoulos, AP. "Essential fatty acids in health and chronic disease," *American Journal of Clinical Nutrition,* Sept 1999.

Storlien, LH, et al. "Fish oil prevents insulin resistance induced by high-fat feeding in rats," *Science,* 1987; 237.

Walsh, GP. "Dietary change and coronary heart disease," *Medical Hypotheses,* Feb 2000; 31(2).

Chapter 41

Blumenthal, Mark. *Herbal Medicine: Expanded Commission, E Monographs,* Integrative Medicine Communications, 2000.

Blumenthal, Mark. "Interactions between herbs and conventional drugs: introductory considerations," *Herbalgram,* 2000; 49.

Davalos, Antoni. *Neurology: American Academy of Neurology,* Apr 25, 2000.

Ernst, E. "Possible interactions between synthetic and herbal medicinal products, part 1: a systematic review of the indirect evidence," *Perfusion,* Jan 2000.

Goldberg, Burton. *Heart Disease, Stroke & High Blood Pressure,* Future Medicine Publishing, 1998.

Haas, Elson. *Staying Healthy with Nutrition,* Celestial Arts, 1992.

Hudson, Tori. *Women's Encyclopedia of Natural Medicine,* Keats Publishing, 1999.

Hudson, Tori. Women's Health Update, *Townsend Letter for Doctors,* Aug-Sept 2004.

Kaufman, MJ, JM Levin, MH Ross, et al. "Cocaine-induced cerebral vasoconstriction detected in humans with magnetic resonance angiography," *Journal of the American Medical Association,* Feb 1998; 279(5): 376–380.

Lininger, Schuyler W, et al. *HealthNotes: A–Z Guide to Drug-Herb-Vitamin Interactions,* Prima Health, 1999.

Liu, My, et al. "The relationship between hyperfibrinogenemia and severity of coronary heart disease," *Zhonghua Nei Ke Za Zhi,* 2004 Nov; 43(11):820–23. [article in Chinese]

Liu, Simin, et al. "Whole grain consumption and risk of ischemic stroke in women," *JAMA,* 2000; 284.

"Low dose oral contraceptives and stroke," editorial, *New England Journal of Medicine,* Jul 4, 1996.

"Migraines in women," *Therapy Weekly,* May 1, 1999.

Miquel, J, et al, "The curcuma antioxidants: pharmacological effects and prospects for future clinical use. A review," *Arch Geontol Geriatr,* 2002 Feb; 34(1): 37–46. [review of studies]

Norred, Carol, et al. "Use of complementary and alternative medicines by surgical patients," *AANA Journal,* Feb 2000; 68(1).

Ockene, Ira, and Nancy Houston Miller. American Heart Association Task Force on Risk Reduction. A statement for healthcare professionals. For a reprint, call (800) 242-8721 and ask for reprint No. 71–0128.

PDR for Nutritional Supplements, Medical Economics, 2001.

Perlmutter, David. *BrainRecovery.com,* Perlmutter Health Center, 2000.

Sahelian, Ray. *DHEA: A Practical Guide,* Avery Publishing Group, 1996.

VanMeurs, J, et al. "Homocysteine levels and the risk of osteoporotic fracture," *New England Journal of Medicine,* May 13, 2004.

Yokoyama, Tetsuji, MD. *Stroke: Journal of the American Heart Association (AHA),* October 2000. (1-888-4STROKE for AHA or www.differentstrokes.co.uk)

Chapter 42

Kamen, Betty. *Betty Kamen's 1,001 Health Secrets,* Nutrition Encounter, 2003.

Sumi, H, et al. "A novel fibrinolytic enzyme (nattokinase) in the vegetable cheese natto85." *Experientia,* 1987, 43:1110–11.

Sumi H, H Hamada, K Nakanishi, et al. "Enhancement of the fibrinolytic activity in plasma by oral administration of nattokinase." *Acta Haematol,* 1990; 84(3): 139–43.

Suzuki, Y, et al. "Dietary supplementation with fermented soybeans suppresses intimal thickening," *Nutrition,* Mar 2003.

Chapter 43

Caulin-Glaser, Teresa. "Primary prevention of hypertension in women," *Journal of Clinical Hypertension,* 2000; 2(3).

Hodgson, JM, et al. "Tea intake is inversely related to blood pressure in older women," *J Nutr,* Sept 2003; 133(9): 2883–86.

Melina, Vesanto and Brenda Davis. *The New Becoming Vegetarian,* Healthy Living Publications, 2003.

Moore, Richard. *The High Blood Pressure Solution,* Healing Arts Press, 2001.

Murray, Michael and Joseph Pizzorno. *Encyclopedia of Natural Medicine,* Prima Publishing, 1998.

Nowson, CA, et al. "Decreasing dietary sodium while following a self-selected, potassium-rich diet reduces blood pressure," *J Nutr,* Dec 2003.

Roberts, James, M. "Magnesium for preeclampsia and eclampsia," *New England Journal of Medicine,* July 27, 1995.

Sata, M, M Kakoki, D Nagata, et al. "Adrenomedullin and nitric oxide inhibit human endothelial cell apoptosis via a cyclic GMP-independent mechanism." *Hypertension* 2000; 36(1): 83-8.

Waknine, Y. "Green, Oolong tea significantly reduce risk of hypertension," *Arch Intern Med,* 2004; 164: 1534–40.

Werbach, Melvyn. *Textbook of Nutritional Medicine,* Third Line Press, 1999.

Chapter 44

Bruce, B, et al. "Isoflavone supplements do not affect thyroid function in iodine-replete postmenopausal women," *J Med Food,* 2003; 6(4).

Divi, RL and DR Doerge. "Inhibition of thyroid peroxidase by dietary flavonoids." *Chem Res Toxicol,* Jan-Feb 1996; 9(1): 16–23.

Horn-Ross PL, KJ Hoggatt, and MM Lee. "Phytoestrogens and thyroid cancer risk: the San Francisco bay area thyroid cancer study," *Cancer Epidemiol Biomarkers Prev,* Jan 2002; 11(1): 43-49.

Kraft. "Crataegus (common Hawthorn) extracts in cardiac failure—are there new promising results and outlooks?" *Perfusion,* 2000.

Messina, Mark. "The Soy Connection," *J Am Diet Assoc,* 2000.

Rice, MM, AB Graves, SM McCurry, et al. "Tofu consumption and cognition in older Japanese American men and women." *J Nutr,* 2000; 130: 676S.

Rister, Robert. *Healing Without Medication,* Basic Health Publications, 2003.

Sardi, Bill. "They're taking the joy out of soy," *Townsend Letter for Doctors & Patients,* Oct 2000.

"What about soy?" *FDA Consumer,* May-June 2000.

White, LR, H Petrovitch, GW Ross, et al. "Brain aging and midlife tofu consumption." *J Am Coll Nutr,* 2000; 19: 242–55.

Zhou, JR, ET Gugger, T Tanaka, et al. "Soybean phytochemicals inhibit the growth of transplantable human prostate carcinoma and tumor angiogenesis in mice." *J Nutr,* Sept 1999; 129(9): 1628–35.

Chapter 45

Block, G, et al. "Epidemiologic evidence regarding vitamin C and cancer," *American Journal of Clinical Nutrition,* Dec 1991; 54(6 suppl).

Clark, LC, et al. "Effects of selenium supplementation for cancer prevention in patients with carcinoma of the skin. A randomized controlled trial." Nutritional Prevention of Cancer Study Group, *JAMA,* Dec 25, 1996; 276(24).

Moffat L, et al. "High dose ascorbate therapy and cancer," NFCR Cancer Research Association Symposium, (2), 1983.

Shibata, A, et al. "Intake of vegetables, fruits, beta-carotene, vitamin C, and vitamin supplements and cancer incidence among the elderly: a prospective study," *British Journal of Cancer,* Oct 1992; 66(4).

Xu, WH, et al. "Soya food intake and risk of endometrial cancer among Chinese women in Shanghai: population based case-control study," *British Medical Journal,* May 29, 2004.

Chapter 46

Cockburn, W. "Breast thermal imaging: the paradigm shift," *IRIE,* 1999.

Gofman, John and Egan O'Connor. *X-Rays: Health Effects of Common Exams,* Sierra Club Books, 1985.

Vaidya, Jayant. "Screening for breast cancer with mammography," *Lancet,* Dec 22/29, 2001: 2166.

Chapter 47

Delanian S, et al. "Striking regression of chronic radiotherapy damage in a clinical trial of combined pentoxifylline and tocopherol," *J Clin Oncol,* 1999; 17: 3283–90.

Moss, Ralph. *Herbs Against Cancer,* Equinox Press, 1998.

Chapter 48

Eliaz, I. "The potential role of modified citrus pectin in the prevention of cancer metastasis. *Clinical Practice of Alternative Medicine,* 2001; 2(3): 177–79.

Guess BW, MC Scholz, SB Strum, et al. "Modified citrus pectin (MCP) increases the prostate-specific antigen doubling time in men with prostate cancer: a phase II pilot study."*Prostate Cancer Prostatic* Dis. 2003; 6(4): 301–04.

Inohara H and A Raz. "Effects of natural complex carbohydrate (citrus pectin) on murine melanoma cell properties related to galectin-3 functions." *Glycoconj J.* 1994; 11(6): 527–32.

Nangia-Makker P, V Hogan, Y Honjo, et al. "Inhibition of human cancer cell growth and metastasis in nude mice by oral intake of modified citrus pectin." *J Natl Cancer Inst.*, 2002; 94(24): 1854–62.

Pienta KJ, H Naik, A Akhtar, et al. "Inhibition of spontaneous metastasis in a rat prostate cancer model by oral administration of modified citrus pectin." *J Natl Cancer Inst,* 1995; 87(5):348–53.

Raz, A and R Lotan. "Endogenous galactoside-binding lectins: a new class of functional tumor cell surface molecules related to metastasis." *Cancer Metastasis Rev,* 1987; 6: 433–52.

Strum S, M Scholtz, J McDermed, et al. "Modified citrus pectin slows PSA doubling time: a pilot clinical trial." Paper presented at the International Conference on Diet and Prevention of Cancer, Finland, 1999.

Chapter 49

Abraham, GE, J Flechas, and JC Hakala. "Orthoiodosupplementation: iodine sufficiency of the whole human body," Optimox Research Info, June 13, 2002. [report]

"Antioxidants do not decrease the efficacy of chemotherapy," *International Clinical Nutrition Review,* Jan 2001: 21(1).

Davis, Devra Lee. "Most cancer is made, not born," *San Francisco Chronicle,* August 10, 2000.

Folkers, K. "Relevance of the biosynthesis of coenzyme Q_{10} and of the four bases of DNA as a rationale for the molecular causes of cancer and a therapy," *Biochem Biophys Res,* 1996; 224(2): 358–361; *Intl Clin Nutr Rev,* July 1997.

Heerdt, Alexandra S, et al. "Calcium glucarate as a chemopreventive agent in breast cancer," *Israel J Med Sci,* Feb-Mar 1995.

Pace A, et al. "Neuroprotective effect of vitamin E supplementation in patients treated with cisplatin chemotherapy," *J Clin Oncol,* Mar 2003; 21(5):927–31.

Portakal, O, et al. "Coenzyme Q_{10} concentrations and antioxidant status in tissues of breast cancer patients," *Clin Biochem,* 2000; *Alt Med Rev,* 2000; 5(6).

Prasad, KN, WC Cole, and JE Prasad. "Multiple antioxidant vitamins as an adjunct to standard and experimental cancer therapies," *Z Onkol,* 1999; 31.

Sagar, SM, "Antioxidants during anticancer therapy," *Focus Altern Complement Ther,* Jun 2004.

Slaga, Thomas J and Judi Quilici-Timmcke. *D-Glucarate: A Nutrient Against Cancer,* Keats Publishing, 1999.

Index

www.ingramcontent.com/pod-product-compliance
Lightning Source LLC
Chambersburg PA
CBHW050225270326
41914CB00003BA/577